D0083181

MADHOUSES, MAD-DOCTORS, AND MADMEN

MADHOUSES, MAD-DOCTORS, AND MADMEN
The Social History of Psychiatry in the Victorian Era

ANDREW SCULL, Editor

 UNIVERSITY OF PENNSYLVANIA PRESS
Philadelphia, Pennsylvania
1981

Cover: *"Mania Succeeded by Dementia"*

A Swiss soldier, aged twenty-seven, admitted to the Charenton in Paris on 5 November 1827. According to Esquirol, his madness followed by a few weeks a dispute with his officers that had led to his demotion. At first "his delirium was general; he talked incessantly, indulged in wild actions, ripped up and broke everything he could lay his hands on." Subsequently he became withdrawn, incoherent, then all but mute. This engraving shows him in the latter state, a period in which "he spent a large part of each day crouching in an armchair, head sunk on his chest, eyes dull, but with a fixed stare."
(Source: Jean Etienne Dominique Esquirol, *Des Maladies Mentales* [Paris: J. B. Baillière, 1838] 2:229–30 and plate 13.)

Cover and illustrations on pp. 120, 200, and 338 are reproduced here by courtesy of the Wellcome Trustees.

Library of Congress Cataloging in Publication Data
Main entry under title:

Madhouses, mad-doctors, and madmen.

   Includes bibliographical references.
   Contents: The social history of psychiatry in the Victorian era / Andrew Scull — Rationales for therapy in British psychiatry, 1780–1835 / William F. Bynum, Jr. — Phrenology and British alienists, ca. 1825–1845 / Roger Cooter — [etc.]
   1. Psychiatry—Great Britian—History—19th century.
2. Social psychiatry—Great Britian—History—19th century.
3. Great Britian—History—Victoria—1837–1901. I. Scull, Andrew T. [DNLM: 1. Psychiatry—History. 2. History of medicine, 19th century. WM 11.1 M181]
RC450.G7M26 1981   616.89 00941   81–3365
ISBN 0–8122–7801–1   AACR2
ISBN 0–8122–1119–7 (pbk.)

Printed in the United States of America

*For my father
and mother*

Contents

Part Three: Changes in the Profession and Its Orientation

Part Four: Psychiatry and the Law

Contents

Illustrations

Contributors

BONNIE ELLEN BLUSTEIN is an Assistant Professor of History at the University of Louisville, Kentucky. She received her Ph.D. from the University of Pennsylvania. She has published articles on the history of neurology and biology and is currently working on a biography of the American neurologist, William Alexander Hammond, M.D.

WILLIAM F. BYNUM, JR., is chairman of the sub-department of the History of Medicine at University College, London, and Assistant Director of the Wellcome Institute for the History of Medicine. He received his M.D. from Yale University and his Ph.D. from Cambridge University. He is the author of numerous articles on the history of medicine and the history of science and is currently working, with Roy Porter and Michael Neve, on a history of British psychiatry from the eighteenth to the twentieth century, to be published by Athlone Press. He is also co-editor of *Medical History*.

MICHAEL J. CLARK is a graduate in Modern History of Linacre College, Oxford, currently researching the role of evolutionary physiological psychology in British psychiatric theory in the late nineteenth century. He has written two forthcoming papers, "Evolutionary Physiological Psychology in Late Nineteenth-Century Britain," and " 'Morbid Introspection' and British Psychological Medicine, ca. 1830–1900," and is also interested in the nineteenth-century history of speech disorders and speech therapy.

ROGER COOTER is presently a Visiting Fellow at the Wellcome Unit for the History of Medicine at the University of Oxford. A social historian, he received his Ph.D. from the University of Cambridge in 1978, was a fellow at the Calgary Institute for the Humanities in 1979–80, and a Killam fellow at Dalhousie University in 1980–81. He has published articles on British social history, the social context of science, and the politics of pseudoscience. His book *The Cultural Meaning of Popular Science: Phrenology and the Organization of Consent in Nineteenth-Century Britain* is to be published by Cambridge University Press. He is currently at work on a study of alternative medicine in the nineteenth century.

PETER MCCANDLESS is an Associate Professor of History at the College of Charleston, South Carolina. His publications include " 'Build! Build!': The Controversy over the Care of the Chronically Insane in England, 1855–1870," in the *Bulletin of the History of Medicine*, 1979. He is currently at work on a social history of insanity in nineteenth-century Britain.

WILLIAM LL. PARRY-JONES M.D., B. Chir., F.R.C. Psych., is Consultant Psychiatrist at the Warneford Hospital, Oxford, and Clinical Lecturer in Psychiatry at the University of Oxford. He is a fellow of Linacre College, Oxford, and the author of *The Trade in Lunacy* (London: Routledge and Kegan Paul/Toronto: University of Toronto Press, 1972).

ANDREW SCULL is an Associate Professor of Sociology at the University of California, San Diego. He previously taught at Princeton and the University of Pennsylvania, and during 1976–77 was an American Council of Learned Societies Fellow at University College, London. Educated at Balliol College, Oxford, and at Princeton University, he is the author of *Decarceration: Community Treatment and the Deviant: A Radical View* (Englewood Cliffs, N.J.: Prentice-Hall, 1977), and *Museums of Madness: The Social Organization of Insanity in Nineteenth-Century England* (London: Allen Lane/New York: St. Martin's Press, 1979). He has also written numerous articles in such fields as social history, the history of sociological thought, the sociology of the professions, and the sociology of social control. He is presently at work on a study of Durkheim's sociology of law and a monograph on English ideas about insanity in the eighteenth and nineteenth centuries.

ELAINE SHOWALTER is a Professor of English at Douglass College, Rutgers University, New Jersey. She is the author of *A Literature of Their Own: British Women Novelists from Bronte to Lessing*, and is currently working on a study of madness, literature, and society in England from 1830 to 1970.

BARBARA SICHERMAN has taught at Hunter, Vassar, and Manhattanville Colleges, and most recently at Barnard College, Columbia University. She received her Ph.D. from Columbia University. She is the author of *The Quest for Mental Health in America, 1880–1917* (New York: Arno, 1980), and, with Carol Hurd Green, edited *Notable American Women: The Modern Period* (Cambridge, Mass.: Harvard University Press, 1980). She is currently completing a book on Alice Hamilton.

ROGER SMITH is a Lecturer in the History of Science in the History Department of the University of Lancaster, England. He received his Ph.D. in 1970 from the University of Cambridge. He has published articles on the nineteenth-century evolutionary debate and on the history of physiological psychology. He serves as the editor of the British Society for the History of Science Monographs and is the author of a forthcoming book on the insanity defense in the nineteenth century, to be published by Edinburgh and Columbia University Presses.

NANCY J. TOMES is an Assistant Professor of History at the State University of New York at Stony Brook. She received her Ph.D. in 1978 from the University of Pennsylvania. She has published articles on British and American social history and is currently working on a book about asylum practice at the Pennsylvania Hospital for the Insane, 1841–1883.

JOHN WALTON is a Lecturer in History at the University of Lancaster, England. He was educated at Merton College, Oxford, and Lancaster University. He is the author of *The Blackpool Landlady: A Social History* (Manchester: University of Manchester Press, 1978) and has written extensively on the holiday industry and seaside towns in Victorian England. He has also published articles on nineteenth-century medical and psychiatric history.

Acknowledgments

Much of the editorial work on this volume of essays was completed during my tenure of a fellowship at the Shelby Cullom Davis Center for Historical Studies at Princeton University. I should like to express my appreciation to Lawrence Stone, the director of the center, and to the other fellows for providing me with such a stimulating atmosphere in which to work. I am also grateful to the Academic Senate of the University of California, San Diego, for helping to defray some of the costs of the research reported in chapters 1 and 6.

ANDREW SCULL

Introduction

Victorians—at least those privileged Victorians to whom that term is usually applied—seem, for the most part, to have viewed their society's response to mental illness with a mixture of pride and complacency. For most of them, one of the clearest indications of the progressive, humane character of the age was to be found in its response to the misfortunes of the insane. On both sides of the Atlantic, the educated classes basked in the reflected glory that emanated from the mid-century achievement of lunacy reform. In the not so distant past, as many were only too ready to recall,

> coercion for the outward man, and rabid physicking the inward man were . . . the specifics for lunacy. Chains, straw, filthy solitude, darkness, and starvation; jalap, syrup of buckthorn, tartarised antimony and ipecacuanna administered every spring and fall in fabulous doses to every patient, whether well or ill; spinning in whirligigs, corporal punishment, gagging, "continued intoxication"; nothing was too wildly extravagant, nothing too monstrously cruel to be prescribed by mad-doctors.[1]

Now, thanks to the philanthropic efforts of the few and the aroused sympathies of the many, madmen and madwomen had at last been rescued from such viciousness and neglect.

The advances thus celebrated were in the first instance perceived as moral and humanitarian. In many quarters, they were also viewed as scientific, an interpretation those segments of the medical profession that were involved in the treatment of lunacy were naturally very keen to promulgate. To alienists and their allies, changes in society's characteristic responses to insanity reflected and depended crucially upon advances in medical knowledge and understanding. It was progress here that made possible more precise and refined diagnosis, as well as more humane and effective treatment. Science and humanity were then united and given visible and concrete form in the network of new, purpose-built, publicly funded asylums, monuments of moral architecture that more than one

I

contemporary commentator was moved to regard as "the most blessed manifestation of true civilization the world can present."[2]

For many years, work on the history of psychiatry tended to reproduce these ideological self-images essentially intact. Historians were all too prone to mistake intention for accomplishment, rhetoric for reality, and to draw a flattering portrait of gradual progress toward ever greater enlightenment. By the late 1960s, however, such interpretations were under sustained assault for their naïveté and inadequacies. For a time, the pendulum swung perhaps too violently to the opposite extreme, with the term *reform* now reinterpreted as the reverse of humane, as, in Michel Foucault's words, "a gigantic moral imprisonment."[3] Still, as the essays in this volume testify, in the longer run and shorn of the excesses of its youth, the new approach did point toward a more complex and nuanced analysis of reform and a more careful examination of the reality of change. In so doing, the new approach has exposed much that had heretofore escaped notice.

It has become apparent that even at the height of Victorian optimism and complacency, a subterranean tradition persisted in which lunacy reform and its products were perceived with a much more jaundiced eye. The refusal to take the asylum authorities' proclamations at face value certainly extended to some of the patients and their families. So far from believing that the asylum was a therapeutic institution, some contemporary observers noted that "nearly all among the lower classes look[ed] upon [it] as the Bluebeard's cupboard of the neighbourhood."[4] Even respectable citizens were suspicious of the criteria used to assess madness and sanity, and less than convinced of many alienists' probity and capacities. By the last third of the century, the asylum superintendents' pretensions to rest their practice on a scientific basis were under attack from still another quarter, a group of disaffected competitors from within the medical profession; and by this time, too, increasing doubts were being expressed about the wisdom of the asylum solution, along with claims for the superior virtues of treatment in the community.

The essays in this book range widely over these issues, as well as others less noted at the time. In reading them, we come to realize that our contemporary "crisis of psychiatric legitimacy"[5] only echoes earlier such crises that were confronted by the profession; that the debate over the merits and demerits of institutional or community treatment of the mentally disordered has a considerable historical ancestry; and that disputes over the boundary between insanity and criminal responsibility and over the wording and implementation of commitment laws have been endemic features of psychiatry's often difficult relationship with the community at large. Similarly, the profession has had a long history of disputes over whether to account for mental illness in physical or psychological terms, as well as an equally long history of defining and treating it somewhat differently according to the sex of the person involved. The persistence of these issues and problems suggests that historical analysis may have something to contribute, if not to their resolution, then at least to a broader understanding of their social roots and significance.

ANDREW SCULL

Notes

1. Charles Dickens and W. H. Wills, "A Curious Dance Round a Curious Tree," *Household Words,* 17 January 1852.
2. G. E. Paget, *The Harveian Oration* (Cambridge, England: Deighton, Bell, 1866), pp. 34-35, cited in Andrew Wynter, *The Borderlands of Insanity*, 2d ed. (London: Hardwicke, 1875), p. 112.
3. Michel Foucault, *Madness and Civilization* (New York: Pantheon, 1965).
4. "Lunatic Asylums," *Quarterly Review* 101 (1857): 353.
5. Charles Rosenberg, "The Crisis of Psychiatric Legitimacy," in *American Psychiatry: Past, Present, and Future,* ed. George Kriegman et al. (Charlottesville: University Press of Virginia, 1975), pp. 135–48.

A N D R E W   S C U L L

1 The Social History of Psychiatry in the Victorian Era

The history of psychiatry has become in recent years an extraordinarily creative and controversial field. One thinks, in particular, of the idiosyncratic and self-consciously opaque pyrotechnics of Michel Foucault, and of the fascinating and sometimes fierce debate between David Rothman and Gerald Grob over the sources and meaning of lunacy reform in nineteenth-century America.[1] The history of English psychiatry remained wedded for a few years longer to a "progressive" metaphysics, whether of administrative historians like Kathleen Jones, or of practicing psychiatrists-cum-historians like Richard Hunter and Ida MacAlpine.[2] But by the mid-1970s, a few Ph.D. dissertations and a handful of published articles marked the spread of a more skeptical viewpoint there too.[3] I must confess that if a Whiggish theory of history is now in rather deserved disfavor when applied to the *subject* these works are grappling with, it seems appropriate, nevertheless, to regard the historiography as progressing. One only has to compare the newer work with that done by Albert Deutsch, Gregory Zilboorg, or Kathleen Jones, or even by Norman Dain to become aware of the much broader array of issues which are now seen as problematic, the greater range of material that is brought to bear on those questions, and the increased epistemological sophistication of the answers provided.[4]

The work of this new generation of historians, leavened (at least I hope it is leavened) by the contributions of an occasional sociologist, has concentrated heavily upon a reexamination of what was once referred to as "the first great psychiatric revolution," the transformation of social ideas and practices vis-à-vis the insane which marked the late eighteenth and the first half of the nineteenth century. In one way or another, the essays in this book are all concerned with this "revolution" and its aftermath as these were experienced in England and the United States.

Juxtaposing developments in these two societies makes it evident that a wealth of fascinating comparisons and contrasts exists between them, some of which I shall explore in this essay. Although the "psychiatric

5

revolution" was by no means a uniquely Anglo-American phenomenon, its impact in both societies was powerful, and its timing remarkably similar. Moreover, the interest aroused by the striking resemblances (as well as divergences) in the two experiences of "reform" is heightened when developments in the history of psychiatry are set in a broader cultural context. For Victorianism, as Daniel Howe has recently reminded us, "was a transatlantic culture" rooted in a common heritage,[5] a heritage whose impact was strengthened and sustained by the efflorescence of printed and other forms of transoceanic communication from the 1830s onward. And if the American variant was at first a largely derivative and provincial version of its English counterpart, it was embedded nevertheless in a very different social matrix, so that by the end of the century, it had become more distinctive, even as the lines of influence between the two societies became more genuinely reciprocal.

The Victorian age saw the transformation of the madhouse into the asylum into the mental hospital; of the mad-doctor into the alienist into the psychiatrist; and of the madman (and madwoman) into the mental patient. And while it would be a grave error to confuse semantics with reality, it equally will not do to treat these verbal changes as no more than a succession of euphemisms masking a fundamentally static reality. As with all mythical representations, the progressive images that this succession of terms is designed to conjure up bear a significant, albeit distorted, relationship to the social order they purport to describe.

We begin, therefore, with the recognition that the advent of the Victorian era coincided to a striking extent with the culmination of a series of dramatic changes in society's responses to madness. Some of the more obvious of these changes were: The state apparatus assumed a much greater role in the handling of insanity; the asylum became almost the sole officially approved response to the problems posed by the mentally disordered; and the nature and limits of lunacy were themselves transformed. Madness was increasingly seen as something which could be authoritatively diagnosed, certified, and treated only by a group of legally recognized experts. And those "experts" were, of course, medical men— increasingly an organized and self-conscious specialism within the profession of medicine, known to their detractors as "mad-doctors" and among themselves as "alienists" or "medical superintendents of asylums for the insane." (The clumsiness of the title at least captures the extent to which their professional identity was bound up with their institutional status.) Henceforth, "the character and course of mental illness [were to be] . . . shaped irrevocably by medical intervention."[6]

It would be foolish, of course, to suggest that medical concern with madness is a uniquely nineteenth- and twentieth-century phenomenon.

Eighteenth-century medicine continued to rely heavily on the Hellenic tradition of a humoral physiology, pathology, and therapeutics. As such, it could invoke classical authority in support of a recognizably medical theoretical account and therapeutics of mental disorder. And there is evidence that the Greek tradition had its adherents even during the Dark Ages and the early medieval period.[7] Still, and despite the lamentable dearth of research into the handling of the insane even so recently as the eighteenth century, certain generalizations may be ventured.[8] First, the medical-humoral view was only one (though perhaps the most intellectually coherent) of the available ways of accounting for madness. Second, the majority of those practicing medicine—with whatever degree of skill or legitimacy—evinced little interest in or concern with the problems of insanity and the insane. Partly as a consequence, "the care of Lunaticks"[9] was generally entrusted elsewhere than among medical men: to the madman's family; to the jailer; to clergymen; or to the workhouse master. Even the emerging "trade in lunacy" in England, which centered around the growth of the private madhouse system, was far from being a uniquely medical enterprise.[10] And if the law was for the most part silent on the issue of insanity, to the extent that lunatics *were* a focus of concern, they were lumped together with other vagrant groups and were dealt with as amateur magistrates saw fit.

By the latter part of the eighteenth century, however, medical interest was clearly on the upswing—a development given further impetus (in England, at least) by George III's "mania."[11] Whether measured by the volume of medical writings on the subject; the inclusion of lectures on the management of insanity in medical-school curricula;[12] or by the number of medical men practicing in the area, it is clear that doctors were attempting to give some practical substance to their profession's traditional, if previously neglected, claim to jurisdiction over the insane. That substance involved an effort to minister to the body rather than to the mind diseased; for in a Cartesian universe, with the concept of mind conflated with that of soul, physicians almost universally asserted that mental disease had an entirely somatic basis, and thus was accessible to physical remedies. This somatic emphasis is particularly unsurprising when we recall that to adopt a perspective which allowed disorders of the mind/soul to be the etiological root of insanity threatened to call into question the soul's immortality and with it the very foundations of Christianity, or to lend substance to the notion that crazy people were possessed by Satan or the subjects of divine retribution—which, of course, made them better candidates for the ministrations of ecclesiastics than for those of physicians.[13]

Still, the growth of medical dominance in the treatment of the insane did not go unchallenged. The early nineteenth century saw the emergence and spread of a new approach to madness, emphasizing the adaptation of treatment to the circumstances of the individual case to a degree which qualitatively distinguished it from more traditional medical therapeutics. Resting upon psychosocial intervention, the new "moral treatment" represented, in Bynum's words, "a rather damning attack on the medical profession's ability to deal with mental illness" and was, implicitly, a challenge to the somatic etiology preferred by physicians. The threat was heightened in England by the fact that the domestic version of moral treatment which drew the widest attention not only called into question the value of standard medical interventions, but was itself a lay inspired development. Further compounding medical vulnerability within a few years were the revelations of asylum "abuses" before parliamentary select committees, for many of the most blatant episodes here involved medical men and medically run institutions. William Bynum's analysis in chapter 2 presents an examination of medical ideas about, and treatments for, insanity, covering the period immediately prior to the introduction of moral treatment, as well as the profession's response to the challenge offered by the new form of treatment.

Elsewhere, I have suggested that the success of that medical response rested in part upon a careful reworking of the claim that insanity was a somatic disorder, and that the response was essentially a political and social process, culminating in claims that *both* moral and medical treatment were essential for the adequate treatment of lunatics.[14] But, as Bynum points out, the medical profession's somatic emphasis threatened to create a series of difficulties for any attempt to assimilate the newly popular moral therapy to the medical armamentarium. His suggestion that phrenology served as a vital theoretical mediation, an intellectual system providing a crucial ideological linkage which smoothed away the logical awkwardness of employing "moral" means to treat a physical disease, is amplified and more carefully specified in chapter 3, where Roger Cooter gives extended treatment to the relationship between phrenology and psychiatry.

But Cooter goes much further than this. He demonstrates the wide influence of phrenology among early nineteenth-century British alienists and suggests some of that doctrine's multiple attractions for the emerging profession. In particular, he points to the broader social resonance of phrenology with the ideas of social reform and progress, and the ideological and social linkage it provided between the work of the asylum superintendents and attempts to respond to other pressing social issues of the day. On these grounds, too, may rest much of phrenology's appeal, not just to many of the leading early American asylum superintendents (such as Amariah Brigham, Isaac Ray, Samuel Woodward, and Pliny Earle), but also among the laymen—Samuel Gridley Howe and Horace Mann in particular—who played such important roles in the state asylum movement in the

United States.[15] And beyond its symbolic and practical association with reform, phrenology provided a clear physiological explanation of the operations of the brain, one which permitted a parsimonious account of both normal and abnormal mental functioning, and which provided a coherent rationale for the application of *both* medical and moral treatment in cases of insanity.[16]

The centrality of moral treatment to any examination of the history of psychiatry in the nineteenth century has long been recognized. However, this theme has been described all too often in mythological portraits of Pinel literally and metaphorically striking the chains from the lunatics in the Bicêtre and (in the midst of the bloodiest excesses of the French Revolution) inaugurating the first rational and humane approach to the treatment of the mentally disordered. The historiography of psychiatry has undergone a profound transformation since 1965, to which this volume testifies. Yet on the central issue of moral treatment, there is, on one level at least, a fascinating convergence between the old-fashioned directionalist histories, which stress its revolutionary impact and importance, and the work of modern revisionists from Foucault onward, which argues that moral treatment represents a decisive epistemological break in the history of Western responses to madness. Having said this, it hardly needs to be emphasized that the two traditions have evaluated this rupture very differently, and have sought to comprehend its origins and analyze its nature in very different ways. At the very least, it seems to me that the revisionists have successfully established the central importance of seeking answers to three interrelated questions: How can we make sense of traditional approaches to the mad, and in what do these consist? What, penetrating beneath the ideological accounts offered by the reformers themselves, are we to make of moral treatment? And, given the importance of the change it represents, how can we grasp its broader social roots and significance? These are obviously complex and difficult issues, and chapter 4 represents a first and somewhat limited and tentative effort on my part to resolve them.

The institution was, of course, the almost exclusive arena in which the new profession plied its trade. The structure of moral treatment was such that the asylum was also perceived by alienists as one of their crucial therapeutic instruments; that is, the asylum itself was a major weapon (perhaps *the* major weapon) in the struggle to cure the insane. Again, this marks a profound contrast with the eighteenth century. Neither the private madhouses nor the charity asylums of that period can be thought of reasonably as *purpose-built* in the sense in which that term becomes applicable in the nineteenth century. Little connection was seen at that time between *architecture* and *cure*, the latter being held to depend (if it were possible at all) on various forms of physical treatments. Apart from its uses for decorative purposes or for show (for example, the exterior of the second Bethlem, built in 1676, was modeled on the Tuileries), the architecture of these places was primarily designed to secure "the safe confinement and imprisonment of lunatics."[17] Consequently, later generations often commented on "the prison-mindedness of eighteenth century insane asylum designers."[18]

The spreading acceptance of moral treatment was paralleled, however, by a growing emphasis among those charged with curing lunatics upon "the improbability (I had almost said moral impossibility) of an insane person's regaining the use of his reason, except by . . . a mode of treatment . . . which can be fully adopted only in a Building constructed for the purpose."[19] The implication, often made explicit, was that the very physical structure of the asylum was "a special apparatus [designed] for the cure of lunacy. . . ."[20] That is, the building was as important as any drugs or other remedies in the alienist's armamentarium. In the words of Luther Bell, a leading American member of the fraternity, "An Asylum or more properly a Hospital for the insane, may justly be considered an architectural contrivance as peculiar and characteristic to carry out its designs, as is any edifice for manufacturing purposes to meet its specific end. It is emphatically an instrument of treatment."[21]

William Tuke, the progenitor of the English version of moral treatment, had stressed a multitude of ways in which the asylum's physical structure and location contributed to its value as a therapeutic tool. Particularly important was the use of design to permit adequate separation and classification of the inmates. In this way, physical barriers could be used to enforce moral divisions in the patient population, and the treatment of the various classes could be precisely calibrated to match their behavior. Moreover, it was not an extravagance to design and build institutions that were cheerful and aesthetically pleasing to the inmates. The insane were very sensitive to their surroundings, and although "some have been disposed to contemn as superfluous the attention paid to the lesser feelings of the patients, there is great reason to believe, it has been of considerable advantage."[22]

In chapter 5, Nancy Tomes examines the concern with asylum construction and management in an American context, focusing on the ideas of Thomas Kirkbride, the acknowledged American expert on these subjects. Historians, as she points out, have tended to be rather dismissive of those who concerned themselves with such mundane and practical matters. But assessments of this sort are mistaken, not just because the implied separation of administrative and therapeutic concerns on which these judgments rest is seriously anachronistic, but also because they involve a failure to grasp the necessary centrality of the legitimation of the asylum to the emerging profession's social standing.

We must remember that during this period, the idea of confining the sick or helpless members of one's family in an institution was far from being a popular one, particularly among the more "respectable" elements of society. Yet if asylum superintendents were to obtain a population consisting of much more than chronic pauper derelicts, then families who had some choice in the matter had to be convinced somehow that the institution should be the place of first rather than last resort. Unless this effort succeeded, asylums would surely remain starved of funds. Moreover, without a significant proportion of upper-class patients, the newly consolidating psychiatric profession could look forward to no more than a dubious status as a barely legitimate branch of medicine. Somehow, close and unremitting contact with the stigmatized and powerless carries with it its own peculiar reward—a share of their stigma and marginality. Obviously, though, it was by no means self-evident that institutional care was preferable to even the best and most solicitous of domestic arrangements. Hence, this notion required elaborate ideological justification. Only by emphasizing the expertise of those who ran the asylums and the positive benefits of asylum treatment could the institutions' advocates make a presumptive case for extending those "benefits" to those not compelled to use the asylums' services.

Psychiatric legitimacy, then, rested heavily on the public's (especially the wealthy public's) response to the asylum. And Tomes emphasizes that while the problem was most acute for those running private asylums, whose clientele was drawn overwhelmingly from the moneyed classes, it was by no means absent for many of those in charge of the new state asylums. For the latter, too, faced the problem of securing financial support from the community—though here the alternatives with which they were competing tended to be other institutions, such as the workhouse and the jail. In the long run, however, as the difference in the clientele and character of the two sets of institutions grew, so the concerns of the two segments of the psychiatric profession increasingly diverged. More and more, those running the public asylums had to worry about anything *but* the issue of how to attract a clientele.[23] However, for their "colleagues" in the private sector, this clearly remained a central issue. It is this, I suspect, which accounts for the continuing impact Tomes sees patients' families (and even, to a more limited extent, patients themselves) having upon the superintendents' claims and activities; for her study, after all, is focused on the superintendent of one of the most prestigious private institutions in America.

Private or corporate asylums of the sort Kirkbride headed played a critical role in the early stages of the lunacy reform movement in the United States, and chapter 6 analyzes their contributions in detail. Part of the corporate institutions' significance lay in their role in the process Tomes has dissected, the conversion of the relevant segments of the public to the merits of institutionalizing the mentally disordered. But they were important for much more besides. William Bynum's essay emphasizes the relationship between the medical profession's strenuous efforts to retain control of psychiatric institutions and their patients, and the emergence of a very pronounced therapeutic optimism in England; and in chapter 4, I have suggested that this account must be broadened to incorporate an understanding of the structural sources of the new emphasis on the possibility and desirability of cure or rehabilitation. It was in the handful of corporate asylums founded in the 1820s and 1830s that this new optimism emerged in an American context. And, as exemplars of the new system of moral treatment, they likewise served as the major vehicle through which the new approach was transplanted across the Atlantic. The corporate asylums were even the site of a rather faint echo of the challenge to medical hegemony in the treatment of insanity that had occurred in England; and in their subsequent convergence upon a system of authority relationships which gave autocratic powers to the medical superintendent, and which defined both medical *and* moral treatment as the physician's exclusive province, they established the model that all subsequent American asylums emulated.

Historians as widely differing in their outlooks as Albert Deutsch, Gerald Grob, and David Rothman have emphasized the importance of the American reformers' unshakable conviction that lunacy was a curable disorder. And while the "cult of curability" scaled heights here scarcely known on the other side of the Atlantic, I have pointed out that an analogous, if more temperate, climate of opinion certainly existed in England. In both countries, of course, expectations of this sort were to prove unfounded, and asylums increasingly degenerated into little more than custodial warehouses. The issues of what caused this development and to what degree it was inevitable, a function of the inherent flaws of the asylum solution, have naturally evoked considerable discussion and controversy in the recent literature on lunacy reform. But with the partial exception of Gerald Grob's work on the Worcester State Hospital in Massachusetts,[24] those scholars exploring this subject have examined it only at the national level, and in general they (and this applies to my own work just as much as to others') have systematically exploited only a portion of the materials that can be brought to bear on these issues. The very breadth of focus has tended to militate against efforts to ground the generalizations about national trends in the specific experiences of particular asylums. Ultimately, of course, the hypotheses suggested in these synthetic works can be adequately tested, refined, and extended only on the basis of careful case studies of a range of asylums: studies which grasp the relationship of local developments to the broader national picture, but which simultaneously exploit the opportunity offered by the possibility of a more intensive examination of the history of an individual asylum to question and, if necessary, to redraw portions of the larger portrait.

John Walton's essay on the Lancaster Asylum could serve as a model in these respects. The county asylum at Lancaster was one of the first built under the permissive English legislation of 1808. Like a number of other mental institutions, its patients at first were subjected to a regime little different from that of a traditional madhouse, an approach which relied heavily upon physical coercion and mechanical restraint. By the time a change in medical officers brought with it an attempt to apply the principles of moral treatment, Lancaster had grown to be one of the largest asylums in England, containing more than twice as many inmates (525) as the reformers claimed was advisable for a curative institution. And it was suffering from the overcrowding that was to be a standard feature of pauper lunatic asylums in the second half of the nineteenth century.

Samuel Gaskell, the new superintendent appointed in 1840, was clearly one of the more energetic and competent asylum superintendents of his day (a distinction recognized in his subsequent appointment, in 1849, as a Commissioner in Lunacy). Given the central role which the size of the institution and its crowding with chronic paupers are usually held to have played in the *collapse* of regimes based on moral treatment, the fate of Gaskell's attempt to *introduce* moral treatment into an asylum already suffering from these ills has an obvious interest and importance. And I think Walton shows that Gaskell's efforts, assisted by those of the visiting physician, De Vitré, did initially have a transformative effect. The crucial questions, of course, are: How deeply into the lives of the asylum and its inmates did the changes penetrate, and how lasting was their impact? Our answer to the first of these questions must be qualified by the limitations of the records themselves. It is clear, though, that the effort was a serious and sustained one, and initially it achieved some notable successes. It is scarcely unique in this respect. In my own work, I have pointed to the existence of a similar regime at the Buckinghamshire County Asylum, and Grob has shown that similar conditions existed for a time at the Worcester State Asylum.[25] But these limited successes were only temporary. In part, the failure of the predicted cures to materialize prompted the asylums' paymasters to cut back still further on expenditures. And while the new approach worked well in the first flush of enthusiasm, in the long run its dependence upon extraordinary dedication and concern made it vulnerable to the perils of routinization. In a pattern that is unsurprising to those who have examined other institutions' fates, following Gaskell's departure from Lancaster in 1849, all but the surface features of moral treatment soon decayed and disappeared. In the long run, therefore, the experience at Lancaster appears to confirm many of the claims made in the national studies, and it is significant that Walton concludes that in all probability even Gaskell himself would have been unable to stem the pressures to adopt a custodial holding operation.

Influenced by the kinds of outcomes Walton discusses, as early as the mid-1850s, in both England and the United States, a few isolated voices were beginning to despair of the asylum's powers as a curative institution. Most "informed opinion" continued to insist that, given early treatment, a substantial majority of the insane could be restored to sanity; but over the next decade or two, such sanguine views became increasingly difficult to sustain. In both societies, the proportion of the inmates "deemed curable" continued to dwindle relentlessly, and the response of the asylum superintendents on both sides of the Atlantic was gradually to redefine success in more limited terms: comfort, cleanliness, and freedom from the more obvious forms of physical mistreatment, rather than the often unattainable goal of cure. In the words of Dr. Cassidy, superintendent of the Lancaster County Asylum, "The care and alleviation of the condition of the general body of the insane is at least as important a function of asylums as is the so-called 'cure' of a small percentage of cases, few of whom remain permanently sane."[26]

Nevertheless, a minority did not view the situation so complacently. In some quarters, the heretical thought was voiced that "the curative influences of the asylum have been vastly over-rated, and . . . those of isolated treatment in domestic care have been greatly undervalued. . . ."[27] Nor was it just curable cases who did not belong in the asylum. Among the chronically insane, "large numbers are needlessly detained. Of the ninety percent of chronic cases, at least thirty, by the admission of the medical superintendents, and probably nearer forty to less official views, are both harmless and quiet, capable of giving some little help to the world. . . . [With such cases] immediately the physician has ascertained that they are past cure they should at once be drafted out into private houses and keeping."[28] Lockhart Robertson, a former superintendent of the Sussex County Asylum, thought at least a third of the chronic patients would benefit by such a program. Although he had previously been a staunch advocate of asylum treatment, his experience as a Chancery Visitor in Lunacy had convinced him otherwise: "I could never have believed that patients who were such confirmed lunatics could be treated in private families, the way Chancery lunatics are, if I had not personally watched these cases."[29]

From across the Atlantic, Edward Jarvis reported that "the thought is entertained and gaining ground in America, that many of the insane may be better managed out of than in hospitals, and this opinion is beginning to be acted on."[30] He seems to have been referring primarily to his home state of Massachusetts. Between 1867 and 1869, the new State Board of

Charities in Massachusetts had used its annual reports to launch powerful attacks on the existing, asylum-based policy, and to suggest that instead of "immuring them in habitations which we ourselves avoid and teach our children to avoid as the worst into which men can fall," the state ought, so far as possible, to place the insane "in private houses."[31] But the attempt to bring about such a fundamental reorientation of policy sputtered and died. Battered by a variety of pressure groups (not the least of whom were the asylum superintendents) and confronted by public hostility, the board felt compelled in its 1870 report to issue a retraction. The policy which in 1869 had been described as both desirable and well tried was now dismissed as impractical and utopian, and as contrary to the best interests of both the insane and the community.[32]

The model to which these and other critics of the asylum were repeatedly drawn was the Geel Lunatic Colony in Belgium. The first to advocate a shift to a system of this sort was John Galt, the superintendent of the Eastern Lunatic Asylum in Williamsburg, Virginia. Something of a maverick among the early asylum superintendents, he used his institution's annual report for 1854–55, as well as an article in the *American Journal of Insanity* for 1855, "The Farm of St. Anne," to recommend that lunatics be spared the asylum's "daily routine proceeding with the inexorable, monotonous motion of a machine," and instead be sent to live in the community under some degree of supervision. In this way, the patients could benefit from the sane influences of a family circle while being spared the harmful ones of their own family. As at Geel, he suggested, the lunatic thus situated "feels himself a free man, and instead of being cut off from society, he mingles with his more fortunate fellow-men." Galt's proposals, however, were met with outright hostility, his aspersions on asylums decried as "wholesale slanders," and his proposals simply ignored by the rest of the profession—a tactic made easier by his personal isolation and lack of friends in their ranks, not to mention his Southern origins.[33]

Nor were subsequent American efforts to adopt the Geel model any more successful. The Massachusetts State Board of Charities, for example, likewise cited Geel as the basis for its proposals for noninstitutional care. Indeed, it provided elaborate and laudatory descriptions of the Belgian system, accounts derived in large part from Samuel Gridley Howe's visit to the colony. (Howe was the dominant figure on the board.) But once again, as we have seen, the gestures toward such an approach proved unavailing.[34]

In his chapter about Geel, William Parry-Jones demonstrates the recurring fascination of the idea of a lunatic colony for some segments of the British psychiatric profession. At the same time, he documents the often vocal opposition of the majority of the profession to any scheme based on the dispersion rather than the concentration of lunatics. As he points out, the British critics of the asylum were no more successful than their North American counterparts, and official policy continued to rely overwhelmingly on the sequestration of the mad, even when dealing with chronic, apparently harmless lunatics.

The continuing reliance on bricks and mortar rested, I think, on something more than the partially self-interested opposition of asylum superintendents who were in alliance with the Lunacy Commissioners, important as that opposition unquestionably was. There is evidence, some of which Parry-Jones cites, that the public viewed any slackening of the rigid segregation of the mad with more than passing trepidation, reasoning that lunatics would scarcely have been locked up in the first place unless it was not safe to leave them at large.[35] And for many different constituencies, ranging from the inmates' families to the community as a whole, the asylum remained a convenient way to get rid of inconvenient people; one of particular importance to the poor for whom, under existing conditions, the difficult and troublesome sorts who were institutionalized would otherwise have often formed a virtually intolerable burden. To a vital extent, a Poor Law based on the principle of less eligibility and a policy toward lunacy resting firmly on the asylum remained inextricably bound together.[36]

Despite their meager influence on nineteenth-century policymakers, Geel, and the British and American flirtations with Geel, have not lost their contemporary fascination. In part, this may reflect our nostalgia for a lost preindustrial Golden Age, probably as mythical as all other Golden Ages have been; in part, it may derive from our own disillusionment with an institutionally based response to mental disorder, and the conviction of many that "the worst home is better than the best mental hospital."[37] But just as today it requires a nice capacity to calibrate human misery if one attempts to choose between the deficiencies of the asylum and those of community care,[38] so what we know of Geel and related family-based systems prompts genuine uncertainty. Were these, as Parry-Jones puts it, "just a Utopian ideal, just a mirage? . . . Or was the vision real, and still awaiting fulfillment?"

While growing pessimism about the value of asylum treatment, or even about the possibility of cure at all,[39] prompted some people to search for alternatives to institutional forms of care, for others it suggested that the more urgent necessity was to try to forestall the development of insanity in the first place. The idea of prevention had long been an attractive one, and a number of leading figures among the founders of the psychiatric profession had proferred advice on this issue.[40] Naturally, however, as the possibility of cure came more and more to seem unattainable, this advice acquired an ever greater urgency and importance.

The theoretical pronouncements of the emerging mental-hygiene movement understandably reflected (and in the process gave further substance to) the by now commonplace notion of a connection between insanity and civilization, and the need to mitigate the problems that "progress" brought in its train.[41] Here was an essentially "pastoral" task, the promulgation of guidelines about how one should live, to be derived, in this positivistic age, not from theology, but from "science." In its performance, as Barbara Sicherman's discussion in chapter 9 brings out, the mental hygienists provided prescriptions for behavior as heavily colored by their own upbringing and outlook as by the broader social and intellectual climate of the age.

Socially, some of the broader significance of the growing emphasis upon mental hygiene lies in its role in the transition of psychiatry away from an exclusively institutional focus and locus of practice. Organized psychiatry originated precisely in a partly entrepreneurial response to the opportunities offered by the creation of an asylum system, rather than as "the logical institutional expression of an expanding body of knowledge or the crystallization of particular [therapeutic] techniques."[42] But the latter part of the nineteenth century marks the genesis, in peculiar and complicated ways, of that fundamental distinction between institutional and office-based psychiatric practice that still divides the profession in the contemporary world. The emphasis of people like Beard, Jacobi, Mitchell, and Hammond on the importance of preventative measures designed to forestall mental illness, or to catch it in its incipient stages, naturally brought with it a new receptivity to the still functioning, though symptom-bearing, patient who could form the basis of an office-based practice.

In the United States, the development of forms of private practice which sought to break sharply with the dominant image of psychological medicine as concerned with the institutional custody of a chronically ill and often economically deprived clientele was inextricably linked with the rise of the new specialism of neurology. With roots in the clinical opportunities presented by the Civil War, the neurologists soon reached far beyond cases of obvious organic disease or trauma of the nervous system, asserting that since the mind itself was to be understood as a physical phenomenon, its diseases, too, fell within their purview. Such professional imperialism was pushed furthest, perhaps, in George Beard's "discovery" of *neurasthenia*, which asserted for whole realms of functional "nervous" disorder a common origin and a respectable status as a genuine disease entity with an underlying somatic basis.[43] With characteristic symptoms as varied as "sick headache, noises in the ear, atonic voice, deficient mental control, bad dreams, insomnia, nervous dyspepsia, heaviness of loin and limb, flushing and fidgetiness, palpitations, vague pains and flying neuralgia, spinal irritation, uterine irritability, impotence, hopelessness, and such morbid fears as claustrophobia and dread of contamination," the diagnosis of neurasthenia promised a large and varied clientele.[44]

Stigmatized by even the next generation of their own profession as "egotistically restless and in their neurological efforts little better than commercial adventurers,"[45] the earliest neurologists nevertheless exhibited an aggressively scientistic attitude and a near-worshipful attitude toward European authority. They were convinced of the superiority of their own training and of its application to the whole range of nervous and mental disorders, from the serious to the trivial. At the same time, they were contemptuous of the abilities and accomplishments of those who already possessed a monopoly of the professional care and treatment of the insane, the asylum superintendents. The mixture proved explosive. By 1878, neurologists had provoked a fierce and bitter quarrel with their professional adversaries over the suitability of the asylum as an arena for treatment of the insane, and, more broadly, over the respective merits of each group's understanding and treatment of mental disorder—a quarrel that is the focus of Bonnie Blustein's analysis in chapter 10.

The dispute continued unabated into the 1880s, provoking legislative inquiries; prompting a temporary alliance between medical and lay critics of the asylum in the form of the short-lived National Association for the Protection of the Insane and the Prevention of Insanity; and spilling over into the popular press. Then, almost as abruptly as it had begun, the steam went out of the controversy, and the two groups of experts settled down to a period of more or less uneasy coexistence—marked, on the neurologists' side by a refocusing of much of their energy and concern away from insanity and toward a greater emphasis on the diagnosis and treatment (if any) of more demonstrably organic forms of nervous disorder and, on the superintendents' part, by a loosening of the rules for membership in their professional association (to allow assistant asylum physicians and even nonasylum specialists in the treatment of mental disorder to join), and by gestures toward the neurologists' emphasis on the importance of the scientific laboratory and the dissecting room. Occasionally, they even went so far as to hire a neurologist to perform this work in the state hospital basement.

A number of factors contributed to this truce, some of them purely adventitious. Perhaps most fundamentally, the neurologists' efforts to secure a dominant position in the treatment of mental disorder foundered upon the weaknesses of their own claims to be *the* only qualified practitioners of a scientific psychology: claims neither their fellow physicians nor the public at large seemed disposed to accept. Moreover, while the neurologists' slashing attacks on the asylum struck some responsive chords among a public always fascinated by tales of the dark underside of asylum life and perpetually fearful of improper confinement in these "Bluebeard's cupboards of the neighbourhood," they ultimately led nowhere, for the neurologists "had little to substitute for the asylum beyond a general charge to the superintendents to behave like doctors."[46] At the same time, the neurologists' willingness to ally themselves with laymen and to air their complaints in popular newspapers and journals angered the medical profession as a whole, which considered such maneuvers dangerously unprofessional. And the tone and tactics of their campaigns began to contribute, in both medical and lay circles, to a perception of the neurologists as irresponsible and sensationalistic individuals—an ironic and deeply threatening development in view of the importance to the latter of their self-perception as men of science. In the circumstances, the decision to opt for a more or less graceful retreat is not to be wondered at; nor can one be surprised to learn that when, three decades later, some neurologists once more sought a major role in the treatment of the mentally disordered, others of their number viewed their endeavors with circumspection, if not outright hostility.

As Blustein reminds us, the rhetoric of the neurologists was, from the outset, characterized by a thoroughgoing materialism. In these terms, neurologists sought to account for a whole spectrum of problems, ranging from normal psychology to functional and organic nervous disorders and insanity. Much of their therapeutics—from the elaborate shiny machines for administering static electricity to S. Weir Mitchell's famous "rest cure" (which involved isolation from one's family, rest, diet, massage, and the absence of all responsibility)—to our eyes depended for its efficacy largely upon its psychological impact on the patient. But while acknowledging that individual suggestibility sometimes played a part in a cure, the neurologists remained deeply antagonistic, not merely to psychological *explanations* of insanity, but to any sustained or systematic attention to mental therapeutics. Mitchell, for example, while acknowledging some similarities between his rest cure and the activities of exponents of religiously based "mind cures," insisted that the fundamental impact of his approach derived from its contribution to building up the patient's "fat and blood."[47]

Thus when George M. Beard read a paper before the American Neurological Association in which he described experiments with the use of "definite expectation," and had the temerity to suggest that "the expectation is itself a curative force" (and one, moreover, superior to electricity or drugs used alone), he met with furious criticism from his colleagues.[48] The idea that one might systematically exploit such techniques was dismissed as little better than "deception." Dr. Putnam and Dr. Amerson decried the experiments as "unscientific," and Dr. Mason denied the very existence of "mental therapeutics." William Hammond was perhaps the most scathing of all. He announced that "if the doctrine advanced by Dr.

Beard was to be accepted, he should feel like throwing his diploma away and joining the theologians," since once the profession took that fateful step, "we should be descending to the level of all sorts of humbuggery."[49] Here was one issue on which the still-divided neurological and psychiatric professions could agree. In the words of John Gray, ordinarily the chief target of the neurologists' barbs, "If insanity be merely a disease of the mind, pure and simple, we can readily admit the all-sufficiency of moral means of treatment. Believing, however, that it is but a manifestation of physical lesion, . . . to which the psychical phenomena are subordinate or secondary, any other conclusion than that which makes medical therapeutics the basis of treatment involves an absurdity."[50]

Michael Clark's paper examines the similar rejection of psychological approaches in late nineteenth-century British psychiatry. In my own work, I have analyzed some of the social and institutional factors which predisposed Victorian psychiatrists in the direction of a heavily somaticist account of mental disorder.[51] Clark extends and deepens this analysis, demonstrating how the lack of receptivity to psychological approaches was rooted in the "deep structures" of Victorian psychiatric theory. The hostility was all the more notable since, as was sometimes acknowledged at the time, somatic-pathological approaches to insanity in apparently critical areas embodied a double failure. On the one hand, they yielded little in the way of increased *scientific understanding* of the etiology and pathology of insanity; and on the other hand, they possessed no clear-cut or decisive *therapeutic advantages* over "moral treatment" or other more purely empirical nonmedical methods when it came to curing the insane. Yet, in light of Clark's analysis, the broader pressures to adopt an orthodox somatic viewpoint seem so powerful that this outcome was almost overdetermined. As he states in his paper in this volume, "The moral and professional authority of the physician, and his unswerving commitment to the practice of orthodox somatic medicine were seen as bound together in a chain of common connection and mutual dependence; and anything which tended to weaken or undermine either of the interdependent elements would, it was firmly believed, eventually tend to weaken or undermine the other as well."

The question of how this resistance to psychological approaches was overcome—however partially—permitting the development of dynamic psychiatry (especially in its Freudian guise) is a fascinating one. For the most part, however, it falls outside the temporal framework of the analyses presented here. One may briefly note, though, that in the United States at least, it is clear that a critical mediating role was played, ironically enough, by the neurological profession, or at least by a portion of the neurological profession. (*Ironically,* not just because of Freud's own neurological training, but more centrally because, as we have just seen, in the prior period the neurologists had been the most vigorous and committed champions of the somatic style, and had attempted to usurp the medical superintendents' established role in its treatment on the basis of the common somatic origins insanity allegedly shared with other nervous afflictions.)

Much research remains to be done in this area, though one can certainly point to a number of factors which contributed to this change. Not the least important was the continuing therapeutic and scientific barrenness of work based on pathological anatomy, and the growing recognition of this state of affairs. In his 1907 Presidential Address to the American Medico-Psychological Association, C. G. Hill complained that "our therapeutics is simply a pile of rubbish"; and two years later, S. Weir Mitchell echoed the point in his address to the neurologists: "Amid enormous gains in our art, we have sadly to confess the absolute standstill of the therapy of insanity and the relative failure, as concerns diagnosis, in mental maladies of even that most capable diagnostician, the post-mortem surgeon."[52]

Many among the rising generation of neurologists resisted the declining sense of optimism with which most of their elders responded to this sense of incapacity.[53] Instead, they cast around for alternative bases of understanding and treatment. External developments contributed powerfully to their search. The extraordinarily rapid proliferation of religiously based mental-healing cults (of which the most notable was Christian Science) had prompted a growing "exodus of patients from the doctor's waiting room to the minister's study."[54] In the face of this competition, many neurologists concluded that the patients must be saved from themselves. Since people were voting with their feet for mental therapeutics, the profession must somehow respond to their demand:

> There ought to be some definite form of psychotherapeutics approved by the profession so that people would not go after "soul massage" or other faked forms of psychotherapeutics. What are we going to do with the large number who won't come to us and will go to anyone who will raise his psychic standard? We must find out the good behind these false methods and organize it into some wise scientific measure which we can prescribe. Until we do this there will be a continual succession of new cults, Christian Science, osteopathy, etc., to the discredit of medicine and more especially of psychiatry and neurology.[55]

Increasingly, many neurologists were led to concede that "it need not be gainsaid that *religious* psychotherapy has effected cures," in cases where traditional medical-somatic approaches had brought neither understanding nor results. They were swift to add, however, that "the cures it may have produced are such as could have and should have been brought about by means of *rational* psychotherapy in the hands of a conscientious physi-

cian."[56] Medicine perforce would have to abandon its traditional "antagonism to methods of treatment which appeal to other than physical
means. . . ."[57] And indeed, a portion of the neurological profession was
clearly willing to do so. Drawing once more, as had the first generation of
neurologists, on the work of European authorities, by 1900 a small but
growing number were experimenting with the psychotherapies of such
men as Dubois and Janet, and, subsequently, of Freud. By the end of the
decade, there were more and more confident claims that one or another of
these forms of psychotherapy offered "certain definite methods of procedure of a rational sort."[58] This confidence derived in part from the way the
new treatments "made sense" of phenomena that the somatic approach left
outside the realm of systematic observation, or which "could not be logically accounted for in its terms."[59] In the hands of the physician, psychotherapy allegedly became far more precise and scientific than it had
hitherto been, and as such was something which belonged only in the
hands of the trained specialist.[60] Indeed, James Jackson Putnam went so
far as to equate psychotherapeutics with "a surgical operation of the most
delicate sort" and to claim that analysis "of subconscious memories [is]
. . . the major surgery of neurological therapeutics."[61]

Unanimity was far from being reached on these issues, however. A
powerful faction among the neurologists remained unalterably opposed to
any but somatic approaches, and continued to stigmatize those who
strayed from the path of scientific virtue as teetering on the brink of
charlatanry. To those who raised the specter of the loss of patients, Bernard Sachs responded, "Let those who want to go to Christian Science go,
we are not seeking patients. A certain number of them will go. There will
be plenty left. We cannot keep people from consulting quacks of every
description." Furthermore, the very attempt risked both the profession's
"dignity and scientific integrity."[62] The afflictions of these people were, in
any event, not central to the neurological enterprise, with its focus on "the
care and treatment of patients suffering from organic nervous diseases.
. . . While hysterical, neurasthenic patients, and others of the same order,
are numerous enough, their ailments and sufferings are, after all, less
important than the sufferings of those who are afflicted with various forms
of organic spinal disease, say tabes, primary lateral sclerosis, and the like.
Let us try to do more for these patients . . . and do not let us waste too much
time and energy on what people are pleased to call psychotherapy."[63]

Ultimately, the split was irreparable. One branch of the profession
remained wedded to orthodox, somatic approaches, even at the cost of
some narrowing of focus and a recognition that diagnostic refinement
continued to go hand in hand with therapeutic impotence. A second group
sought to make psychological theorizing and therapeutics medically respectable. The latter segment argued that this step was essential if the

neurologist were not to "sink into the narrow niche of curator of the scleroses or an appraiser of teratological defects."[64] And, with Morton Prince, they denied that "the sufferings of hysterical and neurasthenic patients are less important than the sufferings of those who are affected with various forms of organic spinal disease. There are one hundred persons suffering from functional disease to one from organic spine disease, and from the point of view of numbers as well as from that of our power to relieve suffering, the former are far more important. We can do little or nothing for organic diseases of the spinal cord; we can do everything for the functional nervous afflictions."[65]

The neurotics who flocked to the offices of the new psychotherapists were predominantly, though far from exclusively, women. But the sexual composition of the psychiatrists' clientele had not always been preponderantly female. Indeed, a change in the ratio of the sexes under treatment and, to a more limited extent, an associated shift in expert estimates of the respective vulnerability of men and women to madness were themselves among the most important transformations that lunacy reform brought in its train. In the early nineteenth century, writers on insanity had with some consistency assumed that madness was more frequently a female disorder. But closer attention to the statistics of insanity (itself partly a product of the reform movement) for a time pushed them toward revising this opinion. The figures for individual asylums in both the United States and England and, in the latter, parliamentary returns for the country as a whole displayed, with relative consistency, a significant excess of males. Given the alienists' tendency to confuse incidence and prevalence with numbers institutionalized, efforts were soon under way to uncover explanations for the "fact" that "men are actually more liable to disorders of the mind than women."[66] Such endeavors were short-lived, however, for the opening of state-run asylums for the poor was matched by an upsurge in the number of female patients, and before long the balance of the sexes corresponded closely to more conventional assumptions. "Private," upperclass lunatics receiving asylum care continued for a time to be disproportionately male, but by 1875 women also made up a majority of their ranks.

Alienists found in these statistics, as in their practice, a new source of confirmation of the traditional medical view: woman was "the product and prisoner of her reproductive system."[67] The constant shock and strain on her system produced by the unsettled character of her reproductive economy brought in its train a heightened susceptibility to emotional disorder and mental disease, and found its natural expression in the nervous invalid of the neurologist's office and the female inhabitant of the asylum. Culturally constructed conceptions of madness and of the female role thus found their mutual support in a portrait of the biological bases of femininity. Among women, commented one physician, "the nerves themselves are smaller, and of a more delicate structure. They are endowed with greater sensibility and, of course, are liable to more frequent and stronger impressions from external agents or mental influences."[68]

Logically enough, for men like Charles Beard, the overstimulation of women's brains, caused by their increased mental activity in the late nineteenth century, represented a primary source of the worrisome increase in neurasthenia. And in Victorian England as well, psychiatrists vied with one another to account for and to offer advice and treatment to those women whose nervous capacities proved unequal to the strain. The Victorian woman's encounter with insanity is thus a peculiarly important and revealing one, and the many dimensions of that encounter in its English context are explored by Elaine Showalter in chapter 12.

During the course of the nineteenth century, the expansion of the asylum system and the associated growth and consolidation of an organized medical concern with the problem of insanity prompted continuing efforts to modify and systematize the law's relationship to lunacy. Increased attention was paid to such issues as testamentary capacity and the capacity to administer one's business and property; but the major arenas of interaction and conflict between psychiatry and law were the criteria and procedures for certifying someone as a lunatic; and the issue of culpability in criminal law, the so-called insanity defense. Both the broader issue of who was mad and who sane, and the more limited question of when insanity could be proferred as a successful defense to a criminal charge were (as they continue to be) profoundly controversial matters for which no fixed resolution could be found. With good reason, different segments of society felt their vital interests were at stake here; and the cognitive and evaluative frameworks of the contending parties being irreconcilable, conflict necessarily remained endemic.

The issue of improper confinement sparked periodic waves of concern on both sides of the Atlantic throughout the nineteenth century. Almost universally, the focus of the contentiousness was not the liberty of the lunatic, but the likelihood (or impossibility) of a sane person's being improperly committed and subjected to "the *living death* of incarceration" in a lunatic asylum—"a fate," as the Pennsylvania Board of Commissioners put it, "next in horror to being buried alive."[69] These concerns were hardly new ones. Allegations of the use of madhouses to confine the sane surfaced repeatedly in the eighteenth century: in Defoe's pamphlets; in petitions to Parliament; and in the polemics of former patients.[70] Recurrently, those who traded in lunacy faced the charge that their desire for profit led them to acquiesce in such schemes. Belcher's image of the madhouse keeper as a "Smiling Hyena" savagely captures this popular image:

This animal is a non-descript of mixed species. Form obtuse—body black—head grey—teeth and prowess on the decline—visage smiling, especially at the sight of shining metal, of which its paws are extremely retentive—heart supposed to be of a kind of tough white leather.

N.B. He doth ravish the rich when he getteth him into his den.[71]

Such fears seem, if anything, to have intensified in the nineteenth century, despite ever-tighter regulation of the mad business, and in the face of persistent legislative attempts to allay them. Indeed, one might well argue that, paradoxically, these efforts fed rather than quieted the anxiety. Periodic moral panics in England forced two major parliamentary inquiries on this issue, in 1858–59 and again in 1876–77. In the United States, the case of Mrs. Elizabeth Packard attracted widespread attention and sparked a crusade (led by Mrs. Packard herself) to tighten commitment laws.[72] And at other times, ex-patients' pamphlets and law suits (not to mention best-selling novels like Charles Reade's *Hard Cash*) played upon and reinforced public suspicion.[73] The development of more formalized commitment procedures and the apparent acceptance by legislators of the new psychiatric profession's claim that the identification of madness was a judgment for experts alone, meant that lay intervention in these matters was held to be necessarily illegitimate. And yet it was precisely the motives and competence of the "experts" that large segments of the public seem to have questioned.

At the same time, both those who supervised the asylum system, and the superintendents themselves, angrily rejected the charges of false confinement, and in some instances, impugned the motives and mental capacity of those who brought them. Historians have generally concurred in this judgment. But, as Peter McCandless argues in chapter 13, this attitude is probably mistaken, not least because of the always labile and uncertain boundary between sanity and madness, and the inescapable moral and social component in all such judgments.[74] It was not that doctors and relatives conspired to incarcerate the sane (though there may have been a few such cases). Rather, the very bases of physicians' judgments were often heavily value laden, so that in their eyes insanity and immorality at times became all but indistinguishable.

Both the issue of medical authority in the certification of lunatics in general, and the role of expert testimony by alienists on the question of the boundary between insanity and criminal responsibility were highly charged and symbolically crucial issues for the professional aspirations of psychiatry. Perhaps this is one reason why they attracted attention out of all proportion to the size of the social problems they represented.

Moreover, as Roger Smith points out in Chapter 14, disputes about these issues implicitly revolve around fundamental philosophical and moral differences over the interpretation of and attribution of responsibility and/or causation for human action. The alienists sought to remove their discourse to a plane where it would be accorded the objectivity of physical science. We have alluded elsewhere to nineteenth-century psychiatry's insistence upon a somatic etiology for insanity, an account pitched in terms of physical abnormalities, structural or functional, in the brain, other nervous tissue, or neural blood circulation. Such medical views played an essential role in disputes about the insanity defense. So far as the physicians were concerned, their privileged access to such knowledge (on the basis of their clinical and diagnostic skill) ought to secure for their judgments a unique and unchallengeable truth status. And given that their account of the relationship between insanity and behavior was deterministic in form, the moral issue of responsibility dissolved in the confrontation with scientific objectivity.

By contrast, legal discourse remained wedded to a commonsense schema wherein will or intention, the voluntary basis of action, assumed a central place. Notwithstanding the claims of the alienists to the contrary, the choice between these two forms of discourse was (and remains) inherently evaluative.[75] And psychiatrists who attempted to dispute this were repeatedly impeached by their own inability to agree on a diagnosis. The embarrassment of having eminent men testify that the same man was both unambiguously mad and unquestionably sane was one the profession felt deeply, but could never adequately resolve.[76]

Ultimately, of course, any increase in the social acceptability of the medical accounts of criminal insanity rests upon the wider adoption of a determinist universe of discourse. As Smith emphasizes, the existence of any movement in this direction, and the sources of that shift, must necessarily be a focal point of future research, one which will undoubtedly contribute to a further rapprochement between medico-legal history and the general history of science and medicine. In the meantime, his essay repeatedly demonstrates the value of close and epistemologically sophisticated attention to the issue of the social location of the boundary between sanity and madness, making use of a class of materials which historians have otherwise examined cursorily.

Notes

1. Michel Foucault, *Madness and Civilization: A History of Insanity in the Age of Reason* (New York: Mentor Books, 1965); Gerald Grob, *The State and the Mentally Ill* (Chapel Hill: University of North Carolina Press, 1966); idem, *Mental Institutions in America* (New York: Free Press, 1973); David Rothman, *The Discovery of the Asylum* (Boston: Little, Brown, 1971); and, on the Grob-Rothman debate, Andrew Scull, "Humanitarianism or Control: Observations on the Historiography of Anglo-American Psychiatry," *Rice University Studies* 67 (1981): 21–41.
2. Kathleen Jones, *A History of the Mental Health Services* (London: Routledge and Kegan Paul, 1972); Richard Hunter and Ida MacAlpine, *Psychiatry for the Poor* (London: Dawsons, 1974).
3. Andrew Scull, "Museums of Madness: The Social Organization of Insanity in Nineteenth Century England" (Ph.D. diss., Princeton University, 1974); Peter McCandless, "Insanity and Society: A Study of the English Lunacy Reform Movement" (Ph.D. diss., University of Wisconsin, 1974); Michael Fears, "The 'Moral Treatment' of Insanity: A Study in the Social Construction of Human Nature" (Ph.D. diss., University of Edinburgh, 1978).
4. Albert Deutsch, *The Mentally Ill in America: A History of Their Care and Treatment,* 2d ed. (New York: Columbia University Press, 1949); Gregory Zilboorg and G. Henry, *A History of Medical Psychology* (New York: Norton, 1969); Kathleen Jones, *Mental Health Services;* idem, *Lunacy, Law and Conscience* (London: Routledge and Kegan Paul, 1955); Norman Dain, *Concepts of Insanity in the United States, 1789–1865* (New Brunswick, N.J.: Rutgers University Press, 1964).
5. Daniel Walker Howe, "Victorian Culture in America," in *Victorian America,* ed. Daniel Walker Howe (Philadelphia: University of Pennsylvania Press, 1976), pp. 3–28.
6. Peter Sedgwick, "Michel Foucault: The Anti-History of Psychiatry," in *Psychopolitics* (London: Pluto Press, forthcoming).
7. Stanley W. Jackson, "Unusual Mental States in Medieval Europe. 1. Medical Syndromes of Mental Disorder, 400–1100 A.D.," *Journal of the History of Medicine* 27 (1972): 262–97.
8. Basil Clark, *Mental Disorder in Earlier Britain* (Cardiff: University of Wales Press, 1975); A. Fessler, "The Management of Lunacy in Seventeenth Century England," *Proceedings of the Royal Society of Medicine, Historical Section* 49 (1956): 901–7; William Ll. Parry-Jones, *The Trade in Lunacy* (London: Routledge and Kegan Paul, 1972); George Rosen, *Madness and Society* (New York: Harper and Row, 1969); and Foucault, *Madness and Civilization* are partial exceptions to this generalization.
9. William Battie, *A Treatise on Madness* (London: Whiston and White, 1758).
10. Parry-Jones, *Trade in Lunacy.*

11. See especially Ida MacAlpine and Richard Hunter, *George III and the Mad Business* (London: Allen Lane, 1969).

12. See William Cullen, *First Lines of the Practice of Physic* (Edinburgh: Bell and Bradfute, 1808).

13. Andrew Scull, "From Madness to Mental Illness: Medical Men as Moral Entrepreneurs," *European Journal of Sociology* 16 (1975): 219–61. Doctors opposed the psychological theories of mental disorder because they thought such theories would give encouragement to a veritable "swarm of religious psychotherapeutists" (C. B. Farrar, "Psychotherapy and the Church," *Journal of Nervous and Mental Diseases* 36 [1909]: 11–24). Opposition may be found even in the early years of the twentieth century. Freud himself, on his visit to Clark University, felt obliged to caution against "this combination of church and psychotherapy" for which the public appeared to have a weakness; he also asserted the necessity of placing operations on "the instrument of the soul" in trained (i.e., nonecclesiastical) hands. Cf. Nathan Hale, *Freud and the Americans* (New York: Oxford University Press, 1971), pp. 226–27.

14. Scull, "From Madness to Mental Illness."

15. Dain, *Concepts of Insanity*, p. 167. American alienists who embraced phrenology explicitly rejected the charge of materialism. In Isaac Ray's words, "Since Locke's attack on the doctrine of innate ideas, people have become so accustomed to attribute the phenomena of mind to the influence of habit, association, etc., that the *mind itself* seems to be entirely lost sight of, and practically, if not theoretically, believed to be what Hume would make it, a mere bundle of perceptions. From such a philosophy, which makes the most wonderful phenomena of our nature the mere creature of the material world, Phrenology delivers us, and presents in its place a rational and intelligible exposition of the mental powers." Cited in Dain, *Concepts of Insanity*, p. 62.

16. On the importance of the latter point in the struggle to reassert medical hegemony over the treatment of insanity, see Scull, "From Madness to Mental Illness." More doubtful, I think, is Cooter's concluding claim that phrenology's collapse somehow accounts for the erosion of moral therapy and the loss of therapeutic optimism among alienists. The evidence he presents in support of this proposition is scanty and unconvincing. For different assessments of these developments, see Andrew Scull, *Museums of Madness: The Social Organization of Insanity in Nineteenth Century England* (London and New York: Allen Lane and St. Martin's Press, 1979), and John Walton's essay in this volume.

17. House of Commons, *Select Committee on Madhouses Report*, 1815, p. 76.

18. A. Thompson and G. Goldin, *The Hospital: A Social and Architectural History* (New Haven: Yale University Press, 1975). In this connection, it is perhaps worthy of note that the architect of St. Luke's Hospital, probably the most influential of eighteenth-century English charity asylums, was George Dance the Younger, who was also responsible for the design of the new Newgate Prison.

19. Robert Gardiner Hill, *A Lecture on the Management of Lunatic Asylums* (London: Simpkin, Marshall, 1839), pp. 4–6.

20. J. Mortimer Granville, *The Care and Cure of the Insane*, 2 vols. (London: Hard-wicke and Bogue, 1877), 1:15.

21. Cited in Dorothea Dix, *Memorial Soliciting the Construction of a State Hospital for the Insane, in the State of Mississippi* (Jackson, Miss.: Fall and Marshall, 1850), p. 20.

22. Samuel Tuke, *Description of the Retreat* (York: Alexander, 1813), p. 102.

23. Cf. Scull, *Museums*, chap. 7.

24. Grob, *State and the Mentally Ill*.

25. Scull, *Museums*, pp. 214–16; Grob, *State and the Mentally Ill*.

26. Lancaster County Asylum, *64th Annual Report*, 1880, cited in Pliny Earle, *The Curability of Insanity* (Philadelphia: Lippincott, 1887), p. 160.

27. John Charles Bucknill, *The Care of the Insane and Their Legal Control* (London: Macmillan, 1880), p. 114.

28. [Andrew Wynter], "Non-Restraint," *Edinburgh Review* 131 (1870): 225, 229.

29. House of Commons, *Report of the Select Committee on the Operation of the Lunacy Laws*, 1877, pp. 53–55.

30. Edward Jarvis to Sir James Clark, 10 March 1869, cited in Clark, *A Memoir of John Conolly* (London: Murray, 1869), p. 101.

31. Massachusetts State Board of Charities, *4th Annual Report*, 1867, pp. xliii, lvi; *5th Annual Report*, 1868; and *6th Annual Report*, 1869, pass.

32. Ibid., *7th Annual Report*, 1870, esp. pp. xl–xlii; see also Grob, *State and the Mentally Ill*, pp. 209–22.

33. Cf. Norman Dain, *Disordered Minds* (Williamsburg, Va.: Colonial Williams-burg Foundation, 1971), pp. 128–34.

34. The best account of the ambivalent American response to Geel may be found in Grob, *Mental Institutions*, pp. 325–36.

35. See, for example, the comments in Henry Maudsley, *The Physiology and Pathol-ogy of the Mind* (London: Macmillan, 1868); Andrew Wynter, "Non-Restraint"; "Statistics of Insanity in Massachusetts," *North American Review* 82 (1856): 78–100.

36. See Scull, *Museums;* and idem, "Humanitarianism or Control?"

37. E. Cumming and J. Cumming, *Closed Ranks* (Cambridge, Mass.: Harvard Uni-versity Press, 1957), p. 55.

38. L. J. Epstein and A. Simon, "Alternatives to State Hospitalization for the Geriatric Mentally Ill," *American Journal of Psychiatry* 124 (1968): 955–61; Robert Riech and Lloyd Segal, "Psychiatry Under Siege: The Chronic Mentally Ill Shuffle to Oblivion," *Psychiatric Annals* 3 (1973): 37–55; F. Arnoff, "Social Conse-quences of Policy Toward Mental Illness," *Science* 188 (1975): 1277–81.

39. Earle, *Curability of Insanity*.

40. See especially Amariah Brigham, *Observations on the Influence of Religion upon the Health and Physical Welfare of Mankind* (Boston: Marsh, Capet, and Lyon, 1835); idem, *Remarks on the Influence of Mental Cultivation and Mental Excitement upon Health* (Philadelphia: Lea and Blanchard, 1845); and the discussion in Grob, *Mental Institutions*, pp. 160–64.

41. See, for example, Isaac Ray, *Mental Hygiene* (Boston: Ticknor and Fields, 1863); S. Weir Mitchell, *Fat and Blood*, 3d ed. rev. (Philadelphia: Lippincott, 1884);

idem, *Wear and Tear: Or Hints for the Overworked* (Philadelphia: Lippincott, 1871); J. S. Jewell, "Influence of Our Present Civilization in the Production of Nervous and Mental Diseases," *Journal of Nervous and Mental Diseases* 8 (1881): 14–17.

42. Scull, "From Madness to Mental Illness"; John A. Pitts, "The Association of Medical Superintendents of American Institutions for the Insane, 1844–1892: A Case Study of Specialism in American Medicine" (Ph.D. diss., University of Pennsylvania, 1978); Constance McGovern, " 'Mad-doctors': American Psychiatrists, 1800–1860" (Ph.D. diss., University of Massachusetts, 1976). See also Rosenberg, "The Crisis of Psychiatric Legitimacy," pp. 135–48.

43. Charles Rosenberg, "The Place of George M. Beard in Nineteenth Century Psychiatry," *Bulletin of the History of Medicine* 36 (1962): 245–59.

44. Barbara Sicherman, "The Uses of a Diagnosis: Doctors, Patients, and Neurasthenia," *Journal of the History of Medicine and Allied Sciences* 32 (1977): 33–54.

45. Frank R. Fry to Smith Ely Jelliffe, 17 March 1924, cited in Bonnie Blustein, "New York Neurologists and the Specialization of American Medicine," *Bulletin of the History of Medicine* 53 (1979): 170–83.

46. "Lunatic Asylums," *Quarterly Review* 101 (1857): 353; David Rothman, *Conscience and Convenience: The Asylum and Its Alternatives in Progressive America* (Boston: Little, Brown, 1980).

47. Mitchell, *Fat and Blood,* 1877 ed., esp. pp. 55–56.

48. Cf. George M. Beard, "The Influence of the Mind in the Causation and Cure of Disease—The Potency of Definite Expectation," *Journal of Nervous and Mental Diseases* 4 (1877): 429–34.

49. See "American Neurological Association," *Journal of Nervous and Mental Diseases* 3 (1876): 429–37.

50. See John Gray, "Editorial," *American Journal of Insanity* 21 (1865): 558.

51. Scull, "From Madness to Mental Illness"; idem, "Mad-doctors and Magistrates: English Psychiatry's Struggle for Professional Autonomy in the Nineteenth Century," *European Journal of Sociology* 17 (1976): 279–305.

52. Charles G. Hill, "How Can We Best Advance the Study of Psychiatry?" *American Journal of Psychiatry* 64 (1907): 6; S. Weir Mitchell, "[Presidential] Address to the American Neurological Association," *Transactions of the American Neurological Association* 35 (1909): 1. For similar comments, see E. Stanley Abbot, "The Criteria of Insanity and the Problems of Psychiatry," *American Journal of Insanity* 59 (1902): 1–16; and F. X. Dercum, "A Clinical Classification of Insanity," *Journal of Nervous and Mental Diseases* 28 (1901): 489–90.

53. Cf. Hale, *Freud and the Americans,* p. 75.

54. Barbara Sicherman, "The Quest for Mental Health in America, 1880–1917" (Ph.D. diss., Columbia University, 1967), pp. 269–70.

55. Charles L. Dana, in discussion of "Rest Treatment in Relation to Psychotherapy," by S. Weir Mitchell, *Transactions of the American Neurological Association* 34 (1908): 217.

56. Edward Wyllys Taylor, "The Attitude of the Medical Profession Toward the Psychotherapeutic Movement" (Summary and Discussion), *Journal of Nervous and Mental Diseases* 35 (1908): 420.

57. Ibid.

58. Hale, *Freud and the Americans,* p. 48. "The satisfaction of having made understandable order out of chaos came to many of the pioneering psychotherapists.

They argued time and again that the order they 'discovered' proved the truth of their assertions." Ibid., p. 132.

59. Hale, *Freud and the Americans,* p. 48.
60. See the discussion of Taylor, "Psychotherapeutic Movement," White and Jelliffe, *Journal of Nervous and Mental Diseases* 35 (1908): 408–9.
61. Ibid., p. 411. Note the choice of metaphor. Freud, too, on his visit to Clark University, insisted to all who would listen that "the instrument of the soul is not so easy to play and my technique is very painstaking and tedious. Any amateur attempt may have the most evil consequence." Interview with Adelbert Albrecht, *Boston Evening Transcript,* 11 September 1909, quoted in Hale, *Freud and the Americans,* pp. 226–27.
62. Bernard Sachs, "Commentary on 'Rest Treatment in Relation to Psychotherapy,' by S. Weir Mitchell," *Transactions of the American Neurological Association* 34 (1908): 218.
63. Bernard Sachs, "Commentary on 'The Attitude of the Medical Profession Toward the Psychotherapeutic Movement,' by E. W. Taylor," *Journal of Nervous and Mental Diseases* 35 (1908): 405. See also the comments by Dercum, J. K. Mitchell, and Collins.
64. Charles L. Dana, "The Future of Neurology," *Journal of Nervous and Mental Diseases* 40 (1913): 755.
65. Morton Prince, "Commentary on 'Psychotherapeutic Movement,' by Taylor," *Journal of Nervous and Mental Diseases* 35 (1908): 413. The optimism, as so often in the history of psychiatry, was misplaced.
66. John Thurnam, *Observations and Essays on the Statistics of Insanity* (London: Simpkin Marshall, 1845).
67. Charles Rosenberg and Carroll Smith-Rosenberg, "The Female Animal: Medical and Biological Views of Women," in Rosenberg, *No Other Gods: On Science and American Social Thought* (Baltimore: Johns Hopkins University Press, 1976), p. 55.
68. Cited in ibid.
69. Pennsylvania Board of Charities, *Annual Report,* 1876, p. 6 (italics in the original).
70. Daniel Defoe, *A Review of the State of the English Nation* (London: Baker, 1706); idem, *Augusta Triumphans: Or, the Way to Make London the Most Flourishing City in the Universe* (London: Roberts, 1728); Alexander Cruden, *The London Citizen Exceedingly Injured: Or, A British Inquisition Displayed* (London: Cooper and Dodd, 1739); idem, *The Adventures of Alexander the Corrector, with an Account of the Chelsea Academies for Such as Are Supposed to be Deprived of the Use of Their Reason* (London: for the author, 1754).
71. W. Belcher, *An Address to Humanity, Containing a Receipt to Make a Lunatic* (London: for the author, 1796), cited in Parry-Jones, *Trade in Lunacy,* p. 226.
72. Cf. Elizabeth Packard, *Great Disclosures of Spiritual Wickedness!! . . . With an Appeal to the Government to Protect the Inalienable Rights of Married Women* (Boston: for the author, 1864); idem, *Modern Persecution, or Insane Asylums Unveiled,* 2 vols. (Hartford: Case, Lockwood, and Brainard, 1873).
73. For American examples, see Robert Fuller, *An Account of the Imprisonment and Sufferings of Robert Fuller of Cambridge . . . in the McLean Asylum for the Insane* (Boston: for the author, 1833); Elizabeth Stone, *Exposing the Modern Secret Way*

of Persecuting Christians. . . . Insane Hospitals Are Inquisition Houses (Boston: for the author, 1859); An American Citizen, *The Hinchman Conspiracy Case, in Letters to the New York Home Journal* (Philadelphia: Stokes and Brother, 1849).

74. Cf. David Morgan, "Explaining Mental Illness," *European Journal of Sociology* 16 (1975): 262–80.

75. Ibid.

76. For a recent analysis of these issues from a legal perspective, see Stephen J. Morse, "Crazy Behavior, Morals, and Science: An Analysis of Mental Health Law," *Southern California Law Review* 51 (1978): 527–654.

PART ONE
Mad-Doctors and Their Therapies

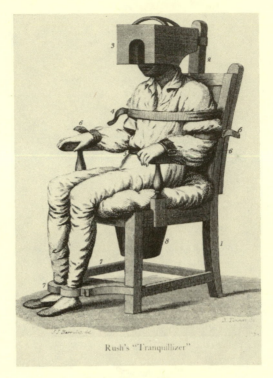

Rush's "Tranquillizer"

Rush's Tranquillizer

Mad-doctors of the early nineteenth century produced some extravagant mechanical devices for the treatment of recalcitrant madmen. Together with the rotary machine or swing, developed by Joseph Mason Cox at Erasmus Darwin's suggestion, Rush's "Tranquillizer" is perhaps the best known of these therapeutic weapons. In a letter of 8 June 1810 to his son James, Benjamin Rush announced:

> I have contrived a chair and introduced it to our [Pennsylvania] Hospital to assist in curing madness. It binds and confines every part of the body. By keeping the trunk erect, it lessens the impetus of the blood toward the brain. By preventing the muscles from acting, it reduces the force and frequency of the pulse, and by the position of the head and feet favors the easy application of cold water or ice to the former, and warm water to the latter. Its effects have been truly delightful to me. It acts as a sedative to the tongue and temper as well as to the blood vessels. In 24, 12, 6, and in some cases in 4 hours, the most refractory patients have been composed. I have called it a *Tranquillizer*.

The spread of moral treatment spelled the demise of Rush's benevolent invention.

(Sources: engraving from *The Philadelphia Medical Museum*, n.s. 1 [1811] 169. Rush's description from Rush to James Rush, 8 June 1810, reprinted in *Letters of Benjamin Rush*, L. H. Butterfield, ed. [Princeton: Princeton University Press, 1951], 2:1052.)

WILLIAM F. BYNUM, JR.

2 Rationales for Therapy in British Psychiatry, 1780–1835

Any general history of psychiatry between, say, the Renaissance and the end of the nineteenth century would likely stress, among other things, the following two points. First, that during this period there was a growing acceptance, both within the medical community and among the general public, that certain behavioral patterns, and certain kinds of mental states, are the result of *disease,* and hence are the proper objects of medical description and treatment; this instead of the ascription of these queer ways of acting or thinking to such things as the possession by demons, a state of sin, or willful criminality. Second, a growing acceptance, again among both physicians and laymen, that the mind is the function of the brain, that a phrase like "mental physiology" is not a contradiction in terms, and that while perhaps it is not equivalent to "cerebral physiology" the two processes are so closely linked that the one cannot be properly understood without reference to the other. This commitment received its fullest expression in the school of German somatic psychiatrists of the last half of the nineteenth century, the school of Griesinger, Meynert, and Wernicke, a group that Ackerknecht has called the "brain psychiatrists."[1]

My end point for this broad summary was the end of the nineteenth century. This was deliberate, for despite the fact that in a general way these two trends have continued to the present day, implicit or explicit challenges to both claims still exist. For example, what might be called the "educational process" among laymen continues unabated: they are told that "mental illness is nothing to be ashamed of," or that "mental illness is just like any other illness." At the same time, within the psychiatric community itself, the whole concept of mental health and mental illness as it is presently formulated has been severely criticized, from the political Left by psychiatrists such as R. D. Laing; while from another vantage

This essay was originally published in *Medical History* (1974) and is reprinted by permission of the Wellcome Trustees.

point, much more to the Right, Thomas Szasz has raised doubts about the "scientific" status of psychiatry, has suggested that our whole notion of "mental illness" is essentially a fiction, and that psychiatrists, instead of being scientific physicians, are actually custodians and public servants, charged with the care of people whom society for various reasons finds intolerable. In some of their roles at least, psychiatrists are thus placed by Szasz in roughly the position of a jailer or poorhouse attendant in the seventeenth and eighteenth centuries, when "lunatics" or "madmen" were identified by law as a species of vagrant whose liberties had to be curtailed in the interest of the safety or convenience of society at large.[2]

The second line of development that I have mentioned, the gradual theoretical shift in thinking about insanity from categories of mind to categories of brain, has also been rechanneled in the twentieth century, and this largely, of course, because of Freud. It is ironic that Freud was the product of German brain psychiatry and that he never lost his belief that mental processes, conscious and unconscious, are completely correlated with physiological changes in the human body. He recognized, however, that the neurophysiology of his day was inadequate to provide an account of psychiatric diseases in neurophysiological terms.[3] His therapeutic measures, notably psychoanalysis, were developed with little reference to his physicalist commitment. Freud adopted a metaphorical language which allowed him to speak about mental phenomena without being simultaneously required to spell out their physiological correlates which he fully believed would be specified in the course of time. The same position has provided other psychiatrists the license to talk as if psychiatric development were independent of neurological development. It was Freud's influence more than anything else which formalized the separation of psychiatry from neurology. At a time when evolutionary biology has undermined the ontological position of the human mind, we still live more or less in a Cartesian world. We recognize diseases of the brain and diseases of the mind, and if the border between is not quite so clear as it might be in the world that Descartes constructed, the number of patients that psychiatrists and neurologists fight over is on the whole rather small. Both of these problems, then, the status of mental disease and the relationship of mental function to brain anatomy and physiology, are still unresolved, which perhaps enables us to appreciate more easily some of the peculiarities which have attended the past theory and practice of psychiatry. In this study, I shall be concerned with aspects of these two problems as they relate to the theoretical and practical implications of moral therapy in British psychiatry of the last decades of the eighteenth and the first decades of the nineteenth centuries.

The development of "moral therapy," as it was frequently called at the time, is, of course, one of the high points in the history of psychiatry.

Although the myth that Pinel struck off all the chains of his patients in one dramatic gesture has been punctured; and although recent research has shown that others besides Pinel were at the time actively engaged in the same kinds of therapeutic experiments, both the drama and the importance of the movement are still recognized in the historical literature. Moral therapy was simultaneously a triumph of humanism and of therapy, a recognition that kindness, reason, and tactful manipulation were more effective in dealing with the inmates of asylums than were fear, brutal coercion and restraint, and medical therapy.[4] It is this last parameter, medical therapy, with which I shall be particularly concerned.

"Broadly constructed, 'moral treatment' included all nonmedical techniques, but more specifically it referred to therapeutic efforts which affected the patient's psychology."[5] This definition of Carlson and Dain adequately reflects the kinds of differences which early nineteenth-century advocates of moral therapy saw between their own approaches and the therapeutic programs of previous generations. Nevertheless, coercion and restraint can operate psychologically just as can liberty and nonrestraint. Benjamin Rush, with his restraining chair, and Erasmus Darwin, with his rotating chair, were presumably just as well intentioned as Pinel or any other advocate of moral therapy. And if these rather brutal eighteenth-century methods "cured," as their inventors claimed they did, we may assume that these cures were "psychological" in precisely the same way as those attained by moral treatment. The modus operandi in both cases was via the patient's mind. The moral therapy of nineteenth-century psychiatrists was admittedly different from the harsher approaches of their earlier colleagues, but much of the change stemmed from the attitudes of the doctors themselves rather than from some entirely new appeal to the patient's psychology.

Nevertheless, if the virtual equation of *moral* with *psychological* blurs some of the distinctions between Pinel's therapeutic endeavors and what went before, the connotations of the phrase "moral therapy" are sufficiently precise to justify its use in describing the reform in psychiatric treatment associated with Pinel, Tuke, and the other late eighteenth-century activists. In fact, the prehistory of the concept of moral therapy appears meager. One can assume that many earlier physicians were tactful enough, humane enough, and perceptive enough to deal with mentally disturbed patients in the quiet, efficient manner which seems to have been the norm at the famous York Retreat, founded by the Quaker philanthropist William Tuke in 1792. Part of the reason for the absence of more objective evidence on this point in the earlier medical literature might be attributed to the lack of many detailed case histories. Obviously, the conditions of the York Retreat never obtained at the large public institutions like Bethlem, but physicians dealing with private, individual, and paying patients may have used different tactics. Perhaps they did, but the evidence is hardly overwhelming. And when we consider the therapy that was meted out for the most famous patient of his day, King George III, we can appreciate the contrast which moral therapy presented. A great deal was at stake with this patient, and there is every reason to believe that Francis Willis, his sons, and other assistants treated the king in a manner which (in Willis's considered opinion) would most likely result in the royal patient's recovery. Yet, as the Countess Harcourt described the situation, "The unhappy patient . . . was no longer treated as a human being. His body was immediately encased in a machine which left it no liberty of motion. He was sometimes chained to a stake. He was frequently beaten and starved, and at best he was kept in subjection by menacing and violent language."[6] He was in addition blistered, bled, and given digitalis, tartar emetic, and various other drugs.

The intimidations and threats technically come under the rubric of *moral therapy,* in the sense that it was his mind which was being appealed to. Perhaps *immoral therapy* is a better description of this approach, but in any case I am less concerned with that than with the blisters, bleeding, digitalis, tartar emetic, and other therapeutic measures. In point of fact, physicians at the time generally decided that George was laboring under a "delirium" instead of a madness.[7] But that little matters, since he was treated by "mad-doctors" (that is, broadly speaking, psychiatrists), and the methods they used with him were not out of the ordinary.

One reason that medical treatment for madness might seem odd is the fact that eighteenth-century theories of mind took far less cognizance of the brain than our theories do. Their universe was more nearly Cartesian than ours in their separation of mind from brain, and, more important, their conflation of the philosophical and medical concept of *mind* with the theological concept of *soul.* This conflation can be seen even in David Hartley's physical model of the mind. Hartley's 1749 *Observations on Man, His Frame, His Duty, and His Expectations* developed an association psychology based on a psychophysical parallelism whereby all mental events have their physical representations in the vibrations of fibers in the brain. Hartley, a devout Christian, introduced a scholium making it against the rules to deduce the materiality of the soul from his physical model of the mind.[8] It is worth noting that in the first volume of Hartley's work (in which he developed his psychology) the word *soul* occurs only in the context of the scholium. The rest of the book is about mind, but the wording of the scholium demonstrates that the two concepts were identical for him. They had been, of course, for Descartes as well; indeed, the French use the word *l'âme* for both. It was the possession of an immaterial soul which distinguished man from the animals, theologically, of course, but psychologically as well. Descartes's strict dualism created a number of philosophical problems; but these were compounded when the same framework was used to talk about mental *disease*. If it is the soul which gives man his reason, is it this same theological soul which is diseased in those individuals who have either lost their reason, or never developed any? The kinds of compromise that had to be made by a physician working within what was essentially a Cartesian framework may be seen in the writings of Thomas Willis. Willis modified the Cartesian picture somewhat in adopting Gassendi's notion that there exist two kinds of soul: sensitive souls which are material and which man shares with animals; and rational souls, immaterial and the possession of man alone. Willis conceived madness to be a disease of the rational soul; but since he also believed in the inviolability of the rational soul, he postulated that in order to function properly, the rational soul is absolutely dependent on the *phantasie*, an attribute of the sensitive soul, possessed by animals and located by Willis in the corpus callosum. Thus Willis could talk about mental disease only by making the rational soul so dependent on the brain that, to modern eyes at least, his distinction between the two kinds of soul becomes for all practical purposes meaningless.[9]

The problem of insanity in the medical literature before the nineteenth century is further complicated by the almost exclusive emphasis on disturbances of *reason*, or the highest intellectual faculties of man. Insanity was conceived as a derangement of those very faculties that were widely assumed to be unique to man; as a matter of fact, we sometimes find in the literature the presumed absence in animals of any condition analogous to insanity taken as proof that man's highest psychological functions result from some principle totally lacking in other animals, that is, the soul. On the surface then, Willis's position seems odd, for he recommends the almost exclusive use of medical therapy to treat a disease the manifestations of which are a malfunctioning of a faculty, reason, which itself results from the operation of an immaterial principle. How, in a Cartesian universe, can physicians cure mental diseases by physical remedies? The answer, of course, is that they don't; they protect the soul, locate the disease in the brain, humors, or elsewhere in the body, and treat that instead. And as long as one conflates the concepts of mind and soul, mental disease is either a misnomer and actually a brain disease indirectly affecting mental functions, or a visitation from the devil or the Deity, that is, possession or retribution. Seen from this perspective, some of J. C. A. Heinroth's rhapsodies make more sense.[10] More common, however, was the opposite position, namely, that the soul or mind is never primarily deranged. Late in the nineteenth century, solid American psychiatrists such as John Gray and Pliny Earle were physicalists in order to protect the soul. Gray wrote in 1885 that insanity is "simply a bodily disease in which the mind is disturbed more or less profoundly, because the brain is involved in the sickness either primarily or secondarily. The mind is not, in itself, ever diseased. It is incapable of disease or of its final consequence, death."[11]

This theological motive thus furnished one reason why a physician of the seventeenth or eighteenth century would not find medical therapy for mental disease odd. Another aspect which I shall not discuss is perhaps more obvious: this was the general inheritance of the humoralism of Greek physiology, pathology, and therapy. On one level at least, humoralism accounted for mental diseases theoretically and dictated the appropriate medical therapy. It provided a traditional rationale for medical therapy, and both of these factors, the theological and the humoral, should be kept in mind when evaluating the reactions of British physicians to moral therapy.[12]

Another factor was more obviously social and economic. Work by historians such as Foucault, Ackerknecht, and Rosen has pointed to the profound changes in social attitudes toward insanity between the sixteenth and nineteenth centuries.[13] Despite the fact that physicians had frequently been concerned with what might be called the disease concept of insanity, the care, or custody at least, of the insane was less frequently in their hands. England's 1744 Vagrancy Act is instructive here. Section 20 of the act dealt with "those who by lunacy or otherwise are so far disordered in their Senses that they may be dangerous to be permitted to go Abroad." Any person could detain such a vagrant, and the consent of two justices of the peace was adequate to "cause such Persons to be apprehended and kept safely locked up in some secure place." No medical certificate was necessary and the decision about ultimate release was in the hands of either the jailer or the local magistrates.[14] This was how the 1744 act left the situation, but during the next half-century or so several significant changes occurred. The medical community began to assume an increased responsibility for the care of the insane, and this phenomenon is reflected in various institutions, in various acts of Parliament, and in a growing medical literature on the subject. The institutions include St. Luke's Hospital, London, founded in 1751, the Manchester Lunatic Hospital, 1766, and the Newcastle Lunatic Hospital, 1767. St. Luke's was conceived by its founders as a rival to Bethlem, and while conditions apparently left something to be desired, they were a definite improvement over those at Bethlem. The physician to the new hospital was, of course, William Battie, whose 1758 pamphlet titled *On Madness* was construed by John Monro, physician to Bethlem, as an attack on the latter's father. Their debate need not concern us here.[15]

This same period also saw the growth in the number of "private madhouses," about which William Parry-Jones has recently written.[16] These private establishments (run by individual entrepreneurs for a profit) have been a feature of English life for several centuries, but in fact their relation to the medical profession itself remained unclear during the eighteenth century. Anyone could open a private madhouse, that is, receive lunatics in his house on a paying basis. Many, and perhaps even most, of these proprietors were medical men, but there was nothing which required them to be, and tacit in the lack of legal regulation was the implication that either (1) their function was custodial rather than therapeutic; or (2) anyone could select and administer the therapy indicated by insanity. The first act aimed at licensing these establishments was passed in 1774. It said nothing about the medical qualifications of the proprietors, keepers, or consultants; but the act did recognize medical jurisdiction in cases of insanity in two ways. First, it set up a commission to inspect private madhouses within the metropolitan area, and this commission was composed of members appointed by the Royal College of Physicians. Second, it required that a medical certificate be obtained before a person could be committed to such an establishment.[17] Before the licensing acts of the nineteenth century were introduced, which better defined who in fact was a "medical man," this second part of the act was of uncertain practical importance.[18] Nevertheless, the social significance of this act lay in its recognition that insanity was a medical issue, rather than, as implied in 1744, a condition which any person could recognize and which any magistrate could formalize.

By the end of the eighteenth century, then, British physicians were playing an increasing role, legal and practical, in the diagnosis and therapy of the insane. A large number of medical works dealing with insanity appeared during the last decades of that century, partly the result of the wide interest aroused by George III's illness, but also the reflection of those more general considerations just mentioned. The best known of these works include Thomas Arnold's *Observations on the Nature, Kinds, Causes, and Prevention of Insanity* (1782–86); sections of John Ferriar's *Medical Histories and Reflections* (1792–98); William Pargeter's *Observations on Maniacal Disorders* (1792); Alexander Crichton's *Inquiry into the Nature and Origin of Mental Derangement* (1798); Andrew Harper's *Treatise on Insanity* (1789); and John Haslam's *Observations on Insanity* (1798).

This growing medical interest in and control over the insane was to some extent challenged by the spread of moral therapy. From the beginning, British commentators identified the emphasis on moral therapy as one of the striking characteristics of Pinel's 1801 *Traité sur l'aliénation*. His English translator, David Daniel Davis (1777–1841), noted in his introduction to the 1806 translation that "this volume is chiefly valuable for the great attention to the principles of the moral treatment of insanity which it recommends."[19] Pinel was not the first to stress psychological factors in the causation of insanity. Indeed, he himself referred to earlier writers on this point, for example, to Alexander Crichton's consideration of the passions in the generation of what Crichton called mental derangement. Pinel, however, explicitly completed the circle: that which is psychologically caused is most effectively psychologically treated. The relationship between causation and treatment is a two-way affair, for "the successful application of moral regimen exclusively, gives great weight to the supposition, that, in a majority of instances, there is no organic lesion of the brain nor of the cranium."[20] For Pinel, insanity was a mental condition, hence logically treated by psychological methods. Such was his success with moral therapy that he completely abandoned medical therapy on most of his patients, giving them a trial of moral therapy and resorting to medicinal (physical) remedies only with those on whom the psychological measures had failed.

Pinel's program achieved impressive results which he thoroughly substantiated in his treatise. Nevertheless, it raised several questions. What, for instance, was the role of the physician to be? The successful application of moral therapy required most of all a willing and sensitive staff, and Pinel's case histories were filled with patient-keeper interactions; much less frequently did he record direct interaction with himself. He further mentioned the "common sense and unprejudiced observation" on which his work was based; again, Pinel paid warm tribute to the principal keeper of the asylum, from whom he had obviously derived a great deal.

The same kinds of questions were implicit in the history and structure of the York Retreat. The Retreat, as it was affectionately known, was founded in 1792, but it was not until 1813 and the years following that its methods were widely discussed. Samuel Tuke's *Description of the Retreat* was published in 1813, and Sydney Smith eulogized Tuke's book and the Retreat in the *Edinburgh Review,* one of the leading periodicals of the day.[21] The Retreat had a ready foil, for Tuke's work emerged from the controversy surrounding the alleged mismanagement of the other York institution for the insane, the York Asylum. Whereas the Retreat was founded and largely run by laymen, the York Asylum was easily recognized as a typical medical concern presided over by a physician, Charles Best. Public attention continued to be focused on the condition of the insane during these years through the hearings of a parliamentary select committee concerned with the "better regulation of madhouses" in 1815 and 1816. The committee accumulated and published some 600 pages of evidence that, according to the *Edinburgh Review,* contained "beyond all question, the most important body of information, that has ever appeared, upon the subject of Insanity."[22] Such was the public esteem accorded to the ideals of the founders of the Retreat that Edward Wakefield in 1815 could think of no higher praise for the private madhouse of Mr. Finch at Laverstock than by remarking, "In this establishment I saw all that Tuke has written realized."[23] After a visit to the Retreat in 1812, Dr. Andrew Duncan had asserted "that the Retreat at York, is at this moment the best-regulated establishment in Europe, either for the recovery of the insane, or for their comfort, when they are in an incurable state."[24]

Tuke's *Description* was hardly polemical in tone; yet the work contained a rather damning attack on the medical profession's capacity to deal with mental illness. Samuel Tuke was not a physician. In fact, he had wanted to become one and, quite naturally, to specialize in the treatment of mental disorders. Family pressure kept him in the family business. Nevertheless, we can presume that Samuel did not possess his grandfather William Tuke's general aversion to the medical profession.[25] It is clear from the *Description* that the experience of the Retreat had convinced Samuel Tuke of the decided superiority of moral over medical therapy.

From the beginning, the Retreat was provided with the usual visiting physician. Kindness and the various trappings of moral therapy were always the aims of the Retreat, but Tuke insisted that the minimization of medical therapy was not built into the institutional structure; it had merely evolved from careful observation. Only gradually had the Retreat's first physician, Thomas Fowler, abandoned the "bleeding, blisters, setons, evacuants, and many other prescriptions, which have been highly recommended by writers on insanity."[26] Fowler was no general therapeutic nihilist; his three major publications all concern therapy, and he compounded and gave his name to the arsenical solution which was so popular in the nineteenth century and which in Britain still has its devotees.[27] Like Pinel's, Fowler's was the therapeutic skepticism of a physician who had simply explained his therapy carefully. As Tuke summarized it, Fowler "plainly perceived how much was to be done by moral, and how little by any known medical means."[28]

At the Retreat, like the Bicêtre, the physician was a shadowy figure, the burden of therapeutic responsibility having fallen on the keepers and other members of the staff whose personal contacts with the patient were much greater than that of the physician. Tuke never proposed to abolish the office of physician to the Retreat. Indeed, he suggested that the physician could be a very important figure: "The physician, from his office, sometimes possesses more influence over the patients' minds than the other attendants." The phrase "the other attendants" is telling; it suggests that very little of the physician's role was dictated by his specific medical training, and that a great deal was dictated by simple benevolence and common sense.

The success of moral therapy thus threatened to change the rather newly established place of the medical man in the treatment of insanity; and, as we have seen, theories of insanity were also at stake. Pinel was explicit in drawing out the theoretical implications of moral therapy, in seeing mental disease as frequently a functional condition unaccompanied by structural changes. However, Pinel's work was somewhat confused by his emphasis on the epigastrium in the origin of many attacks of insanity.[29] Samuel Tuke, on the other hand, refused to commit himself on the ultimate nature of insanity, but he recognized the problem in the terms previously outlined: "If," he wrote, "we adopt the opinion, that the disease originates in the mind, applications made immediately to it, are obviously the most natural, and the most likely to be attended with success. If, on the contrary, we conceive that mind is incapable of injury or destruction, and that, in all cases of apparent mental derangement, some bodily disease, though unknown, really exists, we shall still readily admit, from the reciprocal action of the two parts of our system upon each other, that the greatest attention is necessary, to whatever is calculated to effect the mind." Tuke's attitude was essentially pragmatic; it was enough for him that moral therapy was effective, whatever the reason.

Moral therapy, then, was hardly a straightforward affair; and its implications for both medical theory and medical practice were not lost on the physicians of the early nineteenth century who attempted to assess its true significance. However much they might profess to admire the methods of Pinel or the Tukes, very few were prepared to abandon entirely the medical treatment of insanity. When William Tuke had been asked by the parliamentary committee about the effect of medicine in cases of mental derangement, the venerable old man had replied, "In cases of mental derangement, from what I have learnt, it is thought very little can be done; but when the mental disorder is accompanied by bodily disease of one kind or other, the removal of the complaint has frequently recovered the patient; this comes within my personal observation, having frequently enquired into the effect of medical treatment."[30]

If physicians could do nothing for the lunatic except treat his bodily afflictions, then medical men had no special claims to a unique place in the treatment of mental illness. Their income, prestige, and medical theories were all threatened. So, in some instances at least, was their integrity, for many of the abuses that the parliamentary committee had called to notice involved medical men.

It is not surprising, then, that we find a certain defensiveness in the British psychiatric literature of the 1810s and 1820s. For the doctor at least, the rise of moral therapy was not an unmixed blessing.

The Parliamentary Select Committee that in 1815 and 1816 examined the management of various institutions responsible for the care of the insane was not actively hostile to the medical profession. The committee was particularly concerned with improving the quality of care available for the lunatic in both public and private institutions, and the hearings focused on several specific instances of brutality and neglect that had come to light in the immediate past. William Norris, for instance, had spent the last ten or fifteen years of his life chained in a damp cold cell in Bethlem, no one remembering precisely how long it had been. The committee repeatedly queried the practice of keeping violent or incontinent patients naked and chained. And the odd pregnancy of a female patient or the sudden death of an inmate under mysterious circumstances kept the discourse at a dramatic level. Bethlem and the York Asylum fared badly at the hearings, and the scandals which came out of these institutions put the medical men who controlled them on the defensive. Even the printed transcripts convey the tight-lipped resentment with which Thomas Monro, John Haslam, and Charles Best answered many of the questions put to them during the proceedings.

The committee, for instance, was anxious to determine how frequently Monro visited Bethlem in his capacity as sole physician to the hospital. On 8 May 1815 Bethlem's steward, George Wallet, expressed his opinion that Monro attended "but seldom; . . . I hear he has not been round the house but once these three months; he may have been there without my knowledge, he has been at the Hospital more frequently, but not round the gallery [where the patients generally stayed]."[31] Four days later Haslam informed the committee that Monro visited the hospital "twice a week, Saturday and Wednesday, or Tuesday; he suits his convenience." A week later Monro himself put the figure at "about three times a week."[32]

Patient neglect was of course not a medical monopoly, and one group of madhouses also at fault were those at Hoxton, owned by Sir Jonathan Miles. Miles himself was not a physician, and while each of his madhouses had a regular apothecary, the official limit of the apothecary's responsibility ended with the patient's bodily complaints. Should the patient or his family be concerned about the mental disorder, an outside physician had to be specifically engaged to visit the patient on a consultant basis.[33] That no medical treatment was routinely provided for the psychiatric complaints was obviously viewed by the committee as an abuse. Nevertheless, one of the questions frequently put to the various witnesses concerned just that issue. John Latham, president of the Royal College of Physicians, was asked directly, "Are you of opinion that if medicines were occasionally administered to patients for insanity only, it would be productive of any chance of recovery?" Latham answered, "I think it is probable it would."[34] This is the response that a physician might be expected to make, and Latham's opinion was substantiated by Dr. James Veitch, Dr. John Weir, Sir Henry Halford, and Dr. Thomas Monro.

But was medical therapy to be aimed at the mental disorder itself, or only at bodily conditions accompanying it? Thomas Bakewell, a nonmedical proprietor of a much-respected private madhouse in Staffordshire, told the committee, "I do not look upon medicine as of great importance for the mental disease; but there are bodily complaints connected with it, requiring the application of medicine."[35] Edward Wakefield, a Quaker land agent who was active in exposing the abuses at the York Asylum, Bethlem, and at other asylums, was even more definite about the place of medicine in the care of the insane. Asked whether medical men ought to be "Inspectors and Comptrollers of Madhouses," he replied, "I think they are the most unfit of any class of persons. In the first place, from every enquiry I have made, I am satisfied that medicine has little or no effect upon the disease, and the only reason for their selection, is the confidence which is placed in their being able to apply a remedy to the malady."[36] Wakefield's attitudes had been colored by the unfavorable contrast between the medically orientated York Asylum and the Retreat, where "there are Quakers who are neither medical men or of any Professional class, who are conspicuous for the extraordinary treatment of Insane persons, by the attention and kindness which they pay to them."[37]

It is of interest that in 1816 Wakefield retracted his statements concerning the impotence of medical therapy in the treatment of the insane. Between 1815 and 1816 he had discovered a madhouse that conformed to his warmest expectations on how the insane should be most effectively and humanely treated. This was Laverstock House, near Salisbury, run by a surgeon named William Finch. Finch shared the confidence of the majority of his medical colleagues in the efficacy of medical therapy in cases of insanity, and his success convinced Wakefield that insanity is a disease "which in its incipient state is capable of relief from medicine. . . . I examined the register of the many cases which had come under [Finch's] care, and he has completely proved to my satisfaction, that medical treatment is of the greatest consequence."[38]

Wakefield was an important convert for the medical men, since the reforming activities of laymen like him, William Tuke, and Godfrey Higgins represented a viable alternative to the medical model of insanity reflected in the medical literature of the period. If laymen like the Tukes could operate a more effective asylum than the doctors could, traditional therapeutic regimens and theories of insanity were both jeopardized. The medical witnesses that the committee examined unanimously expressed confidence in the unique role of doctors in the psychiatric situation.

They also spoke for the rest of their profession. Thus George Man Burrows, writing in 1828, praised the moral treatment of the York Retreat, but he "viewed with regret the little confidence professed by the benevolent conductors . . . in . . . the great efficacy of medicine in the majority of cases of insanity."[39] Earlier, Andrew Harper, who had developed a theory of insanity that was essentially mental, rather than corporeal, expressed his regret that the treatment of insanity had fallen "too much into the hands of men who never possessed any great share of physical skill."[40]

Thomas Mayo, who later became president of the Royal College of Physicians, lamented in the name of medicine what he conceived as a growing emphasis of psychological aspects of insanity to the exclusion of the physical changes that always accompanied it. Insanity, he wrote in 1817, is a "subject so interesting in its nature, as almost to have been wrestled by the philosopher out of the hands of the physician. To vindicate the rights of my profession over Insanity, and to elucidate its medical treatment, are the objects at which I have aimed." He went on to point out that hypochondriasis, for example, though at that time frequently referred to as a mental disease, was treated in nosological works where it really belonged, as a "disorder of the body."[41]

John Haslam was even more explicit in his 1817 *Considerations on the Moral Management of Insane Persons.* Haslam in fact was one of the group specifically criticized by Monro for emphasizing psychological features of insanity to the neglect of physical ones. To the extent that he did, we tend to praise rather than censure him. Haslam's writings do contain astute psychological observations, but like Monro, Haslam was in theory a physicalist. Haslam fully admitted that *management,* as he referred to what we are calling moral therapy, could be effective in contributing to the cure of insanity, or at least (and this is an important qualification) to the "comfort and happiness of the lunatic." But, he went on,

> of late it has been seriously proposed, in a great deal to remove both the medical treatment and moral management of insane persons from the care of physicians, and to transfer this important and responsible department of medicine into the hands of magistrates and senators. For the welfare of those afflicted persons, and for the security of the public, it is to be hoped that such transfer may never be established; but that the medical and moral treatment of the insane may continue to be directed by the medical practitioner, under the sanction and superintendency of the College of Physicians. The concurring opinions of all thinking persons allow insanity to be a disease, and those best acquainted with this disorder are most persuaded of the relief to be obtained by a judicious administration of medicine.[42]

Even in admitting the importance of *management,* as opposed to active medical therapy, Haslam insisted on the absolute right of a medical man to take complete charge of the care of the insane. His comments were obviously directed in part at the York Retreat; but of course any nonmedical keeper of a private madhouse might consider himself implicated. Additionally, the investigations of the Parliamentary Select Committee of 1815 and 1816 were still much on Haslam's mind in 1817. One of the features which had emerged from these proceedings was that there was simply no agreement among medical men about the actual details of medical therapy. Haslam and his chief, Thomas Monro, had disagreed on the value of emetics in the treatment of insanity. The third medical officer to Bethlem, the recently deceased surgeon Bryan Crowther,[43] also mentioned in his 1811 book on insanity various routine medical procedures (such as a spring bloodletting) performed on virtually all the Bethlem patients, regardless of their complaints or general condition.[44] Such indiscriminate therapy was hard to justify, especially in the light of moral treatment, for one of its most important features, stressed by both Pinel and Tuke, was that moral therapy was individually tailored to the needs and capacities of the patient. Psychological causation is by definition a highly individual matter, and moral therapy required the therapist to know his patient far more intimately than most medically oriented physicians apparently ever bothered to do.

Medical men could thus neither agree on the specifics of medical therapy nor defend the rigid and indiscriminate therapeutic patterns that sometimes obtained in places like Bethlem. Indeed, when pressed, they could sometimes show a remarkable lack of confidence in all forms of medical therapy for the insane. Thomas Monro once admitted to the Select Committee that management was probably far more efficacious than medicine, that, as a matter of fact, the medical measures probably did not do any good. Later, however, he explicitly insisted that his statement should not be construed to mean that he thought medical therapy was dispensable.

Like the books of Pinel and Tuke, then, the Select Committee's investigations made moral therapy seem more efficacious and more humane at the expense of medical therapy. Haslam's comments must be read in the light of the committee's investigations, for he more than any other individual felt the full brunt of the public outcry at the appalling conditions in certain public and private institutions devoted to the insane. Crowther had died just before the committee opened its hearings. Monro was allowed to "retire," but his son was immediately appointed physician to Bethlem, thus assuring the Monro association with the venerable institution for many years to come. Haslam, on the other hand, was dismissed without a pension after more than twenty years' service. He was then fifty-six years old and probably knew more about mental disorders than any other person in Britain.[45]

With Crowther dead, Monro in retirement, and Haslam and most of the keepers dismissed, the staff at Bethlem almost completely changed in the space of only three years. The institutional policies changed but little, however, and actual reform had to wait until mid-century. The comments of a relatively new staff member at Bethlem describe the situation there after the Select Committee had adjourned. These were by William Lawrence, Crowther's successor as surgeon to Bethlem. Appointed just before the Select Committee opened its investigations, Lawrence survived the public outcry of that earlier occasion only to have a public indignation of a slightly different sort two years later threaten his position at Bethlem, as well as at Bridewell's, and St. Bartholomew's.[46] Lawrence's views on moral therapy, and his stated reasons for holding them, lay at the heart of the matter. Believing that the mind is the function of the brain, he found it difficult to conceive that insanity is other than a primary disease of the brain, secondarily disturbing its functions (that is, mental processes). "The effect of medical treatment [he went on] completely corroborates these views. Indeed they who talk of and believe in diseases of the mind, are too wise to put their trust in mental remedies. Arguments, syllogisms, discourses, sermons, have never yet restored any patient; the moral pharmacopoeia is quite inefficient, and no real benefit can be conferred without vigorous medical treatment, which is as efficacious in these affections, as in the disease of any other organ."[47] These remarks may tell us more about the state of Lawrence's mind, when they were delivered in 1818, than about the real debate on moral therapy, but they show that one member of Bethlem's "new" staff still had more sympathy for the traditional modes of treating insanity.

Lawrence's words remind us that there are two diametrically opposed reasons why a person during this period might believe that psychiatric disorders are primary diseases of the brain. If one held to the theological identity of mind and soul, then, as we have seen, such a belief protected the mind as an ontological entity from the ravages of disease, decay, and mutability. On the other hand, if one held that the mind is the function of the brain, totally dependent on that organ, and that all mental functions result from, or at least are accompanied by, physiological processes, then mental derangements might naturally be thought to have a corresponding structural malformation or derangement. Thus we find Lawrence, widely accused of materialism, holding similar views on the subject of insanity with William Newnham. Writing in the *Christian Observer* for 1829, Newnham explicitly pointed to the theological implications entailed in ascribing disease to the mind: "A great error has arisen, and has been perpetuated even to the present day, in considering cerebral disorder as *mental;* requiring, and indeed admitting, *only* of moral remedies, instead of these forming only *one* class of curative agents; whereas the brain is the mere *organ* of mind, not the mind itself; and its disorder of function arises from its ceasing to be a proper medium for the manifestation of the varied action and passion of the presiding spirit."[48] Like Lawrence, but for opposing reasons, Newnham believed that insanity is always brain disease.

The view that mental derangement is always accompanied by physical derangements of some sort was, of course, not the only position to take on the subject. Among British physicians of the early nineteenth century, however, it was a widely held opinion, and this despite persuasive counterevidence. For almost all of them admitted that no convincing anatomicopathological analysis could always be performed in cases of insanity. There were two aspects to this breakdown between the clinical and pathological correlations. In the first place, no consistent lesion could be found in the brains or skulls of lunatics examined postmortem. Certain kinds of lesions seemed to crop up with regularity, evidences of vascular congestion and general cerebral inflammation, thickening of the skull, and so forth, but there was basic agreement that lunatics frequently died at the height of an attack without having any evidence of pathological changes inside their skulls. In the second place, the whole range of changes most often found at postmortem examinations of lunatics could be demonstrated easily in the brains of persons dying with full possession of their faculties. There was thus no concrete reason to believe that psychiatric disorders are actually brain diseases, and this very lack of postmortem correlation was taken by some as good evidence that the mind is an immaterial essence not ever primarily affected with disease. But as we have noted, that belief itself furnished strong motivation for throwing the lesions of insanity on the brain. Other factors besides convincing empirical evidence led British physicians to their belief that insanity is fundamentally a physical condition. Several of these factors have already been alluded to: the conflation of the concepts of mind and soul, the inheritance of physical explanations from antiquity, the lay threat to medical control of the insane implicit in the milieu of moral therapy and early nineteenth-century institutional reform. In addition to Mayo, Lawrence, Newnham, Haslam, and Monro, other medical men who explicitly subscribed to the physical model of mental illness during the period included Andrew Marshal, George Nesse Hill, David Uwins, Joseph Mason Cox, George Man Burrows, W. A. F. Browne, James Cowles Prichard, Andrew Combe, Sir William Ellis, Francis Willis, and John Conolly. This is a heterogeneous group, united, however, by the proposition that insanity is a condition caused by physical changes and consequently within the reach of medical therapy. Francis Willis, for example, told his audience at the College of Physicians' Gulstonian Lectures of 1822 that "We must lament, it should ever be gravely pronounced from the lips of any medical experience, that 'medicine is of no use in the disorders of the mind'; an opinion highly detrimental to the practice of Physic, and its ulterior happy results! Yet I remember to have heard formerly at a lecture, that furor uterinus was a disease exclusively of the mind, and on that account incurable."[49] Willis's therapeutic optimism about the "happy results" of medical therapy was part of his justification for keeping insanity within the scope of medical theory and practice.

Nevertheless, some dissension existed even within the medical community as a few doctors toyed with the proposition that insanity is always a disease of the mind. In 1789, in his *Treatise on the Real Cause and Cure of Insanity*, Andrew Harper had announced that insanity is a primary disease of mind, "independent and exclusive of every corporeal, sympathetic, direct, or indirect excitement, or irritation whatever." Harper thus separated "true insanity" from melancholia and dementia, assumed by him to be purely corporeal diseases. His reasons for coming to this position were hazy, his language confused, and his therapy did not consistently follow from his theoretical pronouncements. He has been seen as a true psychiatric pioneer for his emphasis on the mental nature of insanity, but his influence during our period was very slim.

A more challenging position was put forward by William Saunders Hallaran, in a book published in 1810. Hallaran suggested that the sensorial changes taking place in insanity may be due to strictly mental causes, or to physical causes. He thus distinguished "mental insanity" from those bodily diseases whose symptoms mimic mental insanity. The importance of identifying the conditions properly lay in the differing therapeutic regimens required for each. Mental insanity could be cured by moral therapy, whereas medical therapy was required in the cases of bodily disease. Hallaran thus took moral therapy at its face value and used it to support his theoretical structures.[50]

I have outlined in this essay three major positions which can be found in the British psychiatric literature of the late eighteenth and early nineteenth centuries: (1) that insanity is always attended by structural changes and hence is ultimately a physical condition; (2) that insanity is always a mental condition, properly differentiated from any physical disease which secondarily produces mental symptoms; (3) that insanity may be caused by either physical disease or by mental aberrations. The majority of British physicians who expressed themselves on the subject of insanity during our period subscribed themselves to the first position, that insanity is a disease of the body. Many of them also supported the increased application of moral therapy. How did they reconcile psychological treatment for physical disease? One way, of course, was by neglecting to examine the issues very closely and merely accepting moral therapy on a pragmatic basis. Another was by distinguishing (as did Haslam) between the value of moral therapy in making patients more malleable and easier to deal with, and its ultimate use in a direct therapeutic sense.

Both of these approaches were essentially negative, but there was a third, more positive rationale for moral therapy which applies to several of the list of sixteen physicalists mentioned in this study. This concerns Gall's phrenology. It is significant that four of these physicians keenly interested in moral therapy were phrenologists: Sir William Ellis, Andrew Combe, John Conolly, and W. A. F. Browne. Ellis is remembered for his work with occupational therapy; Browne, for his judicious use of moral therapy first at the Montrose Lunatic Asylum, and later as superintendent of the Royal Crichton Asylum. Conolly, of course, is famous for his introduction of the no-restraint system at Hanwell, in Middlesex.[51] The phrenological concept of mental functions circumvented the traditional Cartesian framework and permitted phrenologists to refer simultaneously to the experienced mental state and its underlying physiological counterpart. The effectiveness of moral therapy could be understood both in terms of psychological benefit and the concomitant hypertrophy of the stimulated areas of the cerebral cortex.[52]

The peculiar features of phrenological doctrine give an underlying coherence to the activities of various phrenologically inclined psychiatrists. Moral therapy was no phrenological monopoly, however.[53] Many medical superintendents and consultant physicians of the growing number of county lunatic asylums and private madhouses adopted therapeutic programs that relied heavily on management. Increasingly, too, psychosocial aspects of insanity were emphasized in discussions of etiology. In the first few decades of the nineteenth century, however, there was no widespread abandonment of the more strictly medical aspects of psychiatric therapy. Psychiatrists remained what William James once called "medical materialists."[54] Insanity continued to be conceived as a physical disease potentially within the reach of medicinal agents. There was no great movement toward the lay treatment of the insane along the lines of the York Retreat. In fact, the lay reformers who played major roles in the events leading up to the parliamentary investigation of 1815 and 1816 seemed content to allow medical men to retain their central position in the care of the insane. Doctors in turn responded with an exuberant confidence in their capacities to cure a high proportion of the insane who came under their ministrations in the early stages of the disease. Some even claimed a cure rate as high as ninety percent under appropriate circumstances.[55]

In any case, the decades immediately following the parliamentary investigation represent for British psychiatry a period of therapeutic optimism, an optimism founded in part on a concerted medical attempt to retain control of psychiatric institutions and their patients. Both lay reformers and medical men were anxious that insanity be recognized as a disease and that the insane be placed in hospitals and asylums rather than jails and workhouses. The motives of laymen like Edward Wakefield and William Tuke were essentially humanitarian. The motives of the medical men were much more complicated. Professional, social, and economic considerations colored their own judgments and tempered the enthusiasm they showed toward moral therapy. They were prepared to adopt many of the features of the York Retreat into their own therapeutic programs. They were not prepared to jettison their medical models of insanity; nor were they willing to compromise their central roles in the diagnosis and treatment of the mentally ill. They were successful in establishing the medical speciality of psychiatry. Nevertheless, their psychiatric descendants still face many of the same problems, as evidenced by contemporary debates on the nature of mental disease, the status of lay psychoanalysis, or the amount of general medical education necessary for one who intends to specialize in the management of diseases of the mind.

Notes

I am grateful to Prof. E. H. Ackerknecht, Mr. R. S. Porter, and Dr. R. M. Young for their comments on an earlier version of this paper. I also benefited from discussions at the Johns Hopkins Institute of the History of Medicine, University of Western Ontario, University of Pennsylvania, and Oxford University.

The research was conducted at King's College Cambridge, during the tenure of a fellowship from the Josiah Macy, Jr., Foundation, New York City.

1. E. H. Ackerknecht, *Short History of Psychiatry,* trans. S. Wolff (New York: Hafner, 1968), pp. 74ff; Roger Smith, "Background of Physiological Psychology," *History of Science* 11 (1973): 75–123; Otto Marx, "Wilhelm Griesinger and the History of Psychiatry: A Reassessment," *Bulletin of the History of Medicine* 46 (1972): 519–44.

2. E.g., Vagrancy Act of 1744, Section 20, which dealt with lunatics, discussed by Kathleen Jones, *Lunacy, Law, and Conscience 1744–1845* (London: Routledge and Kegan Paul, 1955), pp. 28ff. For Laing, see Robert Boyers, ed., *Laing and Antipsychiatry* (London: Penguin Books, 1972). Szasz's works include *The Myth of Mental Illness,* 1st ed. 1961 (London: Paladin, 1972); and *The Manufacture of Madness,* 1st ed. 1970 (London: Paladin, 1973).

3. See especially Freud's 1895 "Project for a Scientific Psychology," Marie Bonaparte et al., eds., *The Origins of Psychoanalysis* (London: Iago, 1954), pp. 347–445.

4. On moral therapy, see Eric T. Carlson and Norman Dain, "The Psychotherapy That Was Moral Treatment," *American Journal of Psychiatry* 117 (1960): 519–24; J. Sanbourne Bockoven, "Moral Treatment in American Psychiatry," *Journal of Nervous and Mental Diseases* 124 (1956): 167–94; Alexander Walk, "Some Aspects of the 'Moral Treatment' of the Insane up to 1850," *Journal of Mental Science* 100 (1954): 807–37.

5. Carlson and Dain, "Psychotherapy," n. 4, p. 519.

6. Quoted by Kathleen Jones, *Lunacy,* n. 2, pp. 41–42. For a stimulating and thorough consideration of George III's illness, see Ida MacAlpine and Richard Hunter, *George III and the Mad-Business* (London: Allen Lane, 1969).

7. MacAlpine and Hunter, *George III,* esp. chap. 5.

8. David Hartley, *Observations on Man, His Frame, His Duty, and His Expectations.* (London: Richardson, 1749), 1:33.

9. I have discussed this problem in greater detail in "The Anatomical Method, Natural Theology, and the Functions of the Brain," *Isis* 64 (1973): 445–68.

10. Heinroth was the early nineteenth-century German romantic psychiatrist who was one of the first to postulate that insanity is a primary disease of the

mind rather than of the brain. However, he also believed that possession and states of sin were among the causes in insanity. Cf. Otto Marx, "J. C. A. Heinroth (1773–1834) on Psychiatry and Law," *Journal of the History of the Behavioral Sciences* 4 (1968): 163–79.

11. Quoted by Bockoven, "Moral Treatment," n. 4, p. 188. Cf. Charles Rosenberg, *The Trial of the Assassin Guiteau* (Chicago: University of Chicago Press, 1968), esp. pp. 193ff; Gerald Grob, *Mental Institutions in America* (New York: Free Press, 1973); Norman Dain, *Concepts of Insanity in the United States, 1789–1865* (New Brunswick, N.J.: Rutgers University Press, 1964).

12. Cf. Ackerknecht, *Short History*, n. 1, p. 38: "Psychotherapy had after all been theoretically impossible both on the basis of the older somaticism and on the basis of the old beliefs about the soul."

13. Michel Foucault, *Madness and Civilization*, trans. Richard Howard (New York: Mentor Books, 1967); George Rosen, *Madness in Society* (London: Routledge and Kegan Paul, 1968), esp. chaps. 5 and 6.

14. Cf. Jones, *Lunacy*, n. 2, pp. 28ff; Nigel Walker, *Crime and Insanity in England* (Edinburgh: Edinburgh University Press, 1968–73), 1:42ff.

15. Battie's *Treatise* and Monro's *Remarks* have been reprinted with an introduction and annotations by Richard Hunter and Ida MacAlpine (London: Dawson's, 1962).

16. William Ll. Parry-Jones, *The Trade in Lunacy* (London: Routledge and Kegan Paul, 1972).

17. Ibid., pp. 9ff.

18. The Medical Act of 1858 was the most important of the licensing acts. It is discussed by Charles Newman, *The Evolution of Medical Education in the Nineteenth Century* (London: Oxford University Press, 1957), chap. 4.

19. Philippe Pinel, *A Treatise on Insanity*, trans. D. D. Davis (1806; facs. reprint ed., New York: Hafner, 1962), pp. liv–lv. Cf. Evelyn Woods and Eric Carlson, "The Psychiatry of Philippe Pinel," *Bulletin of the History of Medicine* 35 (1961): 14–25.

20. Pinel, *Treatise*, n. 19, p. 5.

21. Samuel Tuke, *Description of the Retreat* (1813; facs. reprint ed., introduced and annotated by Richard Hunter and Ida MacAlpine (London: Dawson's, 1964); [Sydney Smith], *Edinburgh Review* 23 (1814): 189–98.

22. *Edinburgh Review*, 28 (1817): 431–71.

23. *Report of Committee for Better Regulation of Madhouses* (London: Baldwin, Cradock, and Joy, 1815), p. 299.

24. Quoted in MacAlpine and Hunter, *George III*, n. 6, p. 336.

25. Tuke, ed. Hunter and MacAlpine, *Description*, Introduction.

26. Ibid., p. iii.

27. Thomas Fowler, *Medical Reports on the Effects of Tobacco* (London: Johnson, 1785); *Medical Reports on the Effects of Arsenic* (London: Johnson, 1786). John Winslow has recently suggested that Charles Darwin's chronic ill health was secondary to long-term arsenic ingestion via Fowler's Solution. *Darwin's Victorian Malady* (Philadelphia: American Philosophical Society, 1971).

28. Tuke, *Description*, p. iii.

29. Pinel, *Treatise*, n. 19, pp. 40–41.

30. William Tuke, in *Report of Committee*, p. 161.
31. Ibid., p. 59. Cf. the testimony of Elizabeth Forbes, the matron, pp. 74–75.
32. Ibid., pp. 102 and 106.
33. Ibid., pp. 178ff, esp. p. 227.
34. Ibid., p. 265.
35. Ibid., p. 334. For Bakewell's asylum, cf. Parry-Jones, *Trade in Lunacy*, pp. 83–84.
36. Ibid., p. 303.
37. Ibid.
38. *Reports from Committees* (1816), First Report, p. 36. On Finch's madhouse, cf. Parry-Jones, *Trade in Lunacy*, n. 16, pp. 116–18.
39. Quoted by Hunter and MacAlpine, Introduction to Tuke, *Description*, p. 23.
40. Andrew Harper, *A Treatise on the Real Cause and Cure of Insanity* (London: Stalker and Walter, 1789), p. 111.
41. Thomas Mayo, *Remarks on Insanity* (London: Underwood, 1817), pp. v, 4, 80.
42. John Haslam, *Considerations on the Moral Management of Insane Persons* (London: Hunter, 1817), pp. 2–3. Cf. Edward James Seymour, *Observations on the Medical Treatment of Insanity* (London: Rees, Orme, Brown, 1832), p. 6, who deplored the removal of cases of insanity to persons who "limit attention to the mere personal security of their patients, without attempting to assist them by the resources of medicine."
43. Haslam told the committee that "Mr. Crowther was generally insane, and mostly drunk. He was so insane as to have a strait-waistcoat." Such information was not likely to increase the committee's confidence in the medical regimen practiced at Bethlem.
44. *Report of Committee*, pp. 129ff.
45. Denis Leigh, "John Haslam, M.D.—1764–1844, Apothecary to Bethlem," *Journal of the History of Medicine* 10 (1955): 17–44.
46. Owsei Temkin, "Basic Science, Medicine, and the Romantic Era," *Bulletin of the History of Medicine* 37 (1963): 97–129.
47. William Lawrence, *Lectures on Physiology, Zoology, and the Natural History of Man* (London: J. Callow, 1819), p. 114.
48. [William Newnham], "Essay on Superstition," *Christian Observer* 29 (1829): 265. Cf. Newnham, *The Reciprocal Influence of Body and Mind Considered* (London: J. Hatchard, 1842).
49. Francis Willis, *A Treatise on Mental Derangement* (London: Longman, 1823), p. 6. Willis was the grandson of the clergyman/doctor of the same name who supervised the treatment of George III during his bouts of "madness."
50. W. S. Hallaran, *An Enquiry into the Causes Producing the Extraordinary Addition to the Number of Insane* (Ireland: Cork, Edwards and Savage, 1810), esp. pp. 1ff.
51. William Ellis, *A Treatise on the Nature, Causes, and Treatment of Insanity* (London: Holdsworth, 1838); W. A. F. Browne, *What Asylums Were, Are, and Ought to Be* (Edinburgh: Black, 1837); John Conolly, *The Treatment of the Insane without Mechanical Restraints* (London: Smith, Elder, 1856). Selections from these works may be found in Richard Hunter and Ida MacAlpine, eds., *Three Hundred Years of Psychiatry* (London: Oxford University Press, 1963).
52. On phrenology in general, see E. H. Ackerknecht and Henri Vallois, *Franz*

Joseph Gall and His Collection (Madison: University of Wisconsin Press, 1956); Owsei Temkin, "Gall and the Phrenological Movement," *Bulletin of the History of Medicine* 21 (1947): 275–321; R. M. Young, *Mind, Brain, and Adaptation* (Oxford: Clarendon Press, 1970). Andrew Combe, *Observations on Mental Derangement* (Edinburgh: Anderson, 1831), is a good phrenological exposition of insanity.

53. On the question of the influence of phrenology on the American asylum movement of the first half of the nineteenth century, see David J. Rothman, *The Discovery of the Asylum* (Boston: Little, Brown, 1971); and W. David Lewis, *From Newgate to Dannemora* (Ithaca, N.Y.: Cornell University Press, 1965).

54. James's phrase is cited by Owsei Temkin, *Galenism* (Ithaca, N.Y.: Cornell University Press, 1973), p. 88.

55. These statistics were invalid for a number of reasons, such as the common practice of counting each discharge as a "cure." Thus if one patient was admitted and discharged five times during the year, he would represent five "cures."

ROGER COOTER

3 Phrenology and British Alienists, ca. 1825–1845

Converts to a Doctrine

Even in the light of its legitimate claim to be an important stimulant to research in cerebral physiology, phrenology seems to be an unpromising vehicle for understanding the progress of psychiatry in the nineteenth century. Yet, in the first half of that century at least, phrenology *was* important for the progressive development of psychiatry, for it had something to say at each of the required levels: its doctrine could claim to be scientific and somatic; it led to treatments which were moral and were conveyed as such; and it brought the phenomenon of madness into contact with the social world and the progressive social philosophies of the time. Above all, it was comprehensible. Its advocates and its converts promised to provide at a stroke solutions to the mysteries of character, personality, talent or the lack of it, crime, and madness. While the most basic assumptions of phrenology have continued to influence psychology, physiology, neurology, sociology, criminology, and psychiatry, all of the particular claims which led to its pervasive influence prior to 1850 were subsequently considered absurd. My intention in this study is to build up phrenology's transforming influence in psychiatry and then to tear away the phrenological scaffolding. Progress—always assuming that "progress" is "progressive"—often uses strange and fascinating mediators in the advancement of social, political, moral, and scientific ideas. Phrenology, I will argue, was probably the single most important, as well as one of the most curious, of these vehicles for the progress of psychiatry in the second quarter of the nineteenth century.

In this inquiry I will be primarily concerned with exposing how and why phrenology between the 1820s and the 1840s came to dominate psychiatric thought, or how, to quote James Cowles Prichard in the early 1830s,

This essay was originally published in *Medical History* (1976) and is reprinted by permission of the Wellcome Trustees.

"the celebrated system of Gall . . . eclipsed all other attempts to theorise on the functions of the brain."[1] In doing this I will be working between three approaches to psychiatric history: the socioinstitutional, the clinical, and the scientific. On the first of these, the socioinstitutional approach, the criticism made by Alexander Walk almost thirty years ago still remains valid; namely, that there is substantially more to nineteenth-century psychiatry than metropolitan Commissioners in Lunacy and select committees of inquiry, or that psychiatric history must be seen as a set of institutions being driven between the wheels of Utilitarianism and Evangelicalism.[2] Walk's reaction to the institutional approach stemmed from his examination of the diverse contemporary attitudes and opinions on one clinical aspect of early nineteenth-century psychiatry, the "moral treatment." This internal or clinical approach to British psychiatry has since received further attention, most recently by William Bynum,[3] who has expanded the clinical picture to expose the dichotomy that was created by the introduction of moral therapy vis-à-vis the position of medical therapy. On this aspect of psychiatry I shall have more to say further on in this essay.

The third, or what I have called the scientific approach to British psychiatry, has been touched upon by several writers though it has never been thoroughly explored. The reluctance of medical historians to treat phrenology seriously because of its stigma as a "pseudoscience" has been largely responsible for neglecting phrenology in its role as the first "science of brain." The eclecticism of the early nineteenth-century alienists and the obfuscation in much of their writing scarcely increases the appeal of such an investigation. Moreover, in treating phrenology as a major contribution to the scientific evolution of psychiatry, difficulties are further compounded by the fact that it was a uniquely popular science in early Victorian Britain for largely social reasons.[4] Thus while the scientific approach to psychiatry should, prima facie, remove us from the social context and involve us more deeply with an internalist discussion, through phrenology this approach extends beyond neurological, clinical, and institutional aspects to the consideration of far broader social issues. To deal fully with these social ramifications of phrenology is outside the scope of this essay. Nor will it be apposite here to elucidate the social background that would be necessary if we were to comprehend the frameworks in which the superintendents of lunatic asylums operated. It is necessary, however, before entering upon the more specific applications of the phrenological doctrine to psychiatric theory and treatment, to give some attention to the social claims of phrenology, and, in particular, to the relation of these claims to the acceptance of the doctrine by alienists. One of the themes I will be introducing in this essay, therefore, is that the science of phrenology forms an essential starting point for a broader his-

torical synthesis of nineteenth-century psychiatry because the doctrine
was *also* a phenomenon of considerable social significance.

There is abundant evidence to substantiate the claim that
phrenology completely reorientated psychiatric thought. Briefly, this
reorientation can be seen as the shift in psychiatry to an interpretation of
mental illness as related to the physiology of the brain. Franz Joseph
Gall (1758–1828), the founder of what became popularly known as
phrenology, "convinced the scientific community once and for all that
'the brain is the organ of the mind' and argued strongly that both its
structure and functions could be concomitantly analysed by observation
rather than speculation."[5] Despite disclaimers by defensive phrenologists, Gall's doctrine overstepped the limits of orthodox inquiry by
"physiologizing" the mind within the brain so that it could become (as in
Cartesian philosophy it was not) the subject of scientific study. The old
philosophical use of the term *faculties of the mind* was transformed both
medically and popularly into the notion of faculties as the functions of
specific cerebral parts and often made to be synonymous with the parts
themselves. Investigating the derivation of the word *function* as a systematic term in psychology, K. M. Dallenbach concluded that *"phrenology is
the matrix from which our term is derived"*; that only after Gall and Spurzheim had propagated the doctrine did *mental functions* take on its present
meaning.[6] Thus long after phrenology had been abandoned by professional men, the complaint could still be heard that "the old notions promulgated by phrenologists . . . still tend, I fear, to confuse our view, and
to prevent a true scientific conception of the constitution of the intellect."[7] Such a statement only underscores the conclusion of Ackerknecht
that Gall's doctrine was "at least as influential in the first half of the
nineteenth century as psychoanalysis in the first half of the twentieth."[8]

In this essay I want to outline briefly the extent to which phrenology
was involved with the nineteenth-century asylums in Britain; to give some
indication of the alienists[9] and writers involved; and to establish the place
they occupy in psychiatric history. An examination of the advancement of
phrenology among the medical profession generally; reference to the social
implications involved in the contemporary acceptance of the doctrine; and
what exactly the doctrine appeared to be offering to alienists will constitute the remainder of this background material. Further on, I will be
concerned almost entirely with looking at Gall's system in the context of
the then-existing theories and practices of clinical psychiatry in an attempt
to define the place it came to occupy. Turning to subsequent developments
during the twilight of phrenological psychiatry, I will try to place in
perspective the role of phrenology in early Victorian psychiatry and to
assess the particular nature of its historical significance.

For reasons which will become obvious, such an inquiry cannot be conducted superficially; as serious Victorians themselves recorded when they entered upon this subject, "The great question of phrenology is of too important and too comprehensive a character to be thus cursorily discussed."[10]

The very name of the practical phrenologist and itinerant lecturer, J. Q. Rumball, has often been cited as an apt reflection on the sort of person attracted to phrenology. It may seem that a pseudoscience of lumps and bumps is appropriately associated with such a name. Yet Rumball should not be too quickly dismissed. Like so many of his contemporaries, he took his phrenology seriously and fought strenuously to prevent its sabotage by materialists and mesmerists. More significant here is the fact that Rumball was the proprietor and manager of a private madhouse near St. Albans in Hertfordshire and was also the author of one of the addresses to Lord Brougham in 1843 that called for the pardon of Daniel M'Naughton (from whose case the M'Naughton Rules for the criminally insane were formulated) upon phrenological proofs of the murderer's "moral insanity." In his address Rumball observed that "in treating this question Phrenologically, no excuse is required." As he went on to point out, "Most of the Superintendents of our Public [county] Asylums are Phrenologists. Hanwell, Gloucester, Glasgow, Leicester, Nottingham, and Maidstone are thus governed; in them, the spirit of improvement, of amelioration to the Patient in his physical treatment, and philosophy in his cure, is alone apparent. . . ."[11]

The name of James Quilter Rumball is not to be found in the anthologies of psychiatry nor in any dictionary of biography. As with most of the superintendents of the asylums he mentions, little biographical information is obtainable. However, the correspondence which Rumball points to between phrenological alienists and the spirit of improvement is one that can be verified, if not through minor figures such as Rumball himself, then clearly through some of the most distinguished psychiatrists of the period. Rumball noted Hanwell where John Conolly (1794–1866) superintended; he might have also mentioned Conolly's distinguished predecessor, Sir William Ellis (1780–1839), or W. A. F. Browne (1805–1886) of the Montrose and, later, Crichton Royal asylums. To these three eminent figures Rumball could have added the names of contemporaries of often only slightly less influence: Matthew Allen (1783–1845), the owner and superintendent of the first cottage-style asylum in Britain at High Beech in Epping; Disney Alexander, successor to Ellis at the Wakefield Asylum from 1831 to 1836; Richard Poole, successor to Browne at Montrose after 1839; James Davey (1813–1895), house-surgeon at Hanwell under Conolly and later medical superintendent of the female side of Europe's largest and most modern asylum at mid-century, Colney Hatch in Middlesex; James Scott, superintendent of the Royal Navy Asylum at Haslar; and Edward Wright (1791–1859), apothecary and superintendent of Bethlem. Along with phrenological authors of works on insanity who were not themselves involved with the actual care of the insane, most notably, J. G. Spurzheim (1776–1832) and Andrew Combe (1797–1847), these men comprised what can be termed the hard core of phrenological alienists.[12] All of them would have said that they treated their patients on phrenological principles, although their specific interests in the science had differing degrees of emphasis. While Edward Wright was chiefly interested in phrenology's physiological division of brain for locating organic changes in insane patients, Conolly turned to the science more for the assistance it gave in relating cranial shape to specific forms of insanity. All those within the hard core, however, were directly involved in the dissemination and propagation of phrenology. Conolly was a founding member of the Warwick and Leamington Phrenological Society and was later one of the chairmen of the Phrenological Association.[13] Ellis founded a society while superintending the Wakefield Asylum,[14] and Disney Alexander drew up lectures to be delivered at the Wakefield Dispensary.[15] Matthew Allen was the first itinerant lecturer on phrenology in Britain after Spurzheim,[16] while W. A. F. Browne, though not a charter member of the Edinburgh Phrenological Society, was by the 1830s as dominant a figure in the Society as George and Andrew Combe. Browne also established a phrenological society at Montrose and was one of the most popular lecturers on phrenology to middle- and working-class audiences throughout Scotland.[17] Richard Poole was the first editor of the *Phrenological Journal.* James Scott lectured on the science to audiences in Gosport and he and Edward Wright were at one time presidents of the phrenological societies of Hampshire and London, respectively.[18] James Davey was an influential member of the Phrenological Association and a vigorous author of addresses and phreno-medical tracts that ceased only with his death in 1895.[19] Rumball, it might be added, spent time lecturing on phrenology in the Midlands and in the South West, ran a phrenology shop in the Strand, submitted papers to the *Journal of Psychological Medicine,* and made his mark in history by delineating the formidable head of Herbert Spencer.[20]

As lecturers on phrenology and writers of both popular and specialist medical works, these men had a considerable impact on the rest of the profession. The phrenological endeavors of Spurzheim, Combe, Ellis, and Browne, in particular, greatly contributed to the education of students and practitioners alike and their influence on leading American alienists like Amariah Brigham, Samuel Woodward, and Pliny Earle soon resulted in a reciprocal transatlantic influence on British psychiatrists.[21] It is therefore possible to speak of a second line of phrenological alienists who, if less vocal on the subject, were nevertheless strongly influenced by phrenology in their dealings with the insane. The superintendents of some of the asylums that Rumball mentions can probably be included in this category as can Alexander Mackintosh, medical superintendent of the Dundee Royal Lunatic Asylum; David Uwins at the Peckham Asylum; Forbes Winslow, later editor of the *Journal of Psychological Medicine,* who ran two private asylums in Hammersmith; H. A. Galbraith, surgeon to the Glasgow Royal Lunatic Asylum; Samuel Hare, proprietor and medical attendant of the Retreat for the Insane near Leeds; Donald Mackintosh, superintendent of the Newcastle Lunatic Asylum; and John Kitching, medical superintendent of the Friends' Retreat at York in the 1850s. The phrenological views of these alienists can be traced through letters and articles and verified in some cases by membership in a phrenological society, of which there were over thirty in the first half of the century.

Altogether these alienists make up a list as impressive as it is substantial. It numbers ten of the medical superintendents of the twenty-three public asylums in England and Scotland in 1844 and among them all those which were considered most advanced in management and humanity. It includes, too, the proprietors, managers, surgeons, and apothecaries of some of the more highly regarded borough and private asylums of the time. Undoubtedly there were others for whom there is yet no evidence, just as there are marginal figures connected with the asylums whose phrenological influence is not readily ascertained. Charles Augustus Tulk (1786–1849), for instance, was the chairman of the Committee of Management of Hanwell from 1839 to 1847; earlier he had been a friend and correspondent of Spurzheim and had served at times as the president of the London Phrenological Society in the 1830s.[22] More difficult to trace but potentially of more direct influence in encouraging phrenological techniques could have been persons such as the matron who had worked under Browne at Montrose and who subsequently took up appointment under Conolly at Hanwell.[23] On the other hand, it is also apparent that there were some managers of asylums who desired to be considered as operating on phrenological principles though they had, as Andrew Combe discovered in 1836, only a slight awareness of the science's principles and utility.[24] But the fact that these alienists wanted to be seen as being guided by phrenology—apparently to make their management seem respectably fashionable—gives a further indication of the extent of phrenology's influence at the time.

Despite later claims about the immediate revolutionary impact of the phrenological theory, its acceptance by alienists was gradual and cumulative, progressively so as the older generation of alienists died off. Though by 1803 most alienists in Britain had probably heard, along with the readers of the *Edinburgh Review,* of "Dr. Gall and his skulls,"[25] it was not Gall but his contemporaries Pinel and Tuke who were beginning to have a slight

impact on British asylums. Gall's direct influence was in fact almost negli-
gible. His great multivolume work, *Sur les fonctions du cerveau*, did not begin
publication until 1822 and was not translated into English until 1835 and
then only in America. Gall's one visit to England in May 1823 scarcely
received comment and only one London medical journal gave any report
of his lectures.[26] Spurzheim's British tour of 1814 attracted some medical
attention largely due to his demonstration of the new technique of brain
dissection, but it was not until his later visit in 1816 and subsequent tours
in the twenties that a significant amount of interest (both medical and
popular) was drawn to the theory. Thomas Forster, who had coined the
word *phrenology* for the doctrine in January 1815,[27] dedicated a work to
Spurzheim in 1817 and observed that "although you have left Great Britain
without establishing so fully in the minds of British Anatomists the truth
of the doctrines respecting the Organs of the Brain, as the clearness of the
proofs seemed to warrant . . . yet the valuable Observations on Insanity,
and its periodical exacerbations, which you have given to the World in
your late Work, will give rise to a better knowledge and treatment of that
disease."[28]

Forster was referring to Spurzheim's *Observations on the Deranged
Manifestations of the Mind or Insanity* first published in London in 1817. Yet
it is doubtful if this work had much immediate success in bringing British
alienists around to a phrenological point of view. As the *Lancet* later noted,
it was a "complete and excellent treatise on insanity" but it proffered no
specifically phrenological plan of treatment. The *Lancet* concluded its review with the observation that "phrenology has furnished the theory and
argument [of insanity]; reason and experience the practice."[29] However, it
was only after the publication of Andrew Combe's more cogent treatise,
*Observations on Mental Derangement; Being an Application of the Principles of
Phrenology to the Elucidation of the Causes, Symptoms, Nature, and Treatment of
Insanity* (1831), that this "theory and argument" of phrenology really began
to have a decisive impact on British psychiatric thought. Thereafter
phrenological psychiatry can be said to have taken root and reaffirmed the
belief in its revolutionary claim to solve the enigma of Mind. As Forbes
Winslow declared in his *Principles of Phrenology as Applied to the Elucidation
and Cure of Insanity* (1832), "Until the opinions of Drs. Spurzheim and
Combe were published on this subject the definitions of insanity were
vague and contradictory."[30] The opinion now became widely shared that
an "elucidation" had been formulated where none had previously existed.

Since psychiatry formed no separate branch of medical education in
the early nineteenth century, one means of gaining an insight on the
advancement of phrenology in psychiatry can be found in the reception
of the doctrine within the medical profession generally. An important
boost from this direction came in 1821 when the celebrated lecturer on

surgery, John Abernethy, acknowledged the soundness of Gall and Spurz-heim's physiology and admitted that he could offer no rational objection to the system that he believed worthy of medical attention. Abernethy cautioned, though, that he foresaw "nothing but mischief" if the system became generally known and accredited.[31] The outspoken cockney hero of medical students, John Elliotson, had no such reservations and his incorpo-ration of the subject into his lectures and his establishment of the London Phrenological Society in 1823, made the science increasingly difficult for others to overlook. By February of that year the *Weekly Medico-Chirurgical and Philosophical Magazine* was presenting its readers with leader articles and illustrations of the science, and this coverage was soon extended in Wakley's *Lancet* (established in October 1823) where the doctrine was upheld as both "beautiful and useful."[32] In a more literary fashion the science received further promotion in the *Medico-Chirurgical Review*,[33] ed-ited by James Johnson, and in the *British and Foreign Medical Review*, edited by John Forbes, himself a member of the Phrenological Association. By 1833 the subject had obtained sufficient standing among the medical profes-sion to be lectured on at the London Hospital, St. Thomas's Hospital, Grainger's Theatre of Anatomy, Dermott's School of Medicine, and Lon-don University,[34] as well as at such nonmedical clubs as the London Institution and the Philomathic Institution. In the medical schools outside of London phrenology found similar shelter and advancement: in Man-chester, Daniel Noble lectured on the science at the Chatham Street School of Medicine; in Glasgow, the subject found a spokesman in Robert Hunter, professor of anatomy at the Andersonian University; and in Edinburgh, phrenologists looked favorably on the lectures of John Mackintosh, lec-turer on pathology and the practice of physic at the Argyle Square School of Medicine.[35] In the provinces as well, the "Lit. & Phils." and mechanics' institutes along with the phrenological societies further contributed to propagate the doctrine and to make it fashionable among a wide audience.

Not all who wrote or spoke on phrenology, however, were necessarily endorsing the science in all its details. Votaries of Gall differed widely on their acceptance of the principles, particularly with relation to the practi-cal aspects of cranioscopy, and not everyone who took an interest in the science agreed with phrenologists that it was the best or the only system with which to explain the moral and intellectual nature of man. While those alienists designated the "hard core" came closest to accepting all aspects of phrenology, the majority of those in the medical profession who were receptive to the ideas of the phrenologists were often only sharing —publicly at least—the sentiment of James Johnson, that "without sub-scribing to all the details of phrenology, I believe its fundamental princi-ples to be based on truth."[36]

Such reserved statements of acceptance were expedient, for despite phrenology's advancement within certain medical quarters, opposition to the doctrine remained considerable. During the first three decades of the century in particular, there was persistent ridicule of the notion that a man's faculties could be determined by a detailed examination of his cranium and satirical invective was heaped upon the supposed validity of a detailed organology. Added to this was the opposition, mainly from outside the medical profession, that leveled the charges of fatalism and materialism on the science. The details of these debates between phrenologists and antiphrenologists, especially as dramatized in Edinburgh in the early decades of the century, need not detain us here.[37] What *is* worth noting is the social and intellectual climate that surrounded the debated subject during the period under consideration, for this, as much as any direct contact with phrenology in the medical schools and journals, or through the literary societies and phrenological publications, formed an important part of the increasing awareness of the doctrine by alienists. Attacks in leading journals like the *Edinburgh*, the *Quarterly*, and *Blackwoods*, together with the denunciations by men of eminence such as Sir Charles Bell, Dr. P. M. Roget, Dr. John Gordon, Sir William Hamilton, Dr. Thomas Stone, and Dr. John Barclay, to name but a few,[38] were important as much for the serious interest in the doctrine which they displayed, as for their opposition. The audience of these opponents understood well that not only were personal reputations at stake in the debate but, since the antagonists were within the scientific elite, that the elite itself was being threatened by phrenology. Under these circumstances professions of belief in phrenology became symbolic of views antipathic to the accepted canons of the academic establishment in particular and to traditional ideas and institutions in general. Though Gall's doctrine might as easily have lent itself to defending the status quo (Gall, after all, had reacted against Enlightenment thought, especially the Sensationalism of Helvétius, and his concept of innate faculties could have been used to justify the futility of attempting any reform of man's character) the doctrine was deployed as a confrontation with the British academic elite. What emerged from these debates was the characterization of phrenology as a tool for legitimating radical change and reform.

Phrenology thus attracted a body of men who, for a variety of cultural, political, and idiosyncratic reasons, wished to utilize phrenology for specific social purposes. Though many of these men were themselves members of medical and social elites, they shared a common set of assumptions about and liberal approaches to the institutional arrangements of their society. Not unlike the seventeenth-century Puritan scientists described by Robert Merton,[39] most of them maintained an exaggerated contempt for the ancien régime and expressed this in a profound conviction in the future progress and reformation of society through the application of science. Gall's doctrine, as shaped into a more progressive philosophy in

Britain by Spurzheim and George Combe, was easily translated into a scientific legitimation of these reformist ambitions, which became all the more sharply defined by the nature of the opposition. Not surprisingly, young middle-class liberals who resented the political, social, and cultural restrictions still imposed upon them by the ancien régime were strongly attracted to this science, philosophy, and social program that promised such fundamental and sweeping changes to the society about them.

It is necessary to recognize, therefore, that when medical men turned to advocating phrenology or to joining a phrenological society,[40] they did so not merely because they had become convinced intellectually that Gall's doctrine was scientifically sound. Of equal, if not more, significance to them was the fact that the doctrine symbolized that which challenged the traditional values of the establishment in the context of a rapidly emerging new social and economic order. This socially symbolic role of phrenology was as important for the attraction of alienists to the doctrine as it was for any other occupational group. Indeed, two further social considerations might substantiate a claim that alienists were particularly attracted to phrenology for social reasons. First, since asylums in this period were one of the chief targets of evangelical reformers, alienists were already that much more concerned and involved with Victorian reform than other members of the medical profession. As Norman Dain has suggested in his study of American psychiatric thought, this involvement of alienists with social reform might well indicate that it was as reformers rather than as psychiatrists that phrenology made its extensive appeal.[41] The doctrine certainly harbored a set of social values and beliefs with which they could identify and through the science itself these values could be justified. For instance the idea that British phrenologists increasingly stressed, that man had innate faculties that could be gradually modified and improved through a better environment, nicely agreed with reforming aspirations. The medicoscientific insights revealed by Gall's doctrine may thus have only helped to justify preexisting or emergent social motivations. Second, the separateness of the alienists within their asylums might have hastened their adoption of phrenology as a socially engaging doctrine. Although the wide intellectual connections and social involvement of men like Browne, Ellis, and Conolly, both before and after they became alienists, militate against the notion of alienists as *alienated*, with many of the lesser-known figures the separation of the asylum from the rest of society could possibly have been a significant factor in encouraging phrenological positions.[42] Armed with phrenology, the alienist was no longer merely a "mad-doctor"; he became a proto-social scientist studying an aspect of deviance, the knowledge from which was intimately connected with answers to other pressing social issues such as education and criminal reform.

A wide range of social considerations could thus have underpinned the acceptance of phrenology by alienists, and medical education may either have sparked or only fanned that interest. When we observe that, in addition to being solidly middle class in background, the alienists discussed here were, with few exceptions, less than thirty-five years old when they were first attracted to the science; were predominantly nonconformists;[43] were firmly imbued with an Enlightenment faith in progress and the improvement of mankind through the application of science; and were liberals in politics, often playing leading roles in various reform programs, it is difficult to maintain that the social-reformist countenance of phrenology was merely a coincidental feature of their accepting the doctrine. On the contrary, it appears that social considerations were of primary importance for motivating and for perpetuating interest in a doctrine that boldly asserted its dismissal of old theories while holding out the promise of vast reforms in the care and curing of the insane.

Such factors need stressing, for although phrenology's full appeal to British alienists cannot be understood without referring to the specific scientific aspects of Gall's doctrine, it is easy to overlook what phrenology meant in the social currency of the time when discussing the more internalist issues. In turning our attention to phrenology's involvement with clinical psychiatry, it is worth bearing in mind, therefore, that we are not dealing with simply a "scientific" aspect of psychiatry but rather with a body of uninstitutionalized thought that, while being applied in practical psychiatry, was also popular outside its domain. It was supported and advanced by a normally distinguishable social group and was opposed for social as well as scientific reasons by an equally distinguishable traditionalist elite. It is because of this special nature of phrenology and because of the doctrine's significant place in psychiatry that the scientific approach to early nineteenth-century psychiatry is fundamentally as social as it is scientific.

Since Gall had conducted his many years of research with the primary objective of having the "happiest influence on moral institutions, in the treatment of cerebral disease, particularly mental alienation,"[44] there was good reason why his elaborate anatomical and physiological studies should have gained the attention of British alienists, however indirectly. Although the practice of incarcerating lunatics was losing support among mad-doctors in the early nineteenth century, thanks chiefly to the influence of Pinel and Tuke, no equally bold innovation for the understanding of mental derangement had been popularized. Nor was it likely that any new theory would be put forward so long as the Cartesian proscription on the scientific study of the mind prevailed and metaphysics remained divorced from anatomy. With the brain regarded as an organ of sensation and reflection and with the terms of reference based on the speculative faculties of imagination, reason, memory, and so forth, a discussion of the insane mind could seldom be more than an "academical exercise."[45] Gall, though he rejected the anti-Cartesian metaphysics of his Sensationalist contemporaries, nevertheless effectively undermined the Cartesian framework by constructing a *physiological* psychology based on the brain as the organ of the mind. The dichotomy between mind and body was thus endangered, and the study of mind became united with neurology on the one hand and with the biology of adaptation on the other. It was for this reason—this removal of mind from psychology and its replacement in biology—that George Henry Lewes, who was no champion of popular phrenology, felt that Gall had "produced a revolution" and could be styled "the Kepler of Psychology."[46]

Alienists, as practitioners rather than theoreticians, were alive to the inadequacies of faculty psychology for producing any practical insights into the nature and treatment of insanity. Although materialistic explanations of derangement had not actually been sought, alienists *had* been searching "long and anxiously," according to John Haslam in 1817, for an adequate definition of insanity and "these efforts [had] been hitherto fruitless."[47] Haslam felt, along with many fellow alienists, that "whenever the functions of the brain shall be fully understood, and the use of its different parts ascertained, we may then be enabled to judge how far disease, attacking any of these parts, may increase, diminish, or otherwise alter its functions."[48] Gall's doctrine claimed to supply precisely this need. Perhaps it was natural, therefore, that once alienists had been drawn to the doctrine their condemnation of established metaphysics was severe.[49] "With *Phrenology* it is otherwise," wrote Disney Alexander in 1826: "The founders of that Science . . . did not commence their labours with any preconcerted view of creating, or supporting, a favourite hypothesis; but were led . . . into a train of observations on the functions of the brain; from which they, at length, drew those inferences. . . ."[50]

This was where the science of phrenology supposedly divided itself from the woolly metaphysical thinking of the faculty psychologists; its methodology, claimed to be rigorously Baconian, spoke only of facts and repeated observations.[51] The result was a simplistic physiological explanation of mental organization and function which, unlike faculty psychology it seemed, could be readily applied to understanding insanity. This utility of the science was heralded as a further confirmation of its truth, for, as "Bacon inferred that Aristotle's philosophy was false, because it was barren . . . it is a legitimate inference from the same principle, that phrenology is true because it is fruitful."[52] But if the claim seemed sweeping that through phrenology the mysteries of the mind and of lunacy were to fade into insignificance, a closer look at Gall's doctrine showed that it was by no means insupportable. Nor, in view of some of the contemporary advances in the physical sciences, was the claim perhaps so startling.

Gall's first point, that the brain was the organ of the mind, was alone a milestone for clearer thought. Though the idea was not Gall's own, no one before him had argued so specifically or with so much detail in its defense. Gall's major opponent in France, Pierre Flourens, readily acknowledged that "the merit of Gall, and it is by no means a slender merit, consists in having understood better than any of his predecessors the whole of its importance [of the brain being the organ of the mind], and in having devoted himself to its demonstration. It existed in science before Gall appeared—it may be said to reign there ever since his appearance."[53] In linking physiology of function and anatomy with psychology, Gall was correctly identified as the first to establish the brain as the organ of the mind on a scientific basis. The brain thus came to be regarded "as part and parcel of the human organism, and as subject in common with the liver and lungs, etc., to similar organic laws and sympathies."[54]

The second aspect of Gall's doctrine, that the brain was a congeries of organs, had also been expressed long before Gall,[55] but for the first time "Nature's evidence" was marshaled in support of the idea through Gall's extensive labors in comparative anatomy. That Gall had proved himself a neuroanatomist par excellence was, of course, a key factor for the doctrine's credibility among medical men, for anatomy, beyond even physiology, was universally accepted as a firmly established science about which no speculations could exist. A doctrine so empirically based, many believed, must necessarily be grounded in truth. Moreover, in spite of the brain's appearance, the notion of cerebral localization was a logical and desirable one if only by analogy with the functions of the rest of the body's organs. By 1842 even the hostile *Edinburgh Review* was willing to concede this much, while rejecting the details of Gall's organology.[56] Similarly, Gall's third premise, that "each particular cerebral part, according to its development, may modify, in some degree, the manifestation of a particular moral quality, or intellectual faculty"[57] (which would later become the *caeteris paribus* clause that other factors being equal, size is a measure of power) also seemed reasonable through analogies in the natural world and with the rest of the body. As expressed by the Manchester physician Daniel Noble, "Unless rules of investigation apply to the brain's physiology which differ from those relating to the remaining organization," then these principles of Gall's could not possibly be denied.[58]

It is not difficult, therefore, to understand why medical men should have found these concepts attractive on medical grounds alone: in many respects they were simply an extension of the physiological premises they had already come to accept. Gall's organology did not demand a radically new way of understanding function. Nor did some of the other concepts relied upon by phrenologists mark any distinct break with older medical ideas. The division of man into the four basic temperaments as a basis for phrenological delineations was a clear link between the old and the new, while the phrenological explanation of rational behavior as mental organs in a balanced state bore a strong resemblance to the balance of the "passions" in the humoral tradition. John Mackintosh felt obliged to inform his students in 1830 that it was on the basis of his past "experience and observation" that he concluded that there was much truth in phrenology.[59] Similarly, the author of the standard Victorian text on the *Principles of Forensic Medicine* (1843), William Guy, confessed to adopting the principles of phrenology because they composed a theory "best agreeing with reason and experience."[60] The view of man as a rational mechanism influenced by natural laws was also a well established and physiologically supportable concept by the 1820s. In giving a biological context to the organs of the mind, Gall's doctrine logically elevated or extended this paradigm to the brain. For alienists this removed the frustration of not being able to treat the deranged mind as they would localized diseases elsewhere in the body. Gall was thus seen as having produced a scientific framework for an organization of mind and body that would facilitate a physical understanding of the organs of the mind in their healthy and deranged states.

The fourth aspect of Gall's doctrine[61] was never so defensible from nature nor as convincing in principle. That since the cranium was ossified over the shape of the brain, one's organology could be determined by an external examination of the skull, was a point that caused many persons a great deal of doubt and required of others considerable faith. Yet it was craniology that gained for phrenology not only its notoriety but its most zealous converts. To explain this faith we can make few appeals to the logic, analogies, or past medical experience that serve us for the other aspects of Gall's doctrine.[62] But this does not mean that a belief in cranioscopy should be attributed to blind credulity. The comparison with the miraculous insulin cure for schizophrenia in our own time should help our understanding here. In both cases it was subsequently shown that there was virtually no medical foundation for the claims, yet in both cases, and with neither intentional fraud nor deception, the results—cures and accurate delineations—justified the faith in the practice. When Gall and Spurzheim paraded through the asylums and prisons of Germany and described with uncanny accuracy the reasons why each inmate was confined, their entourage of doctors, warders, and civic officials could hardly do otherwise than believe that this was a correct system, however marvelous.[63] Those who saw Spurzheim's demonstrations in Britain, or those of George Combe, were similarly amazed and often totally convinced of the theory thereby. Even more persuasive was an "accurate" delineation of oneself or one's friends. The English authority on brain anatomy, the medical lecturer and Fellow of the Royal Society, Samuel Solly (1805–1871), was only one of countless physicians who, though having ample reason to praise

Gall without reference to cranioscopy, yet headed his list of reasons for believing in phrenology with this confirmation: "I have received from practical phrenologists . . . such accurate characters of individuals known to me, but unknown to them, that I cannot believe the accounts I received could be the result of accident and conjecture, which must have been the case if phrenology is untrue."[64] Solly's second reason, incidentally, was that phrenology alone could account for all the varieties of insanity.

Most of the alienists referred to here and all those within the "hard core" of phrenological alienists were among the cranioscopic enthusiasts, and for them it was no mere arabesque to the doctrine. William Ellis, who was probably attracted to phrenology as a result of Spurzheim's visit to Wakefield in the early 1820s and Matthew Allen's lectures there a few years later, believed very firmly in the practical value of cranioscopy. In a letter from Hanwell of December 1835 he stated that he "examine[d] the heads of all patients on admission & direct[ed] their treatment accordingly."[65] In calling for proper psychiatric education, he further stressed the benefits to be derived from a knowledge of craniology, noting that a "mere examination of the head, without any previous knowledge of or information whatever as to the habits of the patient," can often provide specific information on the type of insanity involved.[66] Where else in fact was a physician more in need of an external guide for internal diseases than in the diagnoses and treatment of the insane? Though Gall, Spurzheim, and Andrew Combe stressed that "in insanity the configuration of heads is neither to be overlooked, nor to be over-rated" since diseases of the brain like diseases elsewhere were subject to "infinite modification," they agreed that "in the greater number of cases" a relationship could be observed between an enlarged organ manifested in the cranial structure and the specific type of insanity.[67]

Ellis's praise and practice of phrenology made a deep impression on others. Alexander Mackintosh, who visited Wakefield as a doubter of the system, returned to the Dundee Asylum converted to Ellis's methods.[68] Harriet Martineau paid a visit to Hanwell in 1834 and, though a scoffer at phrenology, she willingly agreed with almost every other visitor that Ellis's system of classification, "to which he has been led by his adoption of phrenological principles," showed undoubtable wisdom.[69] Conolly also visited Hanwell in that year and was prompted to address the Provincial Medical Association: "There is reason to hope that as a result of the humane and enlightened management of the large lunatic asylum at Hanwell, under the superintendence of Dr. Ellis, this [phrenological] branch of practice may hereafter be more satisfactorily spoken of."[70]

Conolly's acquaintance with phrenology stemmed from as far back as the early 1820s when he had been a student in Edinburgh. It was probably there that he had witnessed George Combe's delineations on some prisoners after which he had little doubt of phrenology's truth.[71] As he told the members of the Royal Institution in 1854, he was still convinced that "although the doctrines of the phrenologists have met with little favour . . . no person not altogether devoid of the power of observation can affect to overlook the general importance of the shape and even the size of the brain in relation to the development of the mental faculties."[72]

Disney Alexander, also following in Ellis's footsteps, considered it "as proved beyond all reasonable contradiction" that it was at least possible to "distinguish men of desperate and dangerous tendencies from those of good dispositions" from the form and size of the brain during life.[73] What the superintendent of the Royal Navy Asylum appropriately called the "almost infallible beacon of Phrenology" was a craniological sentiment wholeheartedly shared by the seven other alienists who contributed testimonials to George Combe and Sir George Mackenzie in 1836.[74] W. A. F. Browne and Matthew Allen, as lecturers and public demonstrators of the science, also made use of their delineating abilities on their patients. Browne did not refer to this method of analysis in his major work of 1837 (ostensibly not to confuse the nonphrenological reader), but he did offer the assurance that "Insanity can neither be understood, nor described, nor treated by the aid of any other philosophy."[75] Matthew Allen was less cautious: in his *Cases of Insanity* (1831) phrenological delineations form a part of the presentation.[76]

Even much later in the century one could find alienists who retained a faith in cranioscopy. One of these was Dr. J. W. Eastwood, medical superintendent of the Dinsdale Park Retreat at Darlington. Like so many other Victorians, Eastwood had witnessed phrenological delineations in which no deceit had been possible and in which "the descriptions were so accurate as to afford striking evidence of the truth of phrenology." In an article about craniology in the *Journal of Mental Science* in October 1871 he noted, from casts taken from his own skull and from those of his patients, that at least some of the organs in Gall and Spurzheim's system were correct. Reiterating the optimism and hopes of the phrenological alienists of the first half of the century, Eastwood concluded his article: "If we are enabled by these means to understand the morbid manifestations of the brain for the classification of its diseases, and for the diagnosis of insanity, we shall render great service to the special branch of the profession in which we are engaged."[77]

That such hope could be seriously expressed by an alienist in 1871 when craniology as a scientific system had been totally discredited, gives perhaps the best insight on the promise that it held for alienists between the 1820s and the 1840s.

But not all alienists were as convinced of the craniological aspects of Gall's doctrine. Obviously they had not witnessed the "striking evidence" that Eastwood had. That sort of conviction came only through personal involvement; second-hand accounts of craniology's worth were never as convincing, whatever the stature of the spokesmen. Concomitantly, these alienists remained skeptical of Gall's detailed location of the mental organs, though this did not necessarily mean that they were any less enthusiastic about the doctrine's other principles. Many of them were, as David Uwins declared of himself, *"bitten* by phrenology" but few of them had either the occasion or the inclination to state, as Uwins did, that "thinking as I do on the applicability of phrenological principle to measures preventive of insanity, I should not do justice to my conscience, were I to shrink from declaring my sentiments, under the apprehension of being stigmatized as a visionary."[78]

The ridicule to which craniology easily lent itself most often prevented those who accepted the other tenets of the doctrine from openly admitting as much. (That the reputations of those who were becoming eminent in the field of psychiatry rarely suffered because of their public statements on phrenology—Conolly's stature only grew in public and medical opinion; Andrew Combe was appointed physician to the King of the Belgians; Ellis was the first superintendent of a lunatic asylum in Britain to be knighted—seems to have made little difference to the more conservative minded critics.) When Andrew Combe—cautioned by friends to dress up and disguise his phrenology for his treatise of 1831—saw the omission of phrenology from the first draft of Browne's treatise, he was understandably disappointed. It "seems to me so improbable that you should omit it," he wrote to Browne; yet Combe understood why such omissions occurred and what the consequences were: "It is true, present popularity is gained; but my conviction is, that truth is retarded in the long-run, and Phrenology itself thrown into the background, branded with the stamp of folly by those who never suspect that what they read is Phrenology. . . . While the fruit is admired and cherished, the tree is cast into the furnace as fit only to be burned up."[79]

As was the case with so many Victorian works on education, the laws of health, penal reform, and anthropology, it was precisely in this inexplicit manner that phrenology was mainly infused into the discussions on insanity. In effect most writers were prepared to agree quietly with the eminent French pathologist Gabriel Andral that the principles of Gall were fairly proven or that there was "not much astray in assigning particular cerebral parts to special instincts or intellectual faculties."[80] In the 1830s and 1840s this view gained increasing favor among those involved with mental derangement, almost all of whom now relied on brain physiology in their definitions of insanity as diseased or disordered function of the organs of the brain. Since a functional understanding of the brain based on physiology could optimistically deal with the patient in terms of a definable disease that was subject to treatment (whereas earlier brain pathology could offer little hope for the patient), the interest in phrenology was certainly justified. There was, however, no need to subscribe fully to Gall's doctrine—and even less need to assume the dogmatism of the phrenologists—in order to share this optimism. William B. Neville, for instance, the medical adviser for a private asylum in Earl's Court, relied completely on the works of Combe and Spurzheim and on the work of the French alienist (and member of the Paris Phrenological Society) Achille-Louis Foville for his treatise *On Insanity; Its Nature and Cure* (1836). Yet Neville expresses no desire to acknowledge a debt to phrenology. It is this sort of general reliance on phrenological authors and on phrenological facts and assumptions that can be found throughout the writings on insanity in the period and not infrequently in the writings of antiphrenologists. Like the loose reliance on Freudian ideas and terms in the twentieth century that only indirectly acknowledges conceptual and methodological debts to Freud, so in the nineteenth century there were a great many persons who, as Browne said, "*think* phrenologically, judge of conduct and character through the medium of Phrenology and employ its phraseology."[81] What separated these persons from most of the "hard core" phrenological alienists was that they had no special cultural interest in utilizing phrenological ideas; since the subject touched "too dangerously upon too many of those subjects upon which mankind rejoice in conventional delusions,"[82] it was more convenient to avoid explicit reference to it. The ideas worked quite as well without the dogma. Hence most authors of works on the insane came to feel that even if phrenology had not yet established itself as a science (that is, even if the organology and craniology could not be completely trusted), it at least provided some excellent conceptual tools with which insanity could be better understood and through which one could be more optimistic in the treatment of the insane.[83] Again, William Guy was speaking for a great many in the profession when he passed the elogium on "Gall and Spurzheim, and their followers" that to them was "due the great merit of having directed attention to those faculties which are the real source of action . . . and to them must be ascribed the praise of having originated the simplest, and by far the most practical, theory of the human mind."[84]

It was this conceptual advantage of phrenology that facilitated its role as a rationale for both the "moral" and the "medical" treatments of the insane that will be discussed next. As we shall see, Gall's essential reification of the mind provided alienists with a reassuringly scientific basis for optimistically believing that in the actual practice of psychiatry they could impose a logic upon madness.

Doctrine and Practice

Social motivations and contemporary medical knowledge and experience provide a broad basis of explanation for why a great many British alienists were attracted to the phrenological doctrine in the second quarter of the nineteenth century. These factors in themselves, however, are conspicuously incomplete. Since alienists were distinguished by the type of illness they confronted and by the place in which their therapy was normally conducted, it is naturally in the realm of practical psychiatry that one might expect to find more specific reasons for the attraction of phrenology. In particular our inquiry must be directed to the two contemporary treatments of the insane: the "moral" and the "medical."

The "moral" or "psychological" treatment of insanity has long been identified as the most important innovation for the development of practical psychiatry in modern times.[85] Celebrated and symbolized by the efforts of Pinel and Tuke at the end of the eighteenth century, the treatment stemmed from the realization that less use of restraints and less resorting to "heroic" medicines rendered patients more tractable and dramatically increased the cures effected. Moral therapy, as distinguished from medical therapy, referred to those therapeutic techniques that affected the patient's psychology.[86] However, as Dr. Bynum has recently pointed out, the moral therapy "was hardly a straightforward affair; and its implications for both medical theory and medical practice were not lost on the physicians of the early nineteenth century who attempted to assess its true significance. However much they might profess to admire the methods of Pinel or the Tukes, very few were prepared to abandon entirely the medical treatment of insanity."[87]

The moral therapy threatened the status and very existence of physicians within asylums: if cures could be effected by nonmedical means, then the administrators of physic were reduced to mere custodians of the insane. What medical superintendents of asylums required, therefore, was a means of legitimating the humanitarianism and utilitarianism of the moral treatment while simultaneously justifying their place in asylums as the purveyors of essential medical expertise. Pragmatic expediency was one means of forcing such a reconciliation. Much more attractive was phrenology, which not only adequately met both these specific needs, but elevated the moral therapy to a scientific status, in much the same manner that Darwin's theory was subsequently employed to give scientific credence to an existing socioeconomic structure. Phrenology's reference to brain physiology for the understanding of psychological therapy reassured physicians that special medical as well as scientific knowledge was required to deal with the insane. The enthusiasm for phrenology by British alienists can thus be seen as the direct result of the doctrine's expedient arrival and popularization at a period when psychiatry, like the larger society, was in an unsettled transitionary stage and openly receptive to theories that seemed to provide order and systemization. In the name of rational science, phrenology supplied just such a comprehensive ordering mechanism, and through the science the moral treatment became a logical and comprehensible system of exact causal relationships between physical and psychological factors.[88]

The phrenological explanation for the moral treatment was made clearest where the science was most alluring: in the discussion on monomania or partial insanity, where the patient appeared to be rational on all subjects but one. According to William B. Carpenter, the physiologist who did most to undermine phrenology's credibility in Britain, it was the evidence from monomania that gave the greatest strength to a belief in the phrenological system.[89] This is hardly surprising in view of the long-debated issue of the proper nosology of insanity. By assigning each mental disorder a specific cerebral organ, phrenology solved the problem of nosology at a stroke. Not unnaturally, phrenologists dwelt more on monomania than on any other aspect of insanity; indeed, they can be said to have brought the term into fashionable usage. Hitherto no explanation for partial alienation had been articulated and Pinel's use of the term *melancholia* for the phenomenon only served to confuse the long train of speculations.[90] With phrenology the phenomenon could be quite simply explained: religious behavior was a result of the organ of Veneration, sex related to the organ of Amativeness, music to the organ of Tune, greed to the organ of Acquisitiveness, and so on for each of the mental organs. Hence those patients who thought themselves Napoleon were manifesting symptoms of the disordered function of self-esteem, just as the erotomaniacs were reflecting the morbid state of their Amativeness. As explained by a German alienist in the *Medico-Chirurgical Review* of 1825, "Phrenology bids fairest to ascertain the nature of insanity (where it depends, as it very generally does) on moral *causes*, by comparing the faculty most disordered with the organ by which the faculty is supposed to be manifested."[91] Phrenologists called in Shakespeare to lend weight to this idea: " 'I am mad,' says Hamlet, 'north-north-west; when the wind's southerly, I know a hawk from a heronshaw [*sic*].' " Had the brain been a single organ, it was remarked, Hamlet would have been mad at every point of the compass.[92] By extension of the theory, a perversion of several or all of the faculties at one time explained the behavior of those patients who alternated from dejection, to violence, to melancholia. Thus a neat mechanical view of the brain divided into organs that functioned somewhat analogous with muscles provided a ready and accessible means for comprehending the basis upon which the psychological treatment might logically be supposed to operate.

Having ascertained the nature of mental illness, phrenologists were able to present the moral treatment of insanity as an easily understood and regularized system: the disturbed organs were to be suppressed by calling the other mental organs into greater action. The nymphomaniac, for example, required greater exercise of her intellectual faculties and higher sentiments that these might come to preponderate over the enlarged Amativeness. To accomplish this, phrenologists required that their advice for schools and prisons should likewise be applied to asylums—that the asylum become a carefully regulated moral hospital whose special environment could be manipulated for redirecting, training, and strengthening specific mental organs. As with illness elsewhere in the body, the correct attention to the individual's disease and the proper application of judicious means were intended to restore the malfunction to health. "The great point," said Gall, "always is, to divert the attention of the patient from the object of his insanity, by fixing it upon other objects."[93] By providing a healthy environment with rational amusements and occupations individually designed, the organs could be restored to their proper balance. Since brutality only aggravated the illness and caused the inferior faculties to be enlarged by the resentment to punishment, benevolence was justified as the keystone of treatment. Phrenology thus hastened the objective regard for the lunatic as a "patient" whose treatment was dependent upon benevolence and kindness. Alienists thereby gained some of the comfort and security that comes with regarding lunacy as "mental illness." In 1831 Andrew Combe wrote that Gall's doctrine "has already divested the subject of madness of much of its obscurity, and . . . some of its terrors."[94]

Without the phrenological jargon in which their instructions were normally couched, the phrenologists were saying little more than to prevent the patient from idly brooding by providing him with a gentle environment that would stimulate his brain to work in other directions. But this much was already known. As Dr. Daniel Pring critically remarked, "There is nothing very new or erudite in this observation of the phrenologists; it is both old and vulgar."[95] What Pring and other critics failed sufficiently to appreciate was that the quintessence of phrenology's appeal was to be found precisely in its ability to shelter and legitimize existing beliefs by recasting them in a scientific mold. This point is further illustrated by looking at the defense of conventional morality implicit in the phrenological explanation of monomania.

Mental health, the phrenologists were arguing, was the result of the daily exercise of all the mental organs. Inactivity of the brain was a predisposition to insanity, as was the overactivity of any mental organ. Slothfulness and overindulgence were alike at the root of much insanity. It was necessary, therefore, that the public should be educated against perpetuating these vices that would damage their health and (because of the belief in social hereditarianism) the mental health of future generations. The virtues of sobriety, chastity, self-improvement, and moderation in all things were thus recommended. One did not have to be a reader of Johnson's *Rasselas* to recognize the ancient wisdom being expressed here; but for the first time at a popular level this wisdom was being sanctified at the altar of science. No longer was morality to be the exclusive province of theology; the laws of physiology were now to share that administration and with an even greater indisputability. Fittingly and expediently, the Reverend John Barlow incorporated this defense of morality into his *Man's Power over Himself to Prevent or Control Insanity* (1843). Quoting from Conolly that "those who most exercise the faculties of their minds are least liable to insanity," he added that "a brain strengthened by rational exercise . . . is but little likely to be attacked by disease . . . and thus the larger half of the evil is removed."[96]

It followed from the phrenological explanation of monomania that an alienist who was adept at cranioscopy could more speedily effect the right type of moral treatment. Comprehending the relationship between structure and function, the alienist employing cranioscopy had a greater command over his patients. For the doctor then knows, said Andrew Combe, "what are the probable points of attack in the mental constitution; when to be on his guard against counterfeit and subterfuge; and what class of motives or line of mental discipline is likely to be attended with the best effects in subduing excitement, and promoting the return of reason."[97]

This a priori knowledge of the organs diseased was seen as particularly useful for the smooth operation of nonrestraint methods, for potentially violent patients could be recognized and given special attention. And just as a public awareness of the proper functions of the brain was seen as crucial in combating any increase in insanity through immorality, so a public knowledge or access to craniology was seen as a useful means for the early diagnosis of insanity. David Uwins, in common with many practical phrenologists, was making much the same point as the Reverend Barlow when he asserted that "the self-condemnation of a character in finding and feeling his skull to bulge out in its bad parts—bad when exercised inordinately—will come also to be an additional motive for arresting his career of folly and vice before the day of probation be past. . . ."[98] If undetected and unarrested, the alternative was lunacy.

As a rationale for moral therapy, then, phrenology's appeal was at three levels at least: first, it offered a scientific framework based on organology that related psychological factors to brain function, including a particularly convincing explanation of monomania; second, in explaining the nature of psychological insanity it suggested measures for its prevention; and third, it made the moral treatment of the insane the apotheosis of conventional morality. Set beside the enviable examples of reform in asylum management effected by phrenological alienists of stature, these factors were a strong inducement for others in the profession to take up the acclaimed doctrine. The many alienists who came to share the optimism or "spirit of amelioration" that was generated by the elevation of the moral management of the insane to a scientific system of physiological psychology, largely qualified such later assertions as: "Phrenology has destroyed the system of brutal torture . . . [and] that INSANITY, by the discovery and promulgation of Dr. Gall's system of Cerebral Physiology, has been stripped of more than half its horrors."[99] By way of comparison, phrenologists pointed to the example of the antiphrenologist Dr. Edward Millingen who succeeded Sir William Ellis as the superintendent of Hanwell. The *Phrenological Journal* was quick to note that Millingen was having problems managing the insane "without the aid of phrenological acquirements," and Conolly later confirmed that in the single year in which Millingen was at Hanwell "the number of instruments of restraint in the asylum appeared to have been increased; and he [Millingen] subsequently professed his dislike of the non-restraint system very strongly."[100] The claim of Gall's doctrine to have a benevolent influence upon the management and cure of the insane had, of course, already been accomplished by the followers of Pinel and Tuke well before phrenology was popularized in Britain. Nor was Gall's doctrine even the first theoretical explanation for psychological factors in the causing and the curing of insanity.[101] Yet the strong influence of phrenological alienists like Ellis, Conolly, and W. A. F. Browne in promoting and firmly establishing the moral management in Britain almost validated the retrospective assertion that the commonsense system of practical kindness toward the insane was, by Gall's discovery *alone*, "enabled . . . to be based on perfectly rational and scientific principles."[102]

Up to this point I have been concerned with phrenology's role in relation to the moral treatment as based upon Pinel's conviction that insanity was a psychological or "emotional" disturbance. Emphasized in this view were the "moral" or "sympathetic" or "exciting" causes of insanity such as irritations, griefs, overindulgences, and anxieties, all of which were seen to result in functional derangement. Pinel came to justify his physical liberation of the lunatic on the basis of this psychological interpretation: his predecessors, he claimed, had abandoned the lunatic because they conceived of insanity as an incurable organic disease. Pinel supposed from the success of the moral treatment that organic lesions in the brain or cranium must be rare and hence little importance should be attached to "fortuitous and ineffective" pharmaceutical remedies.[103]

As we have noted, however, Pinel's opinion and the treatment he based upon it were not entirely acceptable to other physicians whose training in pathology inclined them to seek evidence of disease wherever sickness presented itself and to think in terms of more orthodox medical remedies. Mental factors, these doctors felt, were more closely integrated with physical factors. As the century progressed, the conviction grew stronger that an adequate understanding of physiological psychology was a prerequisite of relevant diagnosis and treatment.[104] While no one wanted to dispute that the moral treatment appeared to effect cures, many physicians by 1826 would have sided with the *Westminster Review* that this was "to mistake the cause, and to attribute to metaphysical means what is truly a natural change in the diseased parts . . . as no one would trust the cure of whooping cough or intermittent to charms or spiders alone, so to rely on moral means only in Insanity, is to abandon medicine and medical analogy. . . ."

By this date, many alienists would have been prepared to agree further with the author of this review that because of the little basis there seemed to be for medical therapy in insanity, "we must cóntinue to think that an opening, and a valuable one, has been made by the much ridiculed Phrenology. Imperfect as the details of that new branch of physiology still may be, we do not hesitate in thinking that it is of more importance than any physiological view that ever was promulgated."[105]

It is here that we can begin to perceive fully why phrenology as a science of brain anatomy, physiology, and localized pathology should have appealed to alienists above and beyond its attractions on social, institutional, and clinical levels. It brought the mind and psychology via the brain fully into the province of somatic medicine just as it had brought the brain in psychiatry into the domain of biology. As most medical historians now recognize, these were to be phrenology's most important and enduring contributions to the study of the mind and its disorders.[106] For the alienist in the early decades of the nineteenth century such a clearly medical understanding of the insane patient allowed him to regain the position that had been undermined by the introduction of the moral therapy.

In explaining mental states in physicalist terms, phrenology presupposed that pathological changes normally occur in the brain during insanity. Though phrenology was able to explain the moral or, to use Spurzheim's term, the "idiopathic" causes of insanity, it assumed that the resulting derangement was physically based. "We continually repeat that the brain is an organic part," said Spurzheim, "and as to anatomy, physiology, and pathology, subject to the same considerations as any other organ."[107] So phrenology not only extended familiar physiological concepts of the body to the brain,[108] it also applied a familiar somatic pathology to the mental organs, "as rational as that offered by any branches of the healing art."[109] This pathological understanding of insanity was a necessary addition to any psychological explanation, for it provided a

logical reason why increasing numbers of patients in the county asylums
were not being cured by moral means alone. In a manner similar to the
application of hereditarian doctrines in the later nineteenth century,
phrenology's somatic emphasis further rendered madness a "less threatening and more manageable reality" when dealing with those who could not
normally be cured.[110] Phrenological alienists could extol and advance the
moral management of the insane as the most useful method of therapy
while affirming that insanity is mainly connected with organic changes
and proposing medical remedies in accordance with the general principles
of pathology. Gall had actually spoken of topical applications and venesec-
tion to that part of the cranium under which the diseased organ was
thought to lie.[111] Ellis, along with other phrenological alienists, noted
distinct rises in temperature in the region around the organ presumed
diseased.[112] This, it was argued, was the result of inflammation, common
to all body diseases.

Unlike Pinel's predecessors, the alienists who adopted this physicalist
view did not lose their confidence in the curability of insanity even though
it justified the inability to cure all patients. On the contrary, as Spurzheim
optimistically declared: since the brain is an organic part, it must be
curable, "Its organization is only more delicate, and requires more attention."[113] Almost reversing Pinel's justification, phrenologists claimed,
"Had insanity been recognised to be a symptom of cerebral disease, the
insane would never have been rejected and excluded from our sympathies
as the detested of Heaven."[114] Through phrenology, alienists could remain
sanguine even when surrounded by mainly incurable cases. Chronic patients only proved that insanity was a physical disease that had advanced
too far before being brought under medical attention. Hence medical as
well as moral factors made phrenologists prominent among those who
argued for the early treatment of mental disease and, since they believed
it to be a disease like any other, the propaganda they disseminated had the
additional motive of demystifying the public conception of lunacy. Aided
by the ease with which phrenology could be translated into layman's
language, phrenologists were largely successful in this campaign, as is
witnessed by the impression made on Harriet Martineau. After Ellis
guided her through Hanwell in 1834, she wrote, with her usual authority:
"There is all possible certainty that inflammation of the brain may be
stopped as easily as any other inflammation, if it is attacked in time; and
when people have learned to consider it in the same light as any other
ailment . . . they will first train their children, as wise parents do, to give
a simple account of any uneasiness that they may feel, and then be ready
to put them . . . under the management most likely to effect their cure.
When those days come, insanity will probably be no more of an evil than
the temporary delirium of a fever is now. . . ."[115] The exploited analogy,

the implicit faith in science, and the qualification of medical expertise in psychiatry combined with the reaffirmation of conventional wisdom and morality are all expressed here. Together they offered, as Martineau illustrates, a source of optimism both for the public and for other alienists.

It followed that if insanity was "a symptom of diseased brain, just as indigestion is of disordered stomach,"[116] then evidence of the morbid condition should be apparent upon postmortem examination. Gall and Spurzheim's unsupported assertions for pathological findings were opposed in the 1820s by such eminent physicians as James Copland and George Man Burrows, who claimed to have found few cases of lesion in maniacal patients.[117] It was, of course, expedient for a defense of morality through the threat of insanity that no organic causes should be involved; if insanity was a natural bodily disease a person could have no more control over it than over smallpox. Writers like the Reverend John Barlow had to minimize the importance of structural change in insanity to support the notion that it was mainly due to the slacking of one's "intellectual force" or a functional disorder dependent on psychological factors.[118] Prima facie any organic direction of phrenology should have undermined the doctrine's defense of morality as used by persons like Barlow. If insanity was organically based then the proper exercise of the mental organs could have had little effect on its cure. Though phrenologists cited such cases as gout being cured by sudden shock as an illustration of a physical disease being cured by psychological means, they recognized that mental disorders could not all be similarly treated. The uniqueness and great advantage of the phrenological theory, however, was that while it established that insanity was a physical/somatic disease of the brain (as opposed to a "mental" disease of the mind or soul), it interpreted that disease as either functional or organic. In other words, every mental derangement was a material manifestation of one or more of the cerebral parts, but those parts might be either structurally damaged or merely disordered "in the mode of action."[119] Functional or psychological disorders were thus reified as pathological conditions of brain matter. As John Elliotson told his students in his lectures on insanity, "A disease may be *corporal,* and yet not be *structural:* —no affection of any organ may take place."[120] Once again, the analogy with disease in other bodily organs and the application of the "laws governing organic matter" were simply extended to the brain. Phrenologists therefore argued that insanity as a manifestation of disordered function without structural change was commonly the case with recent insanity. This conveniently explained why moral methods were always more effective in dealing with new patients. It also explained the lack of organic lesion found in many postmortem examinations.

Phrenological theory then did not present any impediment to the search for organic lesion; it can be said to have hastened this investigation with phrenologists at the forefront of those exposing the evidence. Edward Wright told the Westminster Medical Society in 1828 that he had examined the brains of more than one hundred insane patients at Bethlem and had "found in all these cases palpable proofs of disease." From this he "passed a high eulogium on phrenology, as the only true means of studying the human mind."[121] Ellis confirmed organic lesion in 207 out of 221 cases, and Browne looked to the supporting evidence provided by Dr. Davidson at the Lancaster Asylum, by Haslam at St. Luke's, and by Georget, Falret, and Voisin in France.[122] Insisting that insanity had a physical cause, James Davey presented findings from one hundred examinations he had made while at Hanwell between 1840 and 1844, in only eight of which cases could he find no morbid appearance on dissection.[123] The Glasgow surgeon and phrenological popularizer, Robert Macnish, turned to the findings of William Lawrence, who had stated that in all the postmortems he had conducted on insane persons there was hardly "a single brain in which there were not obvious marks of disease."[124] Where no morbid appearance could be found, the inference was that the competence of the surgeon was lacking or that techniques of dissection had not yet been perfected *or* that the disease had not yet advanced sufficiently for detection of structural change.[125] That Gall and Spurzheim had discovered a superior method of brain dissection naturally added to the credibility of phrenologists finding lesions where none had previously seemed to exist. Though evidence of morbidity in the brains of insane persons remained a contentious issue well into the 1840s, phrenology was seen as having given a direction and great deal of authorization to the search.[126] Alienists anxious to establish the material basis of mental illness found their rationale in phrenology but increasingly overlooked that the phrenological meaning of *disease* also legitimated purely psychological derangement. By 1850 many fewer alienists were willing to admit that insanity was not a disease of the brain and that organic lesion was not there to prove it. Consequently, as the physician to the York Dispensary stated in 1844, "The doctrine that insanity is a disease of the moral and intellectual faculties only, and curable by merely moral treatment, is now little held, and it is generally acknowledged that it is dependent upon some physical change."[127]

But if evidence of organic lesion further proved that insanity was a disease of the brain as the organ of the mind, it was a more difficult task to pinpoint this evidence in support of Gall's organology. Phrenologists recorded innumerable cases reconciling the location of brain tissue impairment to the patient's particular disposition while insane, and this made it impossible, said one surgeon, "for any one acquainted with the principles of the new doctrine . . . to omit observing the striking coincidence and apparent corroboration which Phrenology seems to receive from morbid anatomy."[128] Yet many necroscopic examinations did not point to this correspondence. Alexander Morison, seeing that the brains of those who had labored under monomania seldom had inflammation confined to one convolution, thought that this disproved Gall's organology.[129] Ellis replied to this with the convincing analogy that "every one knows, that when inflammation takes place in any part of the body, it is not confined entirely to the spot which is diseased."[130] Phrenologists observed, moreover, that in mania the whole of the brain was implicated (or several of the organs at one time), and one could not, therefore, expect to find localized disease.

Since asylums in this period provided few research facilities, the phrenological pathology of insanity could not be easily disputed. Even much later in the century when serious testing was undertaken, the findings remained equivocal. In the 1860s, for example, the aspiring superintendent of the Murray Royal Institution for the Insane at Perth, W. Lauder Lindsay, conducted careful investigations to determine the percentage of observable organic lesions in the insane. Along with the cranioscopic examinations he carried out on 173 of his patients, he could only conclude, "That, while there is apparently much truth in Phrenology, especially in regard to some of its general laws or doctrines, there is unquestionably more error."[131] Opponents of phrenology between the 1820s and the 1840s were in an even weaker position: their opposition was random and there was no antiphrenological clearinghouse to compare with the publications of the phrenologists. Since opponents could offer no alternative explanation of insanity as convincing, as comprehensive, or as morally attractive as the phrenologists, they, too, often appeared in the light in which they were cast, as scientific reactionaries. Eventually, however, the psychophysiological work of Carpenter, in addition to that of Rolando, Flourens, Magendie, and others, undermined the specific physiology of phrenology and the system in the face of increased professionalization became generally discredited. Though the later investigations of Broca, Fritsch and Hitzig, Hughlings Jackson, Ferrier, Crichton-Browne, Sherrington, and others would redeem Gall's basic concept of plural faculties and localized function, by the 1850s phrenology was surrounded by too many untenable points. The fact that the cerebellum proved not to be related to sexual function was only one of the major blows that brought the old phrenology to its knees. By mid-century the "humbug" dismissals of phrenology that had been printed in some of the literary journals in the 1820s and 1830s were beginning to assume a medical validity. The best that phrenology could now hope for in the study of mental illness was the admission from alienists of holding what, very broadly speaking, were "partially phrenological views."[132]

A convenient marking post for the historian is provided by the 1853 publication of Daniel Noble's *Elements of Psychological Medicine.* In the 1830s Noble had been the guiding spirit of the Manchester Phrenological Society; he wrote articles for the *Phrenological Journal* and published several short tracts on the science. In 1842 he wrote for the *British and Foreign Medical Review* an article titled "True and False Phrenology" in which he expressed some doubts about certain aspects of phrenology, condemning the pretensions of cranioscopy as well as some of the wilder philosophic claims of phrenologists. Noble remained, however, a solid supporter of Gall's doctrine. His *Brain and Its Physiology* (1846), which was highly recommended by Samuel Solly, was an elaboration of George Combe's attempt to refute Carpenter's physiology.[133] Ironically, it was Carpenter's detailed review of this work that, as Noble later admitted, brought to an end his faith in phrenology. In the *Elements of Psychological Medicine* Noble conceded that Carpenter's views were more soundly and systematically based and that the time had arrived to abandon Gall's specific organology and to part company with the ever more recalcitrant phrenologists.[134]

Further contributing to phrenology's demise in psychiatry was the decline by the 1850s of the original generation of phrenological alienists. Particularly through Ellis's retirement from Hanwell in 1837, and his death two years later, and through the death of Andrew Combe in 1847, the cause of phrenology in the treatment of insanity lost its most influential practitioner and its ablest propagandist. Though John Conolly, Forbes Winslow, and W. A. F. Browne remained at the front of the profession until their deaths in 1866, 1874, and 1885 respectively, none of them continued actively to espouse the phrenological doctrine in their professional capacities. Of the alienists mentioned in the beginning of this essay, only James Davey continued publicly to laud the science with as much enthusiasm as ever.[135]

The dismissal of the "pseudoscience" of phrenology through the advance of neurophysiology, combined with the retirement of the alienists involved, had important implications for the direction of psychiatry in the second half of the nineteenth century. As liberals interested in reforming the care of the insane, phrenologists had found through their explanation of functional insanity a means of rationalizing and hastening the advance of the moral therapy. They established themselves as preeminent in this field. But as physicalists interested in advancing the idea that insanity was a disease of the brain with a specific pathology, the phrenological alienists had simultaneously encouraged the search for organic/structural changes in the deranged organs of the mind. Through this latter pursuit they not only fully justified the position of the physician within the asylum, but did a great deal to make alienists see themselves as "scientists" or "psychiatrists" adhering to the logic of the physical sciences. Phrenological psychiatry, in other words, established a balance between Pinel's psychological approach to lunacy and the totally organic approach that Pinel had reacted against. With the demise of the phrenological doctrine this balance or psychosomaticism was increasingly difficult to maintain. The lack of scientific—as opposed to anecdotal—evidence for Gall's organology and for the simplistic one-to-one relationship of the organs in monomania forced the dismissal of the phrenological interpretation of functional derangement. This did not mean, however, that the physicalist/organic emphasis of phrenology was also undermined. On the contrary, the neuropathological school, which had been inspired by phrenology (in particular by Broca who had set out to test phrenology but, ironically, localized the faculty of language precisely where Gall had claimed it to be) was to grow to an orthodoxy just as the context of biological explanations were beginning to draw sustenance in the wake of evolutionary theory. The idea of mental disease without actual organic causes became increasingly offensive to psychiatrists. What has been labeled the "physical era" of psychiatry was thus initiated.[136] When the *Asylum Journal* made its appearance in 1853 the new emphasis was strongly reflected: "It is quite time to get rid of the absurd division of disease into organic and functional," it claimed. "All diseases are organic, even blood diseases, and secondary diseases from so-called sympathies."[137] It was the practice founded on this interpretation of insanity that was to be deplored by the functional psychologist William McDougall early in the twentieth century.[138]

Consequent upon the rise of the "physical era" was the decay of the moral treatment. The emphasis that phrenologists had placed on individual therapy designed in accordance with each patient's faculty organization (or disorganization) was no longer of much importance if functionalism was discredited. What Andrew Combe had cautioned against, "the practice of subjecting all lunatics to the same regimen,"[139] was precisely what did occur when the phrenological rationale for doing otherwise was invalidated. Successors to the generation of phrenological alienists only understood that by employing patients on asylum works, the patients were made more tractable and administrative costs were greatly reduced. David Skae, superintendent of the Royal Edinburgh Asylum after 1846 and regarded as the founder of the Edinburgh school of psychiatry, typified many of the later alienists who took "moral" to signify simply the humane treatment and thus appeased their ethical standards while gratifying administrative prowess. By 1851 Skae was reporting that by practicing the "moral treatment" his chief attendant (suitably called the "Master of Works") had extracted £2,000 worth of labor from his patients. The logic of individually designed moral therapy was lost in such reports, and it cannot be regarded as insignificant that Skae was fully convinced of the physical basis of all insanity; nor is it merely incidental that in November 1846 he had written the hostile article on phrenology in the *British Quarterly Review.*[140]

The usual explanation for the breakdown of the moral treatment on the grounds that the asylums became overcrowded with incurable pauper lunatics who sapped psychiatric optimism requires, therefore, a great deal of revision. Hanwell was always a pauper asylum in which, as Ellis noted in the 1830s, one could hope for very few cures. It was not pauper incurables that gradually eroded the moral therapy or the optimism around it, but to a large extent, the loss of the rudder or rationale that phrenology had seemed to provide for its advancement. The option of *scientifically* justifying benevolence and kindness was no longer open when phrenological psychology was excluded.

Examined in this light, the phrenologists were right to insist that only their understanding of insanity could promote the moral treatment as originally conceived. When Browne looked about him in 1864 he was critical of what he saw as passing for moral therapy. "There is a fallacy even in conceiving that Moral Treatment consists in being kind and humane to the insane," he said. "It is this, and a great deal more than all this."[141] The moral treatment, he continued, is "*not* the comforts, and indulgences, and embellishments by which the insane are now surrounded, but the reasons upon which these are provided, the objects in view; and that they are not necessarily, general arrangements for *all* cases, but *special* adaptations for particular conditions and stages. . . ."

Browne realized too late that the phrenological alienists had overextended themselves in both their science and in their management. On the one hand, "benevolence and sympathy . . . unfortunately enhanced the employment of moral means, either to the exclusion or to the undue disparagement of physical means, of cure and alleviation." Confessing "to have aided at one time in this revolution," Browne felt that, in the light of what was then passing for moral management, his contribution "cannot be regarded in any better light than as treason to the principles of our profession."[142] On the other hand, Browne also saw that "the recognition of insanity as a bodily disease, while it conferred incalculable benefits upon the patient, contributed to divert the attention of the physician from the psychical side of the diagnosis."[143] Fittingly, Browne paid tribute to the late John Conolly as one who had been "a philosophical advocate—of a medico-psychology founded upon induction" and he praised Conolly's *Indications of Insanity* as a work showing a familiarity with the real laws of the human mind.[144] Only the historian can perhaps share with Browne the loss he was expressing; his audience would have had little idea of how much their present knowledge owed to the abandoned theory of "lumps and bumps" or how much of the theory had unfortunately been lost.

All this suggests that phrenology had actually made some positive contribution to the practice of psychiatry of the sort that can be measured by the historian's yardstick of "progress." With the exception of cranioscopy, however, this is difficult to quantify. Rather, as the *Lancet* perceived in its 1827 review of Spurzheim's treatise, it was to the "theory and argument" of insanity that phrenology's real contribution was to be found.[145] Its role had been to explain, simplify, systematize, and legitimate existing practices, rationalize familiar ideas, and hasten the emerging trends in psychiatry of the late eighteenth and early nineteenth centuries. The moral treatment was being practiced well before phrenology was popularized, and the search for the physical cause of insanity was at least as old as Democritus. The *Journal of Mental Science* was thus justified in asserting that in real terms phrenology had been little more than a "benevolent influence upon . . . the curative management of abnormal states of the brain and nervous system."[146] Yet phrenology had instilled confidence and optimism by allowing alienists to believe that their practices and pursuits could be justified through science in general and through cerebral physiology in particular. It was only later in the century, when phrenology as a science was invalidated, that critics came to realize that much of what the phrenologists had been saying could have been equally serviceable *without* the phrenology.[147]

Phrenology's place then in nineteenth-century psychiatry is perhaps best described as an agent that motivated and rationalized institutional arrangements and clinical procedures and provided a framework for and direction to its scientific evolution. Though Gall's original ideas were put to many uses by British alienists, they cannot be seen as constituting a single monolithic doctrine that became institutionalized in the accepted sense. It was rather as a free-ranging body of ideas based upon principles of broad application that phrenology was able to play a number of socially and medically legitimating roles (and often contradictory roles) at one time. In this form, phrenology's influence upon psychiatry can be seen in hindsight as important chiefly in relating function to structure; showing the importance of environment in causing and for curing insanity; stressing hereditary factors for protection against insanity and for the improvement of the race (in a pre-Darwinian context); forcing insanity to be seen as a disease of the brain and thus bringing psychiatry into the realm of general clinical medicine as well as reducing the amount of emotional involvement with patients whose conditions could now be seen as physically based; and, finally, in giving the first impetus to individual therapy prior to psychoanalysis. These were hardly trivial achievements even if later generations tended to ignore them and then to take up separate issue with them.

Nearly all the aspects of psychiatry/psychology with which phrenology was involved were later to be the centers of schisms and internecine conflicts that have continued to rage to the present day. To modern eyes it seems amazing that such contentious issues could ever have been bundled into one doctrine. It was only possible, of course, because of phrenology's simple yet totally comprehensive explanation of human behavior. The universality facilitated by the ease with which the doctrine could be understood and manipulated attracted it to a vast range of ideas and beliefs which in themselves had little need for Gall's doctrine but under the rational scientific umbrella it provided, appeared to be more soundly qualified and elucidated. It is this eclecticism of phrenology that explains its long period of influence. Hence the various unconnected strands of early nineteenth-century psychiatry and psychology achieve through phrenology an historical unity and coherence which they otherwise lack. Inevitably, this leaves phrenology—the unifying agent—characterized most by the tensions it contained. When the credibility of the doctrine was seriously damaged its function as a hook for suspending and connecting new ideas was no longer possible and what unity had been gained in psychiatry was quickly fragmented. Divergent opinions thereafter followed more independent paths, increasingly so as specialization and professionalization in psychiatry proliferated the number and the complexity of the issues to be dealt with. Never again would there be the wholesale incorporation of contemporary medical, social, scientific, and moral issues that phrenological psychiatry had managed tenuously to contain.

It is only through acknowledging this peculiar nature of the phrenological doctrine, by observing its scope, and by recognizing its protean ability to absorb new ideas and deal flexibly with them, that we can understand why its appeal was so extensive among alienists in early Victorian Britain. Not without reason did phrenologists proclaim their doctrine to be a "universal panacea." It is the breadth of the doctrine, too, that explains why, oxygenlike, phrenology was virtually consumed in the reaction it created: a pervasive doctrine in the first half of the century whose influence was often invisible and unacknowledged, its separate and definable place in psychiatry almost ceased to exist in the later decades of the nineteenth century. Because of this, phrenology has been largely neglected as a means of broadening our understanding of the development of psychiatry in the nineteenth century. Its role in psychiatry, like its roles in other facets of early Victorian science and society, was such as almost to erase those historically perceptible "later influences" upon which we most often rely for our investigations, in spite of our professed contempt for Whig history.

Notes

An earlier version of this essay was delivered to the Science Studies Unit, Edinburgh University, April 1975. I would like to thank the participants in that seminar for their helpful comments. The assistance of the following persons who read the paper over at various stages is gratefully acknowledged: R. M. Young, W. F. Bynum, John Forrester, Bill Luckin, and Geoffrey Cantor.

1. J. C. Prichard, "Temperaments," in *Cyclopaedia of Practical Medicine*, ed. John Forbes, Alexander Tweedie, and John Conolly (London: Piper, 1833–35), 4:167. Prichard was one of the few leading alienists of the period who was not attracted to phrenological views, largely because his research in natural history brought him to different conclusions than Gall's about the development of the brain in lower animals. He also saw, with greater clarity than most, that phrenology appealed because of the "ready explanation which it *seems to afford* of a greater number of phenomena in natural history and psychology." "Supplementary Note on Peculiar Configurations of the Skull Connected with Mental Derangement, with Observations on the Evidence of Phrenology, and Opinions Respecting the Functions of the Brain," in Prichard, *A Treatise on Insanity and Other Disorders Affecting the Mind* (London: Houlston, 1835), p. 464.

2. A. Walk, "Some Aspects of the 'Moral Treatment' of the Insane up to 1854," *Journal of Mental Science* 100 (1954): 807–37.

3. W. F. Bynum, "Rationales for Therapy in British Psychiatry: 1780–1835," Chapter 2 of this volume.

4. See David De Giustino, *The Conquest of Mind. Phrenology and Victorian Social Thought* (London: Croom Helm, 1975). It is a part of other work with which I am presently involved to show how phrenology served as a mediator for social, political, and moral ideas among the British middle and working classes. It is hoped that, ultimately, the conclusions from that material can be united with those on insanity presented here.

5. Robert M. Young, *Mind, Brain and Adaptation in the Nineteenth Century* (Oxford: Clarendon Press, 1970), p. 3.

6. K. M. Dallenbach, "The History and Derivation of the Word 'Function' as a Systematic Term in Psychology," *American Journal of Psychology* 26 (1915): 484 (italics in the original).

7. W. Cave Thomas, *The Limitation of Brain Power or, the Hygiene of Education. A Lecture to the Society for the Development of the Science of Education* (London: Co-operative Printing, 1878), p. 9.

8. E. H. Ackerknecht, *Medicine at the Paris Hospital 1794–1848* (Baltimore: Johns

Hopkins Press, 1967), p. 172. See also E. H. Ackerknecht and Henri V. Vallois, *Franz Joseph Gall, Inventor of Phrenology and His Collection,* trans. Claire St. Leon, Wisconsin Studies in Medical History (Madison: University of Wisconsin Press, 1956); and Owsei Temkin, "Gall and the Phrenological Movement," *Bulletin of the History of Medicine* 21 (1947): 275-321. None of these works pays attention to the practice of British psychiatry.

9. The term "alienist" is used throughout to signify "one engaged in the scientific study or treatment of mental disease," *Century Dictionary* (New York and London: Century, 1889), vol. 1. Along with "mental alienation," the designation was in common usage in the nineteenth century, and it is employed here as more historically appropriate and precise than the modern equivalent "psychiatrist."

10. [Review of] *Bibliothèque du médecin practicien,"Journal of Psychological Medicine* 2 (1849): 539.

11. J. Q. Rumball, *M'Naughten. A Letter to the Lord Chancellor, upon Insanity,* 2d ed. (London: J. Churchill, 1843), pp. iv–v. An advertisement for Rumball's private (and apparently unlicensed) asylum appears on the back page of his *On the Nature, Cause, and Cure of Asthma* (London: Tallant and Allen, 1857). On the phrenological interest in the M'Naughten case see also James George Davey, *Medicolegal Reflections on the Trial of Daniel M'Naughten* (London: Bailliere, 1843); [Thomas Tichborne], *On the Amendment of the Law of Lunacy. A Letter to Lord Brougham by a Phrenologist* (London: H. Renshaw, 1843); *Phrenological Journal* [hereafter cited as *PJ*] 16 (1843): 182–91; and *Zoist* 1 (1843): 397–405.

12. Major sources: *PJ; Zoist; Lancet;* Hewett C. Watson, *Statistics on Phrenology* (London: Longman, 1836); and Margaret C. Barnet, "Matthew Allen, M.D. (Aberdeen) 1783–1845," *Medical History* 9 (1965): 16–28. More specific references are given below.

13. Richard Hunter and Ida MacAlpine, "[Biographical] Introduction"; John Conolly, *An Inquiry Concerning the Indications of Insanity* (1830; reprint ed., London: Dawsons, 1964), p. 33. The Phrenological Association was founded at the time of the British Association meeting in Newcastle in 1835. Conolly's name appears on the committee as printed in *Zoist* 1 (1843): 220.

14. Watson, *Statistics,* n. 12 above, p. 165.

15. D. Alexander, *A Lecture on Phrenology, as Illustrative of the Moral and Intellectual Capacities of Man* (London: Baldwin, Cradock and Joy, 1826). Alexander was elected a corresponding member of the London Phrenological Society on 6 January 1827; the *PJ* noted his paper to the Leeds Philosophical and Literature Society, 2 December 1831, on "A Phrenological Analysis of the Theory of Dreams, Spectral Illusions, and Some of the More Usual Phenomena of Mental Derangement," and on 9 June 1832 his essay to the Glasgow Phrenological Society, *PJ* 7 (1831–32): 189–90, 479.

16. Barnet, "Matthew Allen," n. 12 above; Watson, *Statistics,* pp. 140–41, 144–46, 155; and Matthew Allen, *Essay on the Classification of the Insane* (London: John Taylor, [1837]), pp. viii–ix.

17. For examples of his remarkable success as a phrenology lecturer before and after his appointment at Montrose, see *PJ* 8 (1832–34): 571–72, 662–63; and 11 (1838): 214.

18. J. Scott, *Extracts from Lectures on Phrenology* (Gosport, privately printed, 1838);

on Wright see *New Monthly Magazine* 33 (1831): 28. Wright (M.D. Edinburgh) was appointed resident apothecary superintendent of Bethlem on 24 March 1819, formerly having held the post of apothecary. He was dismissed in 1830 after a long inquiry into his conduct, which included drunkenness. A tribute to Wright appears in *Sketches in Bedlam . . . by a Constant Observer* (London: Sherwood, Jones, 1823), pp. xxix–xxxi. I would like to thank the archivist of Bethlem, Patricia Allderidge, for her assistance in locating information on Wright.

19. See, for example, his essays in *PJ* 15 (1842): 336–40, 20 (1847): 147–56; *Zoist* 1 (1843): 111–19; *Lancet,* 19 March 1842, 1:850–52, 30 April 1842, 2:158–60; *Medical Times* 6 (1842): 291–93, 310–11; *Journal of Psychological Medicine* 6 (1859): 31–38, 10 (1864): 168–94, n.s. 1 (1875): 88–97, n.s. 2 (1876): 252–62, n.s. 5 (1879): 172–204; *British Medical Journal* 1 (1884): 420.

20. See *Journal of Psychological Medicine* 4 (1851): 392–407; n.s. 2 (1862): 12–37; there are many references to Rumball in the *People's Phrenological Journal* 1 (1843); the details of Spencer's delineation are given in Herbert Spencer, *An Autobiography* (London: Williams and Norgate, 1904), 1:200–201.

21. No comprehensive study has been made of the considerable influence of phrenology in American psychiatry. The subject receives partial attention in Eric T. Carlson, "The Influence of Phrenology on Early American Psychiatric Thought," *American Journal of Psychiatry* 115 (1958): 535–38; John D. Davies, "Phrenology and Insanity," in his *Phrenology Fad and Science. A Nineteenth Century American Crusade* (New Haven, Conn.: Yale University Press, 1955), pp. 89–97; Harold Schwartz, "Samuel Gridley Howe as Phrenologist," *American Historical Review* 57 (1951–52): 644–51; and in Norman Dain, *Concepts of Insanity in the United States, 1789–1865* (New Brunswick, N.J.: Rutgers University Press, 1964), pp. 61–63, 87–88. Of related importance see David Bakan, "The Influence of Phrenology on American Psychology," *Journal of the History of the Behavioral Sciences* 2 (1966): 200–20.

22. Mary Catherine Hume, *A Brief Sketch of the Life, Character, and Religious Opinions of Charles Augustus Tulk,* 2d ed. (London: John Speirs, 1890).

23. Walk, "Aspects," n. 2 above, p. 26*n.* This is the Mrs. Bowden (*née* Powell) praised alongside Tulk in John Conolly, *The Treatment of the Insane without Mechanical Restraints* (London: Smith, Elder, 1856), p. 274, and noted in Sir James Clark, *A Memoir of John Conolly, M.D.* (London: John Murray, 1869), p. 26. Another member of Hanwell's Committee of Management, who was also praised by Conolly, was Serjeant Adams, a member of the Phrenological Association.

24. Cited in George Combe, *The Life and Correspondence of Andrew Combe, M.D.* (Edinburgh: Maclachlan and Stewart, 1850), p. 277.

25. [Thomas Brown], "Viller, sur une nouvelle theorie de cerveau," *Edinburgh Review* 2 (1803): 147. For the earliest references to phrenology in British medical journals, see J. S. Streeter's letter to Samuel Solly, April 1847, in Solly, *The Human Brain,* 2d ed. (London: Longman, 1846), pp. xi–xiii.

26. "Dr. Gall's Lectures on the Physiology of the Brain," *Weekly Medico-Chirurgical & Philosophical Magazine,* 24 May to 23 August 1823, 1:241–369, 2:2–68 (serially).

27. Thomas Forster, "Observations on a New System of Phrenology, or the Anatomy and Physiology of the Brain, of Drs. Gall and Spurzheim," *Philosophical Magazine and Journal* 45 (1815): 44–50.

28. T. Forster, *Observations on the Casual and Periodical Influence of Particular States of the Atmosphere on Human Health and Disease, Particularly Insanity* (London: T. & J. Underwood and Baldwin, Cradock & Joy, 1817), pp. vi–vii. Shortly before leaving England in 1817, Spurzheim had been admitted a licentiate of the Royal College of Physicians, London. W. Munk, *Roll of the Royal College of Physicians, London* (London: Royal College of Physicians, 1878), 3:166–68.

29. "Spurzheim, Knight, and Morison on insanity," *Lancet*, 14 April 1827, 12:53–54; 21 April 84, 85. Cf. Andrew Combe, *Observations on Mental Derangement* (Edinburgh: John Anderson, 1831), p. 324, where it is also noted that Spurzheim appears to offer nothing new by way of treating the insane and that his work is best appreciated by those already familiar with phrenology.

30. London, Samuel Highley, p. 11.

31. J. Abernethy, *Reflections on Gall and Spurzheim's System of Physiognomy and Phrenology. Addressed to the Court of Assistants of the Royal College of Surgeons, in London, in June, 1821* (London: Longman, 1821), pp. 48–49, 7–9. The end-of-the-century phrenologist, Ambrose Lewis Vago, was convinced that this expression of Abernethy's did most to make phrenology medically respectable; thereafter, says Vago, "a surgery was considered to be incompletely furnished without such a bust; and a phrenological head was a regular item in the order for an outfit such as supplied to medical men by the firm of Messrs. Maw, Son, and Thompson, surgical instrument makers of London." *Phrenology Vindicated* (London: Simpkin, [1879]), p. 56. Much the same was repeated by the phrenologist Bernard Hollander, *In Search of the Soul* (London: Kegan Paul, [1920]), 1:345.

32. *Lancet*, 16 April 1825, 1:41. Between 1824 and 1851 the *Lancet* devoted over 600 pages exclusively to phrenology, including a full course of eighteen lectures by Spurzheim (April to September 1825) and a course of twenty lectures by François Broussais (June to September 1836).

33. It described phrenology in 1826 as "the most intelligible and self consistent system of mental philosophy that has ever yet been presented to the contemplation of inquisitive men." "Phrenology and Physiognomy," n.s. 5:437. See also, ibid., 4 (1817): 53–63, 117–34; n.s. 4 (1824): 847–82; n.s. 14 (1831): 321–22; n.s. 23 (1835): 361–70.

34. "Account of the Schools of Medicine in London, Session 1833–34," *Lancet*, 28 September 1833, 1:7. See also Dr. J. W. Crane, "State of Phrenology in Great Britain [with notes by the *Lancet* reporter]," *Lancet*, 22 June 1833, 2:407–8; and J. F. Clarke, *Autobiographical Recollections of the Medical Profession* (London: J. Churchill, 1874), pp. 125–26. The first person to deliver a course of lectures on phrenology to a British medical school (other than the lectures of Gall and Spurzheim) was Henry Haley Holm (1806–1846), Spurzheim's closest friend in London. Ironically, these lectures were begun on the day Spurzheim died, 10 November 1832. Obituary on Holm, *PJ* 19 (1846): 286–89.

35. It is worth noting that George Combe gave by request six lectures on insanity to Dr. Mackintosh's class of two hundred students in April 1832. Charles Gibbon, *The Life of George Combe* (London: Macmillan, 1878), 1:254–55.

36. James Johnson to George Combe in *Testimonials on Behalf of George Combe as a*

Candidate for the Chair of Logic in the University of Edinburgh (Edinburgh: John Anderson, 1836), p. 67.

37. For a full discussion of the phrenology debate in Edinburgh see G. N. Cantor and S. Shapin, "Phrenology in Early Nineteenth-century Edinburgh: An Historiographical Discussion," *Annals of Science* 32 (1975): 195–256. Dr. Shapin's contribution to the discussion ("Phrenological Knowledge and the Social Structure of Early Nineteenth Century Edinburgh," pp. 219–43) has been heavily relied upon for sharpening the focus in what follows. I am indebted to both authors for allowing me to make use of their scholarship prior to its publication.

38. For specific references to these better-known events in phrenology's history in Britain see Cantor and Shapin, ibid.; Temkin, "Gall," n. 8 above; de Giustino, *Conquest*, n. 4 above; and T. M. Parssinen, "Popular Science and Society: The Phrenology Movement in Early Victorian Britain," *Journal of Social History* 7 (1974): 1–20.

39. R. Merton, *Science, Technology and Society in Seventeenth Century England*, new ed. (New York: Howard Fertig, 1970).

40. According to the *PJ*, "one-third of the hundred writers on Phrenology [in Britain], and one-sixth of the thousand members of phrenological societies, are physicians or surgeons." *PJ* 2 (1838): 263.

41. Dain, *Concepts*, n. 21 above, p. 167.

42. Even Conolly felt upon first arriving at Hanwell that he had "severed myself from the ordinary ways and customs of men, and from the cheering influences of society." "Recollections of the Varieties of Insanity," *Medical Times and Gazette* 1 (1860): 9.

43. Ellis and Conolly, for example, both belonged to the Church of England, became apostate and then joined, respectively, the Methodists and the Unitarians. Hunter and MacAlpine, "Introduction,"n. 13 above, p. 11. The secular-tending sympathies of W. A. F. Browne, which were common among most phrenologists, may be observed in his *Observations on Religious Fanaticism; Illustrated by a Comparison of the Belief and Conduct of Noted Religious Enthusiasts with Those of Patients in the Montrose Lunatic Asylum* (Edinburgh, privately printed, 1835).

44. F. J. Gall, *On the Functions of the Brain and of Each of Its Parts*, trans. Winslow Lewis, Jr., Nahum Capen ed. (Boston: Phrenological Library, 1835) 1:54. Except where indicated all references are to this edition.

45. Such was Conolly's comment on his medical dissertation on mania and melancholia (Edinburgh, 1821), "Recollections," n. 42 above, p. 9.

46. "Phrenology," in G. H. Lewes, *Biographical History of Philosophy*, rev. ed. (London: Parker, 1857), p. 640, and "Psychology Finally Recognized as a Branch of Biology. The Phrenological Hypothesis," 3d ed. (newly titled) *The History of Philosophy from Thales to Comte* (London: Longmans, 1867), 2:410.

47. J. Haslam, *Medical Jurisprudence, as It Relates to Insanity, According to the Law of England* (London: Hunter, 1817), p. 62.

48. J. Haslam, *Observations on Madness and Melancholy*, 2d ed. (London, privately printed, 1809), pp. 237–38.

49. Dr. William Collin Engledue's remarks on metaphysics before Gall are typical of the more materialistic phrenological view: "crude indigestible masses of metaphysical speculation! What heaps of idle theories! What display of learned ignorance! . . . useless lumber!" *Zoist* 1 (1843): 6.

50. Alexander, *A Lecture on Phrenology*, n. 15 above, p. 2.

51. John Mackintosh, *Elements of Pathology, and Practice of Physic* (Edinburgh: Longman, 1830), 2:5.

52. "[Review of] Spurzheim on Education," *New Edinburgh Review* 1 (1821): 327. This journal was also edited by Richard Poole. It is interesting that the sharp distinction between the metaphysical and scientific stages of a discipline was developed by Comte, who drew heavily on phrenology for his conception of biology, psychology, and the components of knowledge.

53. P. Flourens, *Phrenology Examined*, trans. Charles de Lucene Meigs (Philadelphia: Hogan and Thompson, 1846), pp. 27–28, quoted in Young, *Mind*, n. 5 above, pp. 20–21.

54. James George Davey, *On the Nature, and Proximate Cause, of Insanity* (London: J. Churchill, 1853), p. 26*n*, quoting himself from a decade previous.

55. On the origin and antiquity of Gall's ideas see Madison Bentley, "The Psychological Antecedents of Phrenology," *Psychological Monographs* 21 (1916): 102–15; Edwin Clarke and C. D. O'Malley, *The Human Brain and Spinal Cord. A Historical Study Illustrated by Writings from Antiquity to the Twentieth Century* (Berkeley: University of California Press, 1968); Erna Lesky, "Structure and Function in Gall," *Bulletin of the History of Medicine* 44 (1970): 297–314; H. W. Magoun, "Development of Ideas Relating the Mind with the Brain," in C. Brooks and Paul Cranefield, eds., *The Historical Development of Physiological Thought* (New York: Hafner, 1959); Nicholas H. Steneck, "Albert the Great on the Classification and Localization of the Internal Senses," *Isis* 65 (1974): 193–211; A. Earl Walker, "The Development of the Concept of Cerebral Localization in the Nineteenth Century," *Bulletin of the History of Medicine* 31 (1957): 99–121. While opponents of phrenology took the doctrine's antiquity to argue against its novelty, phrenologists used it to show the doctrine's "respectable heritage." See "The Phrenology of the Middle Ages, to ed.," *Gentleman's Magazine* 103 (1833): 126–28; "Historical Notice of Early Opinions Regarding the Functions of the Brain," *PJ* 2 (1824–25): 378–91; and "Antiquity of Phrenology," *Lancet*, 5 August 1826, 10:599.

56. [Alexander Smith], "Phrenological Ethics," *Edinburgh Review* 74 (1842): 391.

57. Gall, *Functions*, n. 44 above, 2:224.

58. D. Noble, *The Brain and Its Physiology: A Critical Disquisition on the Methods of Determining the Relations Subsisting between the Structure and Functions of the Encephalon* (London: J. Churchill, 1846), pp. 123–24. Noble (1810–1885), F.R.C.S., F.R.C.P., was a leading Manchester physician, a member of the Provincial Medical Association Council, president of the Lancashire and Cheshire branch of the British Medical Association, and visiting physician to the Clifden Hall Retreat and Why House Lunatic Asylum, Buxton.

59. Mackintosh, *Elements*, n. 51 above, 2:4.

60. P. 207. A 6th ed. of this work in 1888, with David Ferrier as editor, still retained the praise for the reasonableness of phrenology.

61. I have presented here the four aspects of Gall's doctrine that were generally

considered in Britain as the most fundamental parts of his theory. It is worth recalling that Gall was not widely read in Britain and that Gall himself listed the four suppositions of his doctrine as "1. That moral and intellectual faculties are innate. 2. That their exercise or manifestation depends on organization. 3. That the brain is the organ of all the propensities, sentiments, and faculties. 4. That the brain is composed of as many particular organs as there are propensities, sentiments, and faculties, which differ essentially from each other." "Advertisement," *Functions,* n. 44 above, 1:55.

62. Craniology can be related, however, to the more general interest in physiognomy, a great many articles on which appear in the *Asylum Journal* (later the *Journal of Mental Science*). An interest in anthropology by many alienists was another path to craniology, as the anthropological and ethnological journals reveal. Conolly was an early member of the Ethnological Society in the 1840s and was president of the Society in 1855–1856. John Thurnam (1810–1873), joint author with Joseph Barnard Davies of the definitive and much acclaimed *Crania Britannica* (1856), was medical superintendent of the Wiltshire County Asylum from 1851 until his death and was twice the president of the Medico-Psychological Association. As the *Journal of Mental Science* was pleased to note in its review of the *Crania,* a "comparatively large number of names of medical officers connected with our English asylums are found in the list of *subscribers*" 10 (1864): 569–70.

63. See Gall, *Functions,* n. 44 above, 6:295–306, where his visit to the prisons of Berlin and Spandau are quoted from *Freymüthige,* May 1805; and [Richard Chenevix], "Gall and Spurzheim—Phrenology," *Foreign and Quarterly Review* 2 (1828): 12–14.

64. Solly, *Human Brain,* n. 25 above, p. 339. Solly's interest in phrenology was inspired by Spurzheim's demonstration of brain dissection at St. Thomas's Hospital in 1823 (ibid., pp. x–xi). Character readings from the cranium were, of course, double-edged: writing on "Insanity" in his *Dictionary of Practical Medicine* (London: Longman, 1858), 2:503*n*, James Copland noted that he had had his head examined by eminent phrenologists and (as was the case with John Stuart Mill) he was dissatisfied with the findings. The opposite result was much more common, however, and a clear case for its effects on an alienist can be seen through Pliny Earle's enthusiasm for phrenology after he had had his head examined by the American practical phrenologist, Lorenzo Fowler. See Madeline B. Stern, *Heads and Headlines, the Phrenological Fowlers* (Norman: University of Oklahoma Press, 1971), p. 42.

65. A photocopy of the letter and transcript appears in Richard Hunter and Ida MacAlpine, *Three Hundred Years of Psychiatry 1535–1860* (London: Oxford University Press, 1963), pp. 819–20.

66. W. Ellis, *A Treatise on the Nature, Symptoms, Causes, and Treatment of Insanity with Practical Observations on Lunatic Asylums and a Description of the Pauper Lunatic Asylum for the County of Middlesex at Hanwell with a Detailed Account of Its Management* (London: S. Holdsworth, 1838), p. 256; see also pp. 220–21.

67. J. G. Spurzheim, *Observations on the Deranged Manifestations of the Mind or Insanity* (London: Baldwin, Cradock and Joy, 1817), pp. 145–46; J. G. Spurzheim, *The Physiognomical System of Drs. Gall and Spurzheim* (London and Edinburgh: Baldwin, Cradock and Joy, 1815), p. 267. See F. J. Gall, "Influence of the Brain upon

Cranium in Mental Diseases," in *Functions*, n. 44 above, 3:55–59, and Combe, *Observations*, n. 29 above, pp. 104–6. See also John Elliotson, *The Principles and Practice of Medicine with Notes and Illustrations by Nathanial Rogers, M.D.* (London: Joseph Butler, 1839), p. 618. For the popularized view that specific forms of insanity may be judged with "wonderful accuracy" from the cranium, see Robert Macnish, *An Introduction to Phrenology, in the Form of Question and Answer*, 2d ed. (Glasgow, Edinburgh, and London: W. R. M'Phun, 1837), p. 202.

68. Mackintosh to George Combe, in *Testimonials*, n. 36 above, p. 53.

69. Harriet Martineau, "The Hanwell Lunatic Asylum," *Tait's Edinburgh Magazine* n.s. 1 (1834): 308. The same somewhat reluctant admission is made by A. M. [? Martineau], "Pauper Lunatic Asylum at Hanwell," *Athenaeum* 3 May 1834, p. 333.

70. *Transactions of the Provincial Medical and Surgical Journal* 3 (1835): 18.

71. Conolly to George Combe, Hanwell, 5 January 1846, printed in Appendix to Andrew Combe, *Phrenology—Its Nature and Uses: An Address to the Students of Anderson's University at the Opening of Dr. Weir's First Course of Lectures on Phrenology in That Institution Jan. 7, 1846* (Edinburgh: Maclachlan and Stewart, 1846), p. 32. There are also several letters from Conolly to George Combe in which he discusses his faith in cranioscopy in the Combe ms, National Library of Scotland.

72. "On the Characters of Insanity, a Lecture Delivered at the Royal Institution of Great Britain, Feb. 17th," *Asylum Journal* 1 (1854): 70. An illustration of Conolly practicing what he preached is recounted in Clarke, *Recollections*, n. 34 above, p. 202, where Conolly's delineation of Edward Oxford (for the case of *Oxford* v. *the Queen* is given. That Conolly's understanding of phrenology went deeper than the cranium is revealed in his *Inquiry Concerning the Indications of Insanity*, n. 13 above, p. 135n. See also Clark, *Memoir*, n. 23 above, pp. 66–75.

73. Testimonial to the practical value of phrenology, Alexander to Lord Glenelg, in *Documents Laid before the Right Honourable Lord Glenelg, by Sir George Mackenzie, Relative to the Convicts Sent to New South Wales* ([Edinburgh], privately printed, April 1836), p. 17.

74. Ibid., p. 14. The others were Ellis, Browne, A. Mackintosh, Alexander, H. A. Galbraith, D. Mackintosh, and Samuel Hare.

75. *What Asylums Were, Are, and Ought to Be: Five Lectures Delivered Before the Managers of the Montrose Royal Lunatic Asylum* (London and Edinburgh: Black, 1837), p. viii. The work was dedicated to Andrew Combe "as an acknowledgement of the benefits conferred on society by his exposition of the application of phrenology in the treatment of insanity and nervous diseases." In its lavish praise of the work, the *Lancet* thought the dedication most appropriate, 8 July 1837, 2:556.

76. M. Allen, *Cases of Insanity with Medical, Moral, and Philosophical Observations and Essays upon Them. Part I—Volume I* (London: George Swire, 1831) (the work was never concluded). See also Allen, *Essay*, n. 16 above. Both works are excellent examples of Allen's feigned erudition. In its otherwise damning review of the

Essay, the *British and Foreign Medical Review* noted, "We are bound to confess that the heads represented in the plates furnish very respectable phrenological testimony" (7 [1839]: 47).

77. *Journal of Mental Science* 17 (1871): 378.

78. D. Uwins, *A Treatise on Those Disorders of the Brain and Nervous System, Which are Usually Considered and Called Mental* (London: Renshaw and Rush, 1833), pp. 95–96. See also pp. 227–28; and D. Uwins, "Phrenology," *New Monthly Magazine* 34 (1832): 445–55.

79. A. Combe to Browne, 28 January 1837, quoted in Combe, *Life*, n. 24 above, pp. 280–81.

80. G. Andral, "Lecture on Medical Pathology, Delivered in the University of Paris 1833, VIII: Insanity Illustrated by Phrenology," *Lancet*, 16 February 1833, 1:653. Andral was one of the central figures of the Paris clinical school of the first half of the nineteenth century. He was also the first president of the Paris Phrenological Society (established in 1831) when Broussais was vice-president and the alienists Lelut, Fossiti, Foville, Voisin, and Vimont were among the members.

81. W. A. F. Browne to A. Combe, Crichton Institution, Dumfries, 3 January 1845, in Appendix to A. Combe, *Phrenology*, n. 71 above, p. 30. Andrew Combe made this point earlier in "Phrenology," *British and Foreign Medical Review* 9 (1840): 193.

82. "Prichard, Esquirol, Allen, Ellis, Ferrarese, Greco, Farr, Crowther, etc. On Insanity," ibid., 7 (1839): 14. The author (most likely Conolly or the coeditor, John Forbes) believed that the phrenologists could give a better account of certain cases than the antiphrenologists, "But upon that debateable ground we have no wish to enter."

83. Many persons undoubtedly shared the view of Arthur Ladbroke Wigan, that the science could be likened to the earlier position of alchemy: as the latter led to chemistry, "so will phrenology perhaps lead in time to a correct knowledge of the brain and the intellectual faculties." "Considerations on Phrenology," in Wigan, *A New View of Insanity. The Duality of the Mind Proved by the Structure, Functions, and Diseases of the Brain, and by the Phenomena of Mental Derangement, and Shewn to Be Essential to Moral Responsibility* (London: Longman, 1844), p. 159.

84. Guy, *Principles*, n. 60 above, p. 207.

85. The usual equation "moral" for "psychological" is not entirely satisfactory; a more accurate definition of Pinel's usage would be "moral" equals "emotions" and/or "passions." On this problem of definition see Kathleen M. Grange, "Pinel and Eighteenth-Century Psychiatry," *Bulletin of the History of Medicine* 35 (1961): 442–53.

86. See Eric T. Carlson and Norman Dain, "The Psychotherapy That Was Moral Treatment," *American Journal of Psychiatry* 117 (1960): 519.

87. "Rationales for Therapy in British Psychiatry: 1780–1835," chap. 2 of this volume.

88. Phrenologists were quite willing to admit to the antiquity of the ideas they claimed to simplify and systematize. See, for example, "[Rev. of] Benjamin Rush, *An Inquiry into the Influence of Physical Causes upon the Moral Faculty*," *PJ*

12 (1839): 276–78, and George Combe's "Introductory Notice" to Rush's work (Philadelphia: Haswell, 1839).

89. *Principles of Human Physiology* (London: J. Churchill, 1842), p. 226. The phrenological explanation of dreaming as mental organs individually activated was also a very attractive hypothesis. See Andrew Carmichael, "An Essay on Dreaming, Including Conjectures on the Proximate Cause of Sleep," *Philosophical Magazine and Journal* 54 (1819): 252–64, 324–35, and Robert Macnish, *The Philosophy of Sleep* (Glasgow: W. R. M'Phun, 1830).

90. In accordance with the earlier view of the mind as an indivisible whole, partial insanity could not theoretically exist. Lord Brougham advanced this view as late as 1849 to argue against the plea of partial insanity in criminal cases. Brougham, "On Partial Insanity," *Journal of Psychological Medicine* 2 (1849): 323–29. Spurzheim believed that Pinel's use of *melancholia* for partial insanity was entirely misleading, but it was left for Esquirol to coin the word *monomania* in a treatise of 1820. On Esquirol, see Richard Hunter and Ida MacAlpine, *Three Hundred Years of Psychiatry 1535–1860* (London: Oxford University Press, 1963), p. 732. Esquirol's insistence that the term implied no system or theory, but was simply an expression of a fact observed by physicians of all ages, suggests that he was thinking of Gall's theory when he chose the word. See "Homicidal Mania," *Journal of Psychological Medicine* 5 (1852): 420; see also *Oxford English Dictionary* on *monomania*.

It is also worth noting that from Condillac's views Pinel acknowledged the basis of what the phrenologists later reified and elaborated, viz., "that to consider the faculties of the mind separately, would equally contribute to facilitate the study of pneumatolygy [*sic*], as well as lead to very important knowledge, in regard to the nature and varieties of insanity." Pinel, *A Treatise on Insanity*, trans. D. D. Davis (reprint of 1806 trans. of the 1801 ed., New York: Hafner, 1962), p. 22.

91. "Dr. M. Newmann of Berlin, on insanity," *Medico-Chirurgical Review* n.s. 3 (1825): 233.

92. Sidney Smith, *The Principles of Phrenology*, 2d ed. (London: Kendrick, 1849), p. 35.

93. *On the Functions of the Brain and of Each of Its Parts*, trans. Winslow Lewis, Jr., ed. Nahum Capen (Boston: Phrenological Library, 1835), 2:284.

94. *Observations on Mental Derangement* (Edinburgh: John Anderson, 1831), p. 73.

95. *Sketch of Intellectual and Moral Relations* (London: Longman, 1829), p. 95. This type of criticism was further employed by antiphrenological pamphleteers; see, for example, John Wayte, *Anti-Phrenology or Observations to Prove the Fallacy of a Modern Doctrine of the Human Mind Called Phrenology* (Lynn Regis, printed for the author, 1829), p. 95.

96. *Man's Power* (London: William Pickering, 1843), p. 35. See also Combe, *Observations*, n. 10 above, pp. 116–17 and A. Combe to John Mackintosh in Mackintosh, *Elements of Pathology and Practice of Physic* (Edinburgh: Longman, 1830), 2:105.

97. Combe, *Observations*, n. 94 above, p. 354; see also William Ellis, *A Treatise on the Nature, Symptoms, Causes, and Treatment of Insanity* (London: S. Holdsworth, 1838), pp. 220–21.

98. *A Treatise on Those Disorders of the Brain and Nervous System, Which Are Usually Considered and Called Mental* (London: Renshaw and Rush, 1833), p. 99.

99. "Preface" to the [1844] and uncompleted edition of Gall, *On the Functions of the Brain* (London: G. Berger and W. Strange), p. i. For a laudatory account of W. A. F. Browne's management of the Crichton Royal Asylum by a non-phrenologist, see the observations by the Belgian, Dr. C. Crammelinck, as quoted in A. Walk, "Some Aspects of the 'Moral Treatment' of the Insane up to 1854," *Journal of Mental Science* 100 (1954): 832–33. Crammelinck believed that Browne's management at the Crichton Royal outshone all other British asylums and considered the York Retreat as falling far short in standard.

100. *PJ* 12 (1839): 109; Conolly, *The Treatment of the Insane Without Mechanical Restraints* (London: Smith, Elder, 1856), p. 187.

101. The Idéologue and friend of Pinel, Pierre Cabanis (1757–1802), was the first person to provide a theoretical explanation for the psychogenic or functional production of disease in a treatise of 1799. See Erwin H. Ackerknecht, *A Short History of Psychiatry*, trans. Sulammith Wolff (New York and London: Hafner, 1959), p. 33.

102. James C. L. Carson, *The Fundamental Principles of Phrenology Are the Only Principles Capable of Being Reconciled with the Immateriality and Immortality of the Soul* (London: Houlston, 1868), p. 33. See also J. G. Davey, "Phrenology and Insanity," *Medical Times* 6 (1842): 292.

103. Pinel, *Treatise*, n. 90 above, pp. 5, 110–11, 132–33, 221.

104. Roger Smith, "The Background of Physiological Psychology in Natural Philosophy," *History of Science* 11 (1973): 81.

105. "[Rev. of Francis] Willis [*A Treatise*] on Mental Derangement" 5 (1826): 152–53, 155. Other nonmedical journals also devoted space to criticizing exclusively moral regimens in asylums. An interesting example is provided by [William Newnham] in the Anglican *Christian Observer* 29 (1829): 266.

106. See E. H. Ackerknecht and Henri V. Vallois, *Franz Joseph Gall, Inventor of Phrenology and His Collection*, trans. Claire St. Leon, Wisconsin Studies in Medical History (Madison, Wisc.: University of Wisconsin Press, 1956); Owsei Temkin, "Gall and the Phrenological Movement," *Bulletin of the History of Medicine* 21 (1947): 275–321; Temkin, "Remarks on the Neurology of Gall and Spurzheim," in *Science, Medicine, and History*, ed. E. A. Underwood (London, New York, and Toronto: Oxford University Press, 1953), 2:282–89; Hunter and MacAlpine on Spurzheim, *Three Hundred Years*, n. 90 above, pp. 711–20; R. M. Young, "Gall and Phrenology," in his *Mind, Brain and Adaptation in the Nineteenth Century* (Oxford: Clarendon Press, 1970), pp. 9–53; Eric T. Carlson and Patricia S. Noel, "Origins of the Word 'Phrenology,'" *American Journal of Psychiatry* 127 (1970): 696; Carlson, "The Influence of Phrenology on Early American Psychiatric Thought," ibid. 115 (1958): 536.

107. *Observations on the Deranged Manifestations of the Mind or Insanity* (London: Baldwin, Cradock and Joy, 1817), p. 141. The assertion that the brain was an organic part was not uniquely phrenological; Gall and Spurzheim borrowed it from the Idéologues.

108. See pp. 68–72 of this chapter.

109. Daniel Noble, "An Essay on the Application of Phrenology to the Investigation of the Phenomena of Insanity," *PJ* 9 (1834–36): 448.
110. Charles E. Rosenberg, "The Bitter Fruit: Heredity, Disease, and Social Thought in Nineteenth-Century America," *Perspectives on American History* 8 (1974): 231.
111. See [Henry Crabb Robinson], *Some Account of Dr. Gall's New Theory of Physiognomy with the Critical Strictures of C. W. Hufeland, M.D.* (London: Longman, 1807), p. 69, and Alexander Morison, *Cases of Mental Disease with Practical Observations on the Medical Treatment. For the Use of Students* (London: Longman; and Edinburgh: Maclachan and Stewart, 1828), pp. 93–94.
112. Ellis, *Treatise*, n. 97 above, pp. 169–70.
113. Spurzheim, *Observations*, n. 107 above, p. 100.
114. Combe, *Observations*, n. 94 above, p. 77.
115. H. Martineau, "The Hanwell Lunatic Asylum," *Tait's Edinburgh Magazine* n.s. 1 (1834): 308.
116. Robert Macnish, *An Introduction to Phrenology, in the Form of Question and Answer*, 2d ed. (Glasgow, Edinburgh and London: W. R. M'Phun, 1837), p. 202.
117. "Westminster Medical Society," *Lancet*, 26 April 1828, 2:107. Other writers in opposition to the organic viewpoint are given in C. M. Burnett, *Insanity Tested by Science, and Shewn to Be a Disease Rarely Connected with Permanent Organic Lesion of the Brain. And on That Account Far More Susceptible of Cure Than Has Hitherto Been Supposed* (London: Samuel Highley, 1848).
118. Barlow, *Man's Power*, n. 96 above, pp. 48–49.
119. Combe, *Observations*, n. 94 above, p. 64. See also Hunter and MacAlpine on Andrew Combe, *Three Hundred Years*, n. 90 above, pp. 812–14.
120. *The Principles and Practice of Medicine with Notes and Illustrations by Nathanial Rogers, M.D.* (London: Joseph Butler, 1839), p. 626. See also William B. Neville, *On Insanity; Its Nature, Causes, and Cure* (London: Longman, 1836), pp. 119–20. Cf. Norman Dain, *Concepts of Insanity in the United States, 1789–1865* (New Brunswick, N.J.: Rutgers University Press, 1964), pp. 69–70.
121. *Lancet*, 26 April 1828, 2:107. Wright's postmortems were probably one of the reasons for his dismissal from Bethlem, for only the authorized surgeon was supposed to carry out such examinations. In November 1830 Wright was refused the key to the Bethlem dead house.
122. Ellis, *Treatise*, n. 97 above, p. 20. Like Combe, Ellis believed that diseased organization of the brain in recent cases was rare and in old cases almost invariable. Browne, *What Asylums Were, Are, and Ought to Be* (London and Edinburgh: Black, 1837), p. 6.
123. James George Davey, *On the Nature, and Proximate Cause, of Insanity* (London: J. Churchill, 1853), pp. 6, 36.
124. Macnish, *Introduction*, n. 116 above, p. 179. Lawrence did the dissections for Bethlem in the 1820s in his capacity as surgeon to the hospital.
125. Cf. David Rothman, *The Discovery of the Asylum: Social Order and Disorder in the New Republic* (Boston and Toronto: Little, Brown, 1971), p. 110; William Neville, *On Insanity*, n. 120 above, p. 134.
126. See Caleb Crowther, "Remarks on Phrenology," in his *Observations on the Management of Madhouses* (London: Simpkin and Marshall, 1838), pp. 114–15.
127. Beverley R. Morris, *A Theory as to the Proximate Cause of Insanity, Together with*

Some Observations upon the Remote Causes of the Disease (London: H. Renshaw; and York: Bellerby and Sampson, 1844), p. 5.

128. Alexander Hood, "Injuries to the Head or Brain Considered as the Cause of Impaired Corporeal and Intellectual Functions, Illustrated by Cases," *PJ* 2 (1824–25): 91.

129. Morison, *Cases*, n. III above, p. 3. The same point was raised in the review of *Bibliothèque du médecine practicien, Journal of Psychological Medicine* 2 (1849): 539.

130. Ellis, *Treatise*, n. 97 above, pp. 169–70.

131. W. L. Lindsay, *33rd Annual Report of the Directors of James Murray's Royal Asylum for Lunatics, near Perth* (Perth: C. G. Sidey, 1863), p. 47; on the lack of organic lesion, p. 21. C. Carter Blake called this report "one of the most trenchant and severe attacks on the tenets of phrenology which has ever appeared." (*Anthropological Review* 1 [1863]: 476.)

132. Henry Monro, "Note on Phrenology," in his *Remarks on Insanity: Its Nature and Treatment* (London: J. Churchill, 1851), pp. 145–50.

133. S. Solly, *The Human Brain*, 2d ed. (London: Longman, 1846), p. 339. According to Charles Gibbon, Noble's book was "to a great extent inspired by [George] Combe, and partly revised by him." *Life of George Combe* (London: Macmillan, 1878), 2:204.

134. *Elements . . . An Introduction to the Practical Study of Insanity, Adapted for Students and Junior Practitioners* (London: J. Churchill, 1853), pp. x–xi, 36–48.

135. See, for example, J. Davey, "G. Combe and His Writings. A Lecture Delivered at Bristol," *Journal of Mental Science* 10 (1864): 168–94.

136. See J. Sanbourne Bockoven, "Moral Treatment in American Psychiatry," *Journal of Nervous and Mental Diseases* 124 (1956): 198; Rosenberg, "Bitter Fruit," n. 110 above, p. 220.

137. "[Rev. of] *Practical Observations on Mental Diseases and Nervous Disorders*, by Alfred Beaumont Maddock," *Asylum Journal* 1 (1854): 77–78.

138. W. McDougal [*sic*], "The Nature of Functional Disease," *American Journal of Psychiatry* n.s. 1 (1922): 335–54.

139. Combe, *Observations*, n. 94 above, p. 360.

140. Frank Fish, "David Skae, M.D., F.R.C.S., Founder of the Edinburgh School of Psychiatry," *Medical History* 9 (1965): 36–53. Skae's attack on phrenology was replied to by George Combe, "Phrenology: Rejoinder to Dr. Skae," *Lancet* 2 (1847): 194–96, and by J. G. Davey, "Reminiscences of Lunacy Practice," *Journal of Psychological Medicine* n.s. 1 (1875): 205–6.

The same shift in psychiatric emphasis in France is seen in the single generation between the alienists Felix Voisin and his son Auguste. The father was one of the keenest propagators of phrenology in Europe; the son accepted his father's phrenological somatic pathology of the brain but on the basis of it rejected the sufficiency of the moral treatment his father had extolled. Auguste Voisin, *Leçons cliniques sur les maladies mentales professées à la Salpêtrière* (Paris, 1876), reviewed in *Journal of Mental Science* 22 (1876): 131. On Felix Voisin's work at the Bicêtre and at the Vanvres asylums see Gibbon, *Life*, n. 133 above, 2:257–58.

141. W. A. F. Browne, "The Moral Treatment of the Insane; a Lecture (Read before Professor Laycock's Class of Medical Psychology, at Their Visit to the Crichton Institution, Dumfries, July 9, 1864)," *Journal of Mental Science* 10 (1864): 311–12.

142. Ibid., p. 311.

143. "Address; on Medico-psychology," *Journal of Mental Science* 12 (1866): 312.

144. Ibid., p. 326.

145. "Spurzheim, Knight, and Morison on Insanity," *Lancet,* 14 April 1827, 12:53–54, 84–85.

146. Commenting on phrenology in "[Rev. of Joseph] Swan, *The Brain in Relation to the Mind,"Journal of Psychological Medicine* 8 (1855): 322. By 1925 alienists could state more bluntly, "Phrenology has done little to help us." Theo. B. Hyslop, *The Borderland, Some of the Problems of Insanity,* pop. ed. (London: Philip Allan, 1925), p. 289.

147. See, for example, "Dr. Davey's Mental Pathology," *Journal of Psychological Medicine* 3 (1850): 330–31.

A N D R E W   S C U L L

4 Moral Treatment Reconsidered: Some Sociological Comments on an Episode in the History of British Psychiatry

What most sharply distinguishes a propagandistic from an ideological presentation and interpretation of the facts is . . . that its falsification and mystification of the truth are always conscious and intentional. Ideology, on the other hand, is mere deception—in essence self-deception—never simply lies and deceit. It obscures truth in order not so much to mislead others as to maintain and increase the self-confidence of those who express and benefit from such deceptions.

Arnold Hauser

Tuke and Moral Treatment

We are all familiar with that traditional version of psychiatric history which celebrates it as a not always continuous, but ultimately triumphal, procession toward the rational and humane forms of treatment presently practiced. In such accounts, the introduction of moral treatment always occupies a central place of honor: the legendary decision by Pinel to strike the chains from the raving maniacs in the Bicêtre; and the less dramatic but equally significant endeavors of William Tuke to provide humane care for insane Quakers at the York Retreat. It is with moral treatment that I shall be concerned in this essay. I shall try to explicate some of the central dimensions of its English version, and to explore some of its broader social roots and significance. For I take it that one of the more important contributions that a sociologist can make to the history of psychiatry is to break down some of the parochialism that marks most treatments of the subject and to show some of its connections with larger social movements and processes.

This essay was originally published in *Psychological Medicine* (1979) and is reprinted by permission of Cambridge University Press.

One should note, of course, that even restricting our attention to England, Tuke's development of moral treatment was not an isolated achievement. A number of other practitioners in the "mad-business" were experimenting with essentially similar approaches by the end of the eighteenth century. John Ferriar of the Manchester Lunatic Asylum had become convinced that "the first salutary operation in the mind of a lunatic" lay in "creating a habit of self-restraint," a goal that might be reached by "the management of hope and apprehension, . . . small favours, the show of confidence, and apparent distinction," rather than by coercion.[1] And to cite just one other example, Edward Long Fox, from whose Bristol madhouse Tuke recruited Katherine Allen (the Retreat's first matron), independently developed a system of classification and mild management that allowed the elimination of most of the "barbarous" and "objectionable" features found in most contemporary asylums.[2] But it was Tuke's version of moral treatment that attracted attention, first from a stream of visitors, both English and foreign, and then from those parliamentarians and others who had taken up the cause of lunacy reform. So it is to his work that I wish to give most of my attention, while recognizing that it forms part of a much broader shift in the methods used to comprehend and cope with madness.

Traditional Approaches to Madness

From a number of perspectives, I think Tuke's admirers are quite right to stress that his approach marked a serious rupture with the past, rather than simply a refinement and improvement of existing techniques. They go astray, however, when they accept at face value the account that Tuke and his followers provide of their activities. The advent of moral treatment is both something more and something less than the "triumph of humanism and of therapy, a recognition that kindness, reason, and tactful manipulation were more effective in dealing with the inmates of asylums than were fear, brutal coercion and restraint, and medical therapy."[3] It will not do simply to assert that Tuke replaced immoral with moral therapy, or to attribute the reformers' achievements to their superior moral sensibilities, while consigning their opponents to the status of moral lepers, men devoid of common decency and humanity.

On the contrary, the perception that the traditional ways of coping with lunatics in madhouses (even such things as the use of whips and chains to maintain a semblance of order) were inherently cruel and inhumane is by no means as simple and self-evident a judgment as both the reformers and later generations came to believe. The practices of the eighteenth-century madhouse keepers seem so transparently callous and brutal that we tend to take this judgment as unproblematic, as immediately given to any and all who have occasion to view such actions. But cruelty, like deviance, "is not a quality which lies in behaviour itself, but in the interaction between the person who commits an act and those who respond to it."[4] Consequently, whether or not a set of practices is perceived as inhumane depends, in large part, on the world view of the person who is doing the perceiving. Practices from which we now recoil in horror were once advocated by the most eminent physicians and cultured men of their day. That madmen were chained and whipped in asylums in the eighteenth century was well known at the time. How could it be otherwise when, throughout the century, the doors of Bethlem were open to the public, and the inmates exhibited before the impertinent curiosity of sightseers at a mere penny a time, and when every treatise on the management of the mad advocated such treatment? Certainly, such practices were not something of which magistrates only became aware at the turn of the century. Yet it was only then that protests began to be heard that such treatment was cruel and inhumane.

To be sure, some of the treatment meted out to lunatics in private madhouses was the natural product of an unregulated free market in madness—the consequence of the unchecked cupidity of the least scrupulous, of the incentives to half starve and neglect pauper inmates, of the temptation to rely on force as the least troublesome form of control. But there is more to it than that. Even in situations where such factors were obviously inapplicable, lunatics were treated in ways which later generations were to condemn as barbaric and counter-productive—in ways which they (and we) find virtually incomprehensible and almost by default attribute to an underdeveloped moral sensibility, if not outright inhumanity.

The treatment of George III during his recurrent bouts of "mania" perhaps makes this point most dramatically and unambiguously. No doubt Francis Willis, who was charged with treating the king, earnestly sought the monarch's recovery. But to modern eyes, he went about the task in a distinctly peculiar fashion. In the words of the Countess Harcourt, "The unhappy patient . . . was no longer treated as a human being. His body was immediately encased in a machine which left no liberty of motion. He was sometimes chained to a stake. He was frequently beaten and starved, and at best he was kept in subjection by menacing and violent language."[5]

Willis's approach was scarcely atypical. The eighteenth-century "trade in lunacy"[6] attracted a motley crew; but despite the heterogeneity of those engaged in the business, certain traditional approaches and techniques were widely employed—by medical and nonmedical men alike. As with the king, intimidation, threats, and outright coercion were commonly used to cow and subdue the madman, whose condition was viewed as "a display of fury and violence to be subdued and conquered by stripes, chains, and lowering treatments."[7] Most madhouse keepers operated on the assumption that "fear [was] the most effectual principle by which to reduce the insane to orderly conduct,"[8] on the grounds that it was "a passion that diminishes excitement . . . particularly the angry and irascible excitement of maniacs." As eminent a man as William Cullen argued that it was "necessary to employ a very constant impression of fear . . . awe and dread"—emotions which should be aroused by "all restraints that may occasionally be proper . . . even by stripes and blows."[9] Together with a more elaborate and sophisticated intellectual rationalization of these procedures, medicine simply provided its practitioners with a wider variety of tools for "coercing patients into straight thinking and accepting reason . . . : vomits, purges, . . . surprize baths, copious bleedings and meagre diets."[10]

Within a few years of the Retreat's practices obtaining national attention, such treatment (or at least its open avowal) had come to seem unthinkable. The fundamental basis of this whole approach—the subjugation of the madman, the breaking of his will by means of external discipline and constraint, the almost literal battle between reason and unreason—had lost its former appearance of self-evidence and was now seen as wholly inappropriate. I would suggest that a necessary condition for the emergence of such a changed perspective (and of the moral outrage which did so much to animate the lunacy reformers' activities) was a change in the cultural meaning of madness. And I think that such a change can be shown to have occurred.

If, in seventeenth- and eighteenth-century practice, the madman in confinement was treated no better than a beast, that merely reflected his ontological status. For that was precisely what, according to the prevailing paradigm of insanity, he was. One of the most notable features of the pre-nineteenth-century literature on madness is

> its almost exclusive emphasis on disturbances of the *reason*, or the higher intellectual faculties of man. Insanity was conceived as a derangement of those very faculties which were widely assumed to be unique to man; as a matter of fact, we sometimes find in the literature the presumed absence in animals of any condition analogous to insanity taken as proof that man's highest psychological function results from some principle totally lacking in other animals, that is, the soul.[11]

But this was to imply that in losing his reason, the essence of his humanity, the madman had lost his claim to be treated as a human being.

Intellectually, such notions did no violence to the dominant world view of the period. Indeed, they could be viewed as a confirmation of perhaps its critical organizing principle—the idea of the continuity and gradation of nature in what Arthur Lovejoy[12] has termed "the Great Chain of Being." The very idea of a chain, with no discontinuities or gaps, implied that no rigid barriers existed between one part of creation and another, that there always existed intermediate forms. The division between apes and men was a permeable, not an absolute, one in eighteenth-century conceptions of nature—an assumption which was exemplified in a number of different ways: in the denial of the concept of common humanity to the slave; the ready identification of apes and savages (even extending to speculation on fertile copulation between blacks and apes); the portrayal of criminals in animalistic terms; and the assimilation of the mad to the ranks of brute creation. As Bynum puts it, such notions were "built into the analytic tools with which eighteenth-century Europeans classified man."[13] And in the case of lunatics, the apparent insensitivity of the maniac to heat or cold, hunger or pain, his refusal to abide clothing, and so forth were simply taken as confirmation of the correctness of the basic explanatory schema.

If a sociologist may be permitted to cite literary evidence in support of his case, it may be noted that Ophelia, in her madness, is described as,

Divided from herself and her fair judgment,
Without which we are pictures [i.e., no more than
external facsimiles of human beings] or mere beasts.[14]

In a similar vein, Pascal informs us, "I can easily conceive of a man without hands, feet, head (for it is only experience which teaches us that the head is more necessary than the feet). But I cannot conceive of a man without thought; that would be a stone or a brute."[15] "Expert" opinion concurs. John Monro,[16] the physician to Bethlem from 1751 to 1791 and one of the two most eminent mad-doctors of the mid-eighteenth century, speaks of madness as involving "a total suspension of every rational faculty"; just as Andrew Snape, almost half a century earlier, had lamented "those unhappy People, who are bereft of the dearest Light, the Light of Reason." In a revealing passage, Snape then goes on to say, "Distraction . . . divests the rational Soul of all its noble and distinguishing Endowments, and sinks unhappy Man below the mute and senseless Part of Creation: even brutal Instinct being a surer and safer guide than disturb'd Reason, and every tame Species of Animals more sociable and less hurtful than humanity thus unmann'd."[17]

Eminent mad-doctors of the early nineteenth century continued to adhere to this position, arguing that "if the possession of reason be the proud attribute of man, its diseases must be ranked among our greatest afflictions, since they sink us from our preeminence to a level with the animal creatures."[18]

I suggest that the resort to fear, force, and coercion is a tactic entirely appropriate to the management of "brutes." Thus, when we look at the treatment of the insane prior to "reform," we must realize, as Foucault points out, that

> the negative fact that the madman is not treated like a "human being" has a very positive meaning. . . . For classicism, madness in its ultimate form is man in immediate relation to his animality. The day would come when from an evolutionary perspective this presence of animal-ity in madness would be considered as the sign—indeed the very essence—of disease. In the classical period, on the contrary, it manifes-ted the very fact that *the madman was not a sick man.* Animality, in fact, protected the lunatic from whatever might be fragile, precarious, or sickly in man. . . . Unchained animality could be mastered only by *discipline* and *brutalizing.* [19]

The Rupture with the Past

It was this world view that the nineteenth-century reformers and, indeed, society as a whole were in the process of abandoning. Much of the reform-ers' revulsion on being exposed to conditions in contemporary madhouses derived from this changed perspective. For them, the lunatic was no longer an animal, stripped of all remnants of humanity.[20] On the contrary, he remained in essence a man, a man lacking in self-restraint and order, but a man for all that. Moreover, the qualities which he lacked might and must be restored to him, so that he could once more function as a sober, rational citizen.

The beliefs which lie at the heart of the new approach to the insane —Tuke's moral treatment, as well as the less well-known equivalents de-veloped by his contemporaries—differ so profoundly from those underly-ing traditional practices as to lend some credence to Michel Foucault's notion of a *rupture épistémologique.* At the core of the eighteenth-century approach, as we have seen, was its view that the essence of madness was the absence, or the total perversion, of reason. "In the new system of moral treatment," by contrast, "madmen are not held to be absolutely deprived of their reason."[21] Tuke's whole system crucially depends upon "treating the patient as much in the manner of a rational being as the state of his mind will possibly allow"—a change so striking that it attracted much contemporary comment. In Sydney Smith's words, "It does not appear to them that because a man is mad upon one subject, that he is to be consid-ered in a state of complete mental degradation, or insensible to feelings of gratitude."[22]

The emphasis on the lunatic's sensitivity to many of the same induce-ments and emotions as other people was associated, whether as cause or consequence, with other equally profound alterations in his treatment.

What was seen as perhaps the most striking, both at the time and subsequently, was the emphasis on minimizing external, physical coercion—an emphasis which has had much to do with the interpretation of moral treatment as unproblematically kind and humane. William Cullen articulated the eighteenth-century consensus when he contended that

> restraining the anger and violence of madmen is always necessary for preventing their hurting themselves or others; but this restraint is also to be considered as a remedy. Angry passions are always rendered more violent by the indulgence of the impetuous notions they produce; and even in madmen, the feeling of restraint will sometimes prevent the efforts which their passion would otherwise occasion. Restraint, therefore, is useful and ought to be complete.[23]

Tuke's dissent from this position was sharp and unequivocal: "Neither chains nor corporal punishment are tolerated, on any pretext, in this establishment."[24] Less objectionable forms of restraint might be necessary to prevent bodily injury, but they ought to be a last resort, and must never be imposed solely for the convenience of the attendants. As a routine policy, those running an asylum ought "to endeavour to govern rather by the influence of esteem than of severity." The insistence upon "the superior efficacy . . . of a mild system of treatment," together with the elimination of "gyves, chains, and manacles"[25] had a profound effect on contemporary reformers, who saw Tuke's success at the Retreat as proof that the insane could be managed without what were now seen as harshness and cruelty.

This was no kindness for kindness' sake. From its architecture to its domestic arrangements, the Retreat was designed to encourage the individual's own efforts to reassert his powers of self-control. For instead of merely resting content with the outward control of those who were no longer quite human (which had been the dominant concern of traditional responses to the mad), moral treatment actively sought to *transform* the lunatic, to remodel him into something approximating the bourgeois ideal of the rational individual. From this viewpoint, the problem with external coercion was that it could force outward conformity, but never the necessary internalization of moral standards. The change in aim mandated a change in means. Granted, "it takes less trouble to fetter by means of cords, than by assiduities of sympathy or affection."[26] But "the natural tendency of such treatment is, to degrade the mind of the patient, and to make him indifferent to those moral feelings, which, under judicious direction and encouragement, are found capable, in no small degree, to strengthen the power of self-restraint."[27] On purely *instrumental* grounds, then, "tenderness is better than torture, kindness more effectual than constraint. . . . Nothing has a more favourable and controlling influence over one who is

disposed to or actually affected with melancholy or mania, than an exhibition of friendship or philanthropy."[28] Only thus could one hope to reedu-
cate the patient to discipline himself. By acting as though "patients are
considered capable of rational and honourable inducement," and by making use of the vital weapon of man's *desire for esteem* (which even lunatics
were now seen as sharing), inmates could be induced to collaborate in their
own recapture by the forces of reason. "When properly cultivated," the
desire to look well in others' eyes "leads many to struggle to conceal and
overcome their morbid propensities: and, at least, materially assists them
in confining their deviations within such bounds, as do not make them
obnoxious to the family."[29]

The staff played a vital role in this process of reeducation: they must
"treat the patients on the fundamental principles of . . . kindness and
consideration." Again, this was not because these were goods in themselves, but because "whatever tends to promote the happiness of the patient, is found to increase his desire to restrain himself, by exciting the
wish not to forfeit his enjoyments; and lessening the irritation of mind
which too frequently accompanies mental derangement. . . . The comfort
of the patients is therefore considered of the highest importance in a
curative point of view."[30]

Here, too, lay the value of work, the other major cornerstone of moral
treatment, since "of all the modes by which patients may be induced to
restraint themselves, regular employment is perhaps the most generally
efficacious."[31]

By all reasonable standards, the Retreat was an outstandingly successful experiment. It had demonstrated, to the reformers' satisfaction at least,
that the supposedly continuous danger and frenzy to be anticipated from
maniacs were the consequence of rather than the occasion for harsh and
misguided methods of management and restraint; indeed, that this reputation was in large part the self-serving creation of the madhouse keepers.
It apparently showed that the asylum could provide a comfortable and
forgiving environment, where those who could not cope with the world
could find respite, and where, in a familial atmosphere, they might be
spared the neglect that would otherwise have been their lot. Perhaps even
more impressive than this was the fact that, despite a conservative outlook
which classified as cured no one who had to be readmitted to an asylum,
the statistics collected during the Retreat's first fifteen years of operation
seemed to show that moral treatment could restore a large proportion of
cases to sanity.

The Social Roots of the New Approach

But if one must grant the importance of the changing conceptions of
insanity and its appropriate treatment as an intervening cause in the rise

of the lunacy reform movement, one must also recognize that ideas and conceptions of human nature do not change in a vacuum. They arise from a concrete basis in actual social relations. Put slightly differently, the ways men look at the world are conditioned by their activity in it. The question which we must therefore address—albeit briefly and somewhat speculatively—is what changes in the conditions of social existence prompted the changes we have just examined.

In a society still dominated by subsistence forms of agriculture, nature rather than man is the source of activity. Just as man's role in actively remaking the world is underdeveloped and scarcely perceived—favoring theological and supernatural rather than anthropocentric accounts of the physical and social environment—so too the possibilities for transforming man himself go largely unrecognized and the techniques for doing so remain strikingly primitive. In a world not humanly but divinely authored, "to attempt reform was not only to change men, but even more awesome, to change a universe responding to and reflecting God's will" —to embark on a course akin to sacrilege.[32] And where the rationalizing impact of the marketplace is still weak, structures of domination tend to remain *extensive* rather than intensive—that is, the quality and character of the work force are taken as a given rather than as plastic and amenable to improvement through appropriate management and training.

But under the rationalization forced by competition, man's *active* role in the process presents itself ever more insistently to people's consciousness. This development is further accelerated by the rise of manufacturing —a form of human activity in which nature is relegated simply to a source of raw materials, to be worked on and transformed via active *human* intervention. More than that, economic competition and the factory system are the forcing house for a thoroughgoing transformation in the relation of man to man. For industrial capitalism demands "a reform of 'character' on the part of every single workman, since their previous character did not fit the new industrial system."[33] Entrepreneurs concerned to "make such machines of men as cannot err"[34] soon discover that physical threat and economic coercion will not suffice: men have to be taught to *internalize* the new attitudes and responses, to discipline themselves. Moreover, force under capitalism becomes an anachronism (perhaps even an anathema) save as a last resort. For one of the central achievements of the new economic system, one of its major advantages as a system of domination, is that it brings forth "a peculiar and mystifying . . . form of compulsion to labour for another that is purely economic and 'objective.' "[35]

The insistence on the importance of the internalization of norms, the conception of how this was to be done, and even the nature of the norms which were to be internalized—in all these respects we can now see how the emerging attitude toward the insane paralleled contemporaneous shifts in the treatment of the normal and other deviant elements of the population. It coincides with and forms part of what Peter Gay has dubbed "the recovery of nerve"[36]—a growing and quite novel sense that man was the master of his destiny and not the helpless victim of fate; and it has obvious links with the rise of "the materialist doctrine that people are the product of circumstance."[37] "Is it not evident," asked James Burgh (and certainly it *was* to an ever-larger circle of his contemporaries), "that by management the human species may be moulded into any conceivable shape?"[38] The implication was that one might "organize the empirical world in such a way that man develops an experience of and assumes a habit of that which is truly human."[39]

This faith in the capacity for human improvement through social and environmental manipulation was translated in a variety of settings—factories, schools, prisons, asylums—into the development of a whole array of temporally coincident and structurally similar techniques of social discipline.[40] Originating among the upper and middle classes, for example, there emerged the notion that the education and upbringing of children ought no longer to consist in "the suppression of evil, or the breaking of the will."[41] With the growth of economic opportunity and social mobility, the old system of beating and intimidating the child to compel compliance came to be viewed as a blunt and unserviceable technique, for it badly prepared one's offspring for the pressures of the marketplace. The child needed to be taught to be "his own slave driver," and with this end in view, "developing the child's sense of emulation and shame" was to be preferred to "physical punishment or chastisement."[42] John Locke, the theoretician of these changes, said,

> Beating is the worst, and therefore the last Means to be used in the Correction of Children. . . . The *Rewards* and *Punishments*, . . . whereby we should keep Children in order *are* of quite another kind. . . . *Esteem* and *Disgrace* are, of all others, the most powerful Incentives to the Mind, when it is once brought to relish them. If you can once get into Children a Love of Credit and an Apprehension of Shame and Disgrace, you have put into them the true principle.[43]

The essential continuity of approach is equally manifest in the methods and assumptions of the early nineteenth-century prison reformers. Crime had been seen as the product of innate and immemorial wickedness and sin. Now, however, the criminal was reassimilated to the ranks of a common humanity. As Fine puts it, "The prisoner was to be treated as a person, *who possessed a reason in common with all other persons,* in contrast to animals and objects. However hardened the prisoner was, beneath the surface of his or her criminality an irreducible reason still remained."[44] In consequence, as lunatics were for Tuke, they were "defective mechanisms" that could be "remoulded" through their confinement in a peni-

tentiary designed as "a machine for the social production of guilt."[45] And
for such purposes (again the parallel with moral treatment is clear) prison
reformers plainly perceived that "gentle discipline is more efficacious than
severity."[46]

The new practices, which had their origins in the wider transformation of English society, were shared, developed further, and given a somewhat different theoretical articulation in the context of the lunatic asylum.
As in the wider world, so too in the lunatic asylum: one could no longer
be content with the old emphasis on an externally imposed and alien order,
which ensured that madness was controlled, yet which could never produce self-restraint. Control must come from within, which meant that
physical violence, now dysfunctional, became abhorrent.[47] The realization
of the power that was latent in the ability to manipulate the environment
and of the possibility of radically transforming the individual's "nature"
was translated in the context of madness into a wholly new stress on the
importance of cure. It represents a major structural support of the new
ethic of rehabilitation. As the market made the individual "responsible"
for his success or failure, so the environment in the lunatic asylum was
designed to create a synthetic link between action and consequences, such
that the madman could not escape the recognition that he alone was responsible for the punishment which he received. The insane were to be
restored to reason by a system of rewards and punishment not essentially
different from those used to teach a young child to obey the dictates of
"civilized" morality. Just as the peasantry who formed the new industrial
work force were to be taught the "rational" self-interest essential if the
market system were to work, the lunatics, too, were to be made over in the
image of bourgeois rationality: defective human mechanisms were to be
repaired so that they could once more compete in the marketplace. And
finally, just as hard work and self-discipline were the keys to the success
of the urban bourgeoisie, from whose ranks Tuke came, so his moral
treatment propounded these same qualities as the means of reclaiming the
insane.

Notes

A version of this essay was originally presented at a symposium on "History and Mental Disorder" under the auspices of the Wellcome Trust, April 1978.

1. John Ferriar, *Medical Histories and Reflections,* 3 vols. (London: Cadell and Davies, 1795), 2:111–12.
2. Edward Long Fox, *Brislington House, an Asylum for Lunatics, Situate Near Bristol* (Bristol: for the author, 1806).
3. William Bynum, "Rationales for Therapy in British Psychiatry, 1780–1835," chap. 2 of this volume.
4. Howard S. Becker, *Outsiders: Studies in the Sociology of Deviance* (Glencoe, Ill.: Free Press, 1963), p. 14.
5. Cited in Bynum, "Rationales for Therapy."
6. William Parry-Jones, *The Trade in Lunacy* (London: Routledge and Kegan Paul, 1972).
7. Richard A. Hunter and Ida MacAlpine, *Three Hundred Years of Psychiatry* (London: Oxford University Press, 1963), p. 475.
8. Samuel Tuke, Manuscript memorandum of a visit to St. Luke's Hospital, reprinted in Daniel Hack Tuke, *Chapters in the History of the Insane in the British Isles* (London: Kegan Paul and Trench, 1882).
9. William Cullen, *First Lines in the Practice of Physic,* 4th ed., 4 vols. (Edinburgh: Elliot, 1808), cited in Hunter and MacAlpine, *Three Hundred Years,* p. 478. Where such physical force was deemed necessary, he cautioned that stripes, "although having the appearance of more severity, are much safer than strokes or blows about the head."
10. Hunter and MacAlpine, *Three Hundred Years,* p. 475.
11. Bynum, chap. 2 of this volume.
12. Arthur O. Lovejoy, *The Great Chain of Being* (New York: Harper and Row, 1960).
13. William Bynum, "Time's Noblest Offspring: The Problem of Man in the British Natural Historical Sciences" (Ph.D. diss., University of Cambridge, 1974), p. 344.
14. William Shakespeare, *Hamlet,* act 4, sc. 5.
15. B. Pascal, *Oeuvres Complètes* (Paris: Gallimard, 1954), p. 1156.
16. John Monro, *Remarks on Dr. Battie's Treatise on Madness* (London: Clarke, 1758).
17. Andrew Snape, *A Sermon Preached Before the Lord Mayor, the Aldermen, Sheriffs, and Gouvenors of the City of London, April 16, 1718* (London: Bowyer, 1718). Elsewhere, he speaks of madmen who, with their "apish Gestures," prove that

"something with a Human Shape and Voice may for many years survive all that was human besides."

18. J. M. Cox, *Practical Observations on Insanity*, 3d ed. (London: Baldwin and Murray, 1813), p. ix.

19. Michel Foucault, *Madness and Civilization* (New York: Mentor Books, 1965), pp. 66, 69.

20. Compare John Reid's complaint that in "either the public, or the minor and more clandestine Bethlems, . . . such a mode of management is used with men, as ought not to be, although it too generally is, applied even to brutes." *Essays on Hypochondriasis and Other Nervous Affections*, 3d ed. (London: Longman, 1823), pp. 304–5.

21. G. de la Rive, *Lettre Addressée aux Redacteurs de la Bibliothèque Britannique* (Geneva: for the author, 1798).

22. Sydney Smith, "An Account of the York Retreat," *Edinburgh Review* 23 (1814): 189–98.

23. Cullen, *First Lines*, cited in Hunter and MacAlpine, *Three Hundred Years*, p. 478.

24. Samuel Tuke, *Description of the Retreat* (York: Alexander, 1813), p. 141.

25. Ibid., pp. vi, 171.

26. Reid, *Essays*, p. 303.

27. Tuke, *Description*, pp. 159–60.

28. Reid, *Essays*, pp. 303–4.

29. Tuke, *Description*, p. 157.

30. Ibid., p. 177.

31. Ibid., p. 156.

32. H. Soloman, *Public Welfare, Science, and Propaganda in Seventeenth Century France* (Princeton: Princeton University Press, 1972), pp. 29–30.

33. Sidney Pollard, *The Genesis of Modern Management* (Harmondsworth, Middlesex: Penguin, 1965), p. 297.

34. Josiah Wedgwood, cited in Neil McKendrick, "Josiah Wedgwood and Factory Discipline," *Historical Journal* 4 (1961): 46.

35. Maurice Dobb, *Studies in the Development of Capitalism* (New York: International Publishers, 1963), p. 7.

36. Peter Gay, *The Enlightenment: An Interpretation*, vol. 2 (New York: Knopf, 1969).

37. B. Fine, "Objectification and the Bourgeois Contradictions of Consciousness," *Economy and Society* 6 (1977): 431.

38. J. Burgh, *Political Disquisitions*, 3 vols. (London: Dilly, 1775), 3:176.

39. Helvetius, quoted in Fine, "Objectifications," p. 431.

40. Michael Ignatieff, "Prison and Factory Discipline 1770–1800: The Origins of an Idea" (Paper presented at the annual meeting of the American Historical Association, Boston, 1976); Foucault, *Madness and Civilization;* idem, *Discipline and Punish* (London: Allen Lane, 1977).

41. J. H. Plumb, "The New World of Children in Eighteenth Century England," *Past and Present* 67 (1975): 69.

42. Ibid., pp. 67, 69.

43. John Locke, *Educational Writings* (London: Cambridge University Press, 1968). Note the stress on putting them *into* children. Locke's educational doctrines

acquired an ever greater popularity among the upper and middle classes in the latter half of the eighteenth century. J. H. Plumb draws attention to the fact that "by 1780 John Browne could make one of the principal virtues of the expensive academy for gentlemen's sons that he proposed to set up a total absence of corporal punishment" (Plumb, "Children"). (Interestingly, one of William Tuke's early philanthropic endeavors, prior to setting up the York Retreat, had been the establishment of Ackworth, a school for girls.) Seen in the context of these slightly earlier changes, Tuke's comment that "there is much analogy between the judicious treatment of children and that of insane persons" takes on a new significance. In practice, the analogy was to extend even further. When Locke's doctrines (and their intellectual descendants) were modified to accommodate the children of the poor, they spawned the rigidities of the monitorial system: Andrew Bell's "steam engine of the moral world," and Joseph Lancaster's "new and mechanical system of education." When the techniques of the small, upper-class Retreat were adapted to the "requirements" of the mass of pauper lunatics, moral treatment was transformed into a set of management techniques for a custodial holding operation.

44. Fine, "Objectification," p. 429.
45. Michael Ignatieff, *A Just Measure of Pain: Penitentiaries in the Industrial Revolution in England* (New York: Pantheon, 1978).
46. John Howard, *The State of the Prisons* (Warrington, Lancashire: for the author, 1778), p. 8.
47. Compare Michel Foucault's comment on the attractions of the Panopticon to the bourgeoisie: "It is not necessary to use force to constrain the convict to good behaviour, the madman to calm, the worker to work, the schoolboy to application, the patient to the observation of the regulations . . . no more bars, no more chains, no more heavy locks" (Foucault, *Discipline and Punish,* p. 202).

PART TWO
Institutions and the Inmate Experience

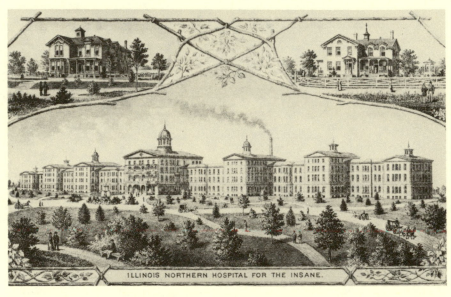

ILLINOIS NORTHERN HOSPITAL FOR THE INSANE.

Illinois Northern Hospital for the Insane

Engravings like these characteristically adorned the annual reports of lunatic asylums on both sides of the Atlantic. The Illinois Northern Hospital for the Insane opened in 1872 and was initially designed for some 300 patients. Like most state hospitals of the period, it was built in a modified version of Thomas Story Kirkbride's linear plan.

(Source: *Annual Report of the Illinois Northern Hospital for the Insane*, reproduced in George A. Tucker, *Lunacy in Many Lands* [Birmingham ? 1885].)

NANCY J. TOMES

5 A Generous Confidence: Thomas Story Kirkbride's Philosophy of Asylum Construction and Management

In 1855, John Galt, a Virginia asylum doctor, criticized his colleagues in the richer hospitals of the North for their preoccupation with asylum construction. As long as "those entrusted with the supervision of the insane, and particularly those at the head of the most richly endowed asylums, shall deem the true interests of their afflicted charge(s) not to consist in aught on their part but tinkering gas-pipes and studying architecture, in order merely to erect costly and at the same time most unsightly edifices ... so long may we anticipate no advancement in the treatment of insanity as far as the United States is concerned," Galt wrote.[1] Historians have echoed this evaluation of early psychiatry's concern with asylum construction and management by dismissing the hospital superintendents' lengthy discussions of ventilation, bathroom fixtures, and window screens as misguided detours from the mental hospital's true purpose, the study and treatment of mental disease. Unlike many issues broached by the early profession which are still of contemporary concern, such as the etiology of mental disorders, the public provision for the poor and criminally insane, and the legal problems surrounding the commitment process, the asylum superintendents' avid interest in the more mundane details of their work has suggested to modern observers a narrowness of perspective. In studying psychiatry's historical development, the literature of asylum construction and management has received only perfunctory and often deprecatory consideration from historians.[2]

While sharing in the low estimation of the superintendents' professional priorities, David Rothman has given the most serious attention to their concern with asylum design and administration. In his book, *The Discovery of the Asylum*, Rothman argues that nineteenth-century reformers believed that institutional forms had "clear and important applications to

121

the wider society." At a time when traditional methods of social control seemed to be failing, they looked to "moral architecture," the science of producing "great moral changes" through appropriate design, as a means to restore social stability. Rothman sees the asylum superintendents' concern with hospital planning as part of this movement. They believed that the asylum, by embodying regularity, discipline, and precision, would serve as a model for the reordering of society. In this fashion, Rothman explains the superintendents' preoccupation with asylum construction and management as a response to and remedy for social disorder.[3]

Rothman correctly perceives a link between the superintendents' concern with asylum design and the larger role in society they envisioned for the institutions they headed. Yet in viewing this concern solely as a response to social disorder, Rothman has misinterpreted the source of the asylum doctors' preoccupation with institutional forms. The error is rooted in Rothman's misconception of early psychiatry's status. Rather than the powerful, indeed monolithic, authorities the doctors appear to be in *The Discovery of the Asylum,* the first generation of asylum doctors were *moral entrepreneurs* struggling to establish their own legitimacy.[4] The precarious situation of their emerging specialty provided a much more concrete cause for anxiety than the state of the social order. Consequently, they devoted their best efforts not to the rehabilitation of society but to the legitimation of the asylum and their position within it.

To argue that the superintendents, by their attention to asylum construction and management, strove to build a strong institutional base for their specialty is hardly original. In *Mental Institutions in America,* Gerald Grob has demonstrated that asylum doctors used their hospital affiliation to advance claims for power and authority over others interested in social policy toward the insane. He sees the superintendents' preoccupation with asylum design and management as unifying (as well as isolating) them in their professional battles with neurologists and lay reformers.[5] Yet the exigencies of professionalization, as described by Grob, do not explain fully the asylum's importance for the superintendents, for he neglects the most immediate objects of their professional exertions: the families and friends of the insane. Before asylum doctors could consider rival doctors or reformers, this segment of the public had to be convinced of the asylum's virtues. Without the financial and moral support of the families and friends of patients, the doctors' claims to expertise would have been meaningless. To understand the establishment of psychiatric legitimacy in the early nineteenth century, then, the emphasis on the asylum must be seen as a response to the public as well as to professional competitors.

From this perspective, the priority given to asylum construction and management by the early superintendents becomes much more comprehensible. The asylum in the early nineteenth century was not an established feature of the social landscape. Its advocates had to convince the public that insanity was a curable disease, best treated in a mental hospital. In the campaign to promote the asylum and the medical specialty associated with it, asylum construction and management played a key role. The hospital's unique appearance and regimen offered proof to the families of the afflicted that these doctors were making use of a radical new treatment for a dreaded ailment. In distinguishing themselves from competitors, the asylum was by far the most impressive item in the superintendents' therapeutic armamentarium. The mental hospital served as their professional showcase, their most effective public advertisement. Therefore, the asylum's success, as measured by its impressive appearance and orderly administration, mattered vitally to their enterprise.

The need to establish legitimacy through asylum design concerned the superintendents of private hospitals more than their colleagues in state institutions. Unlike public asylums, where securing enough patients was never a critical issue, the success of a private establishment depended directly upon its ability to attract a well-paying clientele that required superior accommodations and an impressive regimen. John Galt's bitter remarks about "tinkering gas-pipes and studying architecture" expressed a sentiment shared by other superintendents, that some asylum matters frequently discussed by the heads of "richly endowed" institutions had little relevance to public hospitals. The attention given to asylum construction and management in the superintendents' meetings and publications may have reflected the dominance of private asylum doctors in shaping the profession's agenda of concerns, rather than a real consensus within the specialty on the importance of hospital design.

While the preoccupations of private asylum doctors may have in part determined the direction of professional activity, the avid interest many state-hospital superintendents showed in asylum matters belies so simple an explanation for early psychiatry's concern with institutional forms. The state superintendents' interest sprang from problems of procuring public support, problems which were similar in kind if not degree to those encountered by their counterparts in private institutions. Many public asylums took in a percentage of paying patients, sometimes as much as one-half the total, whose board rates made a crucial difference to the institution's financial stability. In addition, paying patients were often of a class and mental condition that made them desirable inmates in the superintendents' estimation. To secure such patronage, state asylums had to have the same persuasive assets as a private institution. Furthermore, heads of public hospitals had to win the financial support of local officials and state legislators, who judged the asylum by its appearance and good order. With the almshouse and jail as inexpensive alternatives, the state hospital had to project a strong image of its own in order to obtain needed appropriations. Thus the problem of legitimacy affected both state and private hospital superintendents, albeit in different degrees.[6]

The profession's investment in asylum construction and organization as a means to establish its legitimacy with potential patrons, whether family members or state legislators, can nowhere be illustrated better than in the career and writings of Thomas Story Kirkbride. As one of the thirteen founders of the Association of Medical Superintendents of American Asylums for the Insane (now the American Psychiatric Association), which was formed in 1844, Kirkbride played a leading role in the profession until his death in 1883. After eleven years of service as its secretary and treasurer, Kirkbride served the association as president from 1862 to 1870, the longest term accorded to any superintendent of his generation. Never the intellectual match of his fellow superintendents Isaac Ray or Pliny Earle, Kirkbride's considerable reputation rested squarely on his expertise in asylum practice. For over forty years, he headed one of the most prestigious private hospitals in the country, the Pennsylvania Hospital for the Insane. Through his writings on asylum construction, Kirkbride's influence extended far beyond his own hospital. His book, *On the Construction, Organization and General Arrangements of Hospitals for the Insane*, remained the standard text on the subject for thirty years. State mental hospitals all over the country were built according to the "Kirkbride plan" that it detailed. More than any other superintendent, Kirkbride's prestige reflected early psychiatry's respect for excellence in asylum construction and management.

Kirkbride's professional concerns reveal his conviction that the "moral architecture" and moral order of the new hospital were the most powerful means he possessed to summon up belief in the new asylum treatment. His reputation as a healer of mental disease depended almost entirely on his ability to inspire confidence in his most persuasive asset, the hospital. To this end, Kirkbride sought to control every aspect of the hospital environment. Every detail, from the design of the window frames to the table settings in the ward dining rooms, had to be arranged to sustain the impression that here was an institution where patients received kind and competent care. Kirkbride believed that after one visit to his carefully managed institution, his patrons could not fail "to see that neither labor nor expense is spared to promote the happiness of the patients"; consequently, they would be led "to have a generous confidence in those to whose care their friends have been entrusted and readiness to give a steady support to a liberal course of treatment."[7]

In developing this "generous confidence," Kirkbride showed a keen awareness of the needs and attitudes of that segment of the public most important to his undertaking as head of a private asylum: the family and friends of patients. During his treatment of the insane over several years, he had developed a thorough understanding of their motives and reservations in seeking asylum treatment.[8] Kirkbride's desire to win their support shaped both his therapeutic conception of the asylum and the methods he used to sustain that conception through proper design and management. Therefore, the significance of Kirkbride's concern with institutional forms cannot be understood without first examining the therapeutic image he wished to project for the asylum.

Kirkbride clearly delineated this therapeutic image for his patrons in his *Annual Reports*. Although written for several audiences, including the asylum's managers, his professional brethren, and potential contributors, Kirkbride's *Reports* functioned primarily as brochures designed to attract and inform readers who might be considering asylum treatment for an insane relative or friend.[9] He received frequent requests for copies from both prospective patrons and patients' families, and composed his discussions of insanity and its treatment with them in mind. Reserving issues of any complexity for professional journals, Kirkbride aimed his *Reports* at "those interested in knowing the character of our hospitals, and desirous of learning something of the general principles of treatment now adopted." In this audience, he particularly wanted to reach the kind of intelligent but uninformed people he frequently encountered among his patients' families. The relatives of the insane often came to him, he wrote, "for counsel, with feelings of depression and utter hopelessness, far beyond what are commonly connected with the occurrence of any ordinary malady." He observed that "while prepared to make every sacrifice to secure the restoration of the patient, before doing so, they [the relatives] very properly desired some explanation of the nature of the disease, the chances of a recovery, and the reasons for plans of treatment so different from what are commonly adopted in the management of ordinary sickness." In his *Annual Reports*, Kirkbride provided general answers to all these questions, and attempted to overcome, point by point, the most common reservations about hospital treatment.[10]

In format, the *Annual Reports of the Pennsylvania Hospital for the Insane* covered the same topics every year: the cause and nature of insanity, improvements to the building and grounds, amusements, restraint, classification, care of the chronic insane, a short financial statement, and statistical tables describing the patient population. From Kirkbride's repetitive discussions of these topics emerge a clearly articulated set of beliefs and attitudes. The asylum image he sought to project in these discussions bears closer inspection, since it formed the rationale for his philosophy of asylum construction and design.

The *Annual Reports* regularly included elementary information about the nature of insanity. Kirkbride defined insanity simply as a "functional disease of the brain," but offered no detailed discussion of its pathology, preferring instead to elaborate on the proper attitude to be taken toward the disease. Couched in soothing, nonjudgmental tones, his explanations presented insanity as a disease which might affect anyone. "Insanity is truly the great leveler of all the artificial distinctions of society," he frequently told his readers. He minimized the sufferer's personal responsibility for the disease, characterizing it as "an accident . . . to which we are all liable, and especially, if without any direct agency of our own, or certainly without anything on our part that was dishonorable or criminal . . . no reproach to anyone." (Note the use of the inclusive pronoun.) While "prudence and a good constitution" might ward off mental disease successfully, even respectable, morally irreproachable people might be stricken with it; "it is found among the purest and the best of all dwellers upon earth, as well as those who are far from being models of excellence," he wrote. Kirkbride also denied that heredity played a major role in most mental disease. Feeling that medical and lay thinking accorded too much importance to hereditary propensities, he urged the families of the insane not to scrutinize anxiously all their relatives for signs of some ancestral taint.[11]

Kirkbride seemed particularly concerned to present insanity as a disease which did not spare the educated or wealthy. Although he rarely made special reference to his patients on the free list, he frequently mentioned the number of "persons of cultivated and refined minds" in the hospital. He cautioned his readers that "high social position, exalted intellectual endowment, (and) the most abundant wealth" did not guarantee an individual against insanity. On the contrary, he explained, some forms of mental disease particularly affected the better classes. For example, the neglect of physical exercise by many "studious men and women, and . . . others with different sedentary occupations," often led to a variety of "nervous affections." He concluded that a "high state of civilization, with all its benefits, is . . . likely to bring in its train a host of ailments . . . serious and distressing in their character." Kirkbride thus implied to his readers that the more cultured an individual, the more vulnerable he or she would be to mental disease. He also gave them the impression that the hospital was patronized by the "best sort" of people, thereby making it more acceptable to both the wealthy and their less fortunate neighbors.[12]

Having reassured prospective patrons that insanity did not necessarily result from wrongdoing, and affected the most "civilized" classes, Kirkbride still had to provide an explanation for its onset. People needed to make sense of the unexpected and often disruptive mental illness of a friend or relation. Therefore, he frequently enumerated what he believed to be the principal causes of insanity: ill health (which he said accounted for the majority of cases); loss of property; unemployment; grief; intense application to study or business; disappointed expectations; "mental anxiety" (such as nursing the sick); intemperance; and masturbation.[13] Again, with the exception of the last two, none of these explanations for the disease implied any reproach to the patient or family. Within such a broad framework, insanity could be accounted for in relatively comprehensive terms; few individuals would not have experienced at least one of these stresses before developing the mental disturbance, thus providing all concerned with a convenient explanation for its onset.

The most difficult and demanding portion of Kirkbride's arguments sought to convince the family that the mental patient must be treated in the hospital rather than in the home. Kirkbride acknowledged that most families found the decision to commit a relative very difficult. He continually tried to allay their anxiety and sense of guilt by providing arguments to justify the action as well as refute the objections he knew "misguided friends" would make. First, Kirkbride assured his readers that home treatment never benefited the insane, however kind and competent their care. "All the devotion of the tenderest friendship and everything that wealth can furnish," he told them, "are often powerless to afford relief." Without ever implying that the family situation itself might be exacerbating the patient's symptoms, he stated that "simple removal from familiar scenes and associations, with changed habits of life, is often, of itself, sufficient to modify favorably the diseased manifestations." While acknowledging the prevalent belief that "the friends of the insane are disposed unnecessarily to remove them from home and place them in institutions," he insisted that the opposite was, in fact, true; families usually waited too long to commit a patient to the asylum, thus missing the opportunity to arrest the disease in its early stages. Kirkbride also refuted the notion that families acted frequently from improper motives in committing relatives. Although he acknowledged the widely held belief that people sent family members to asylums in order to steal their fortunes or obstruct their happiness, Kirkbride insisted that "as far as my knowledge extends, nothing of the kind has ever been attempted here."[14] Absolved of accusations of undue haste or selfish considerations, his readers could begin to consider hospital treatment seriously.

Having attempted to persuade his prospective patrons that hospital treatment for insanity represented the family's wisest, most benevolent course, Kirkbride discussed the prognosis of the disease. The reward for prompt action, he assured them, might very well be a complete recovery. His experience had shown that eighty percent of all recent cases of insanity recovered in the asylum. The longer the disease had been established, the longer a cure might take; cases of long-standing often proved incurable, he cautioned. For recent and chronic cases alike, Kirkbride alerted his prospective patrons that the patient's hospital stay might be a long one. The family must possess "a determination to persevere in the treatment when once commenced, even under what seems to be the most discouraging circumstances." He condemned any "vacillating course of treatment" which might weaken the patient's cooperation with the hospital regimen. "Let no temporary discouragement, no suggestions of officious friends, no histories of wonderful recoveries by marvelous appliances, no importunities from the patients themselves," he warned, "lead to the suspension of a course deliberately adopted, till after a fair and full trial."[15]

Kirkbride's remarks on the chronic insane also made clear to his audience that should a relative's disease prove incurable, he or she would still receive kind and competent care. His *Annual Reports* continually presented the presence of the chronic cases as an asset to the institution; anyone familiar with the wards, he would aver, knew that chronic cases were among the most intelligent and agreeable persons in the asylum, exercising a "beneficial influence" on all their fellow patients. As long as they could "conduct with propriety," they had all the privileges of the institution. Yet Kirkbride did not advise removing them from the asylum. No case was absolutely incurable, he argued; seemingly chronic cases did recover after years of treatment. If the patient was removed uncured, he or she might quickly deteriorate without the hospital's influence, and again become a burden to the family. Thus Kirkbride encouraged those families with incurably ill relatives to give them a trial at the hospital, and let them remain, even when the case looked hopeless.[16] Although few chronic cases may have exercised the "beneficial influence" Kirkbride claimed for them, he obviously wanted to make the incurable patient's situation appear as attractive as possible to his audience.

Yet Kirkbride could not leave prospective patrons with the impression that recent and chronic cases lived side by side in the hospital. He knew that many families' objections to institutional care arose from their fear that in the hospital "all classes of invalids are mingled together." They had to be convinced that "a thorough separation of the different classes of patients might be effected." Kirkbride's regular discussions of classification provided reassurance to each family that their relative would not have a room next door to a shrieking, filthy lunatic. He explained to his readers that he assigned patients to the wards on the basis of mental condition and "social traits"; in other words, both the degree of the patient's disorder and class affiliation were taken into account. Wealth alone would not entitle a disagreeable or "repulsive" patient to a room on the best ward, he stated. Kirkbride developed several analogies to explain hospital classification in a convincing manner. The hospital, he often said, resembled "a community made up of distinct and congenial families." Each ward resembled a family, "select in itself." While thus enjoying the benefits of properly selected acquaintances, a patient was not obliged to associate with undesirable individuals outside the ward. Like families of different status living on a city block, he explained, "in walking along the streets, it is their own fault, if their attention is directed especially to what is unpleasant rather than to the agreeable sights that are constantly before them."[17]

Kirkbride had another understandable prejudice to overcome: many people could not see the benefit to be obtained by gathering all the insane into one institution, when it seemed only logical that they would make each other worse. He insisted that this was not the case. Patients had such varied symptoms that no process of emulation or imitation took place. Instead, they helped one another to recognize their own delusions. "Every one who has been much about institutions for the insane," Kirkbride wrote, "will acknowledge that certain patients are constantly exercising the most beneficial influence on others." Again, as in his characterization of chronic cases, Kirkbride emphasized the salutary effect certain patients had on others. He mentioned, for example, the increasing number of voluntary admissions, who as "intelligent, sympathizing" patients led others "to take views of their own cases which had not before occurred to them." He assured his readers that a "real interest in the troubles and sorrows" of fellow patients often became an individual's "best means of getting rid of [his] own."[18]

Yet this beneficial patient interaction did not extend to relations with the opposite sex. Kirkbride felt that no benefits and many disadvantages resulted from the mingling of the sexes at social events, having decided from early experiments with such gatherings that they exercised a poor influence on both patients and attendants. He characterized as "among the sacred things confided" to him as the hospital's chief physician, the duty to see that patients "be prevented from forming while there, any acquaintances . . . with the opposite sex, that would be unpleasant to their friends, and after recovery, no less so to themselves." The only "true mode of securing to the male patients, the humanizing influence of female society" he concluded, was to have as female attendants, "ladies of suitable age and character with cultivated minds and attractive manners."[19]

Kirkbride presented the patients' accommodations in the most attractive terms. He well understood the importance of first impressions in securing a patient's confidence and willingness to submit to the hospital regimen, and continually worked to give the buildings "a pleasant and cheerful" character. To this end he regarded "all the aids of external improvements, a certain degree of architectural embellishment, spacious halls, large and well-furnished parlors, and comfortable chambers" as among the "legitimate objects" of his expenditures. Each *Report* invariably included some pleasant description of the building or the pleasure grounds surrounding it, which Kirkbride continually characterized as "highly cultivated and improved." One early *Report,* for example, lovingly detailed the ornamental trees, shrubs, flower borders, and walks surrounding the hospital. "These walks," Kirkbride elaborated, "have been so located as to embrace our finest and most diversified views, to wind through the woods and clumps of trees which are scattered through the enclosure."[20]

Having sketched in the hospital's comfortable accommodations, Kirkbride reassured his prospective patrons that the patients were kept amused constantly. Every *Report* included a list of their entertainments, which grew longer and longer each year. Outdoor exercise and games, excursions to the city, teas and dinner parties, church services, all were detailed in such a way that the reader would have difficulty imagining a patient ever bored or unoccupied. One memorable year, Kirkbride listed over fifty different activities that were available to the patients, ranging from light gymnastics to "fancywork." The centerpiece of the hospital's offerings was its celebrated lecture series and magic-lantern displays, given by a succession of assistant physicians. By reading over the list of topics covered in the series, including discussions and scenes of foreign countries, demonstrations in natural science, and illustrations of new inventions like the telegraph or steam engine, families would be convinced that hospital treatment included the equivalent of a lyceum series.[21]

Kirkbride gave an equally encouraging impression of the constant attention patients received from their attendants. The readers learned of the high standards he used in selecting these members of his staff, who, as he pointed out, spent the most time with the patients. The perfect attendant, according to Kirkbride, possessed "a pleasant expression of face, gentleness of tone, speech and manner, a fair amount of mental cultivation, imperturbable good temper, patience under the most trying provocations, coolness and courage in times of danger, cheerfulness without frivolity, industry, activity, and fertility of resources in unexpected emergencies." Such an individual would be "able to act as the guide and counsellor and friend of all the patients in their varying conditions." Despite their excellent personal qualities, he acknowledged that the regular attendants were not of a class that could be expected to engage the intellectual and artistic interests of the more cultivated patients. To fill this need, the patients enjoyed the services of companions or teachers, "intelligent and educated individuals with courteous manners, and refined feelings, genuine Christians" who encouraged reading, music, and handiwork in the wards. Never hinting that he might have difficulty hiring attendants or companions of such saintly virtue, Kirkbride left his audience with the impression that the hospital's attendants conformed to the high standards he set for them.[22]

Kirkbride insisted that his attendants used only kindness and persuasion in controlling the patients, and repeatedly expressed in the *Reports* his aversion to any form of physical restraint. He warned prospective patrons that he could not dispense with it altogether, however, for at times patients became violent with others, or tried to harm themselves. To ensure that restraint was used only when all other methods had failed, Kirkbride told his readers that he kept the restraining apparatus in his office, and always supervised its use himself. He wrote, "I do not approve of a great variety of apparatus being kept in the wards of a hospital." The constant presence of the "strong chairs, muffs and other fixtures of the kind" has an "unpleasant influence" on both the patients and their attendants. Kirkbride felt that the free use of restraint encouraged the attendants to "think of their own ease, rather than the welfare of the patients." This tendency was not to be countenanced in his hospital.[23]

Through his discussions of such topics as restraint, classification, and attendants, Kirkbride projected a reassuring set of beliefs about insanity and hospital treatment, which helped families and friends make sense of the disease and encouraged their patronage of the hospital. Kirkbride had to do more than simply convince them of these truths through the *Annual Reports*, however. The asylum itself had to confirm his arguments whenever family members came to commit a patient, or returned later to visit. By comparing the hospital image created in his *Reports* with his professional writings on asylum construction and management, it is possible to see how Kirkbride's professional priorities were shaped by his desire to impress and reassure his lay patrons. From the perspective of his lay clientele, his attention to particular aspects of the hospital's appearance and function take on a new significance. One can begin to see how he worked to have the building's design and organization reinforce his patrons' beliefs about the hospital, and eliminate certain realities of institutional life that might undermine such confidence.

Kirkbride's concern with asylum construction began literally from the ground up, with the choice of a good site. He advised that the hospital be located outside a city of some size, easily accessible by train and good roads. Such a location would ensure plentiful supplies and employees, as well as varied excursions for the patients. The hospital itself, he instructed, should be in a secluded area, to provide the patients with ample privacy. The soil had to be tilled easily, so that the farm and gardens would produce food for the patients' table, and the area around the hospital itself could be improved extensively. "The surrounding scenery should be of a varied and attractive kind, and the neighborhood should possess numerous objects of an agreeable and interesting character," he wrote. The building itself should be placed so that the views from every window, especially the parlors and rooms occupied during the day, had pleasant prospects and "exhibit life in its active forms." The choice of a good site thus determined some of the hospital's most desirable features for its patrons: its accessibility, its attractiveness, and its supply of fresh food.[24]

The style of the building had to be considered carefully. "Although

it is not desirable to have an elaborate or costly style of architecture,"
Kirkbride wrote, "it is, nevertheless, really important that the building
should be in good taste, and that it should impress favorably not only the
patients, but their friends and others who may visit it." Any resemblance
to a prison had to be carefully avoided. "The means of effecting the proper
degree of security should be masked," he advised, and the building's custodial appearance camouflaged by ornamenting its grounds with gardens,
fountains, and summer houses. These external improvements cost considerable money, Kirkbride acknowledged, but played such an important role
in convincing patients and their families to support the institution that
they could not be neglected. Every detail made a difference, he warned, for
"no one can tell how important all these may prove in the treatment of
patients, nor what good effects may result from first impressions thus made
upon an invalid on reaching a hospital."[25]

The good impression made by the building's exterior arrangements
had to be sustained by the appearance and practicality of its interior. "No
desire to make a beautiful and picturesque exterior should ever be allowed
to interfere with the internal arrangements," Kirkbride wrote. The building had to sustain the cheerfulness of its exterior. As he advised one asylum
superintendent, "Have your parlors and rooms large and airy, with high
ceilings, your corridors wide," and the overall impression of the building
will be sustained.[26]

The "linear" or "Kirkbride" plan incorporated several fundamental
prerequisites of a good building design. It had wings radiating off the
center section (see Figure 1) so that each ward had proper ventilation and
an unobstructed view of the grounds. By leaving open spaces at the end
of each wing, "the darkest, most cheerless and worst ventilated parts" of
the hospital could be eliminated, Kirkbride explained. He also advised
inserting bay windows in the long halls, so that more light and air could
enter. By not having the wings close together, there was "less opportunity
for patients on opposite sides seeing or calling to each other, and less
probability of the quiet patients being disturbed by those who are noisy."[27]

The linear plan also allowed for the maximum separation of the
wards, so that the undesirable mingling of the patients might be prevented.
Male and female patients had separate wings. Within the wings, each ward
had its own staircase, so that the patients might proceed directly outside
to the pleasure grounds or to the center building without marching
through another ward. Eight wards, the minimum Kirkbride felt desirable, could be established in each wing. He advised that the worst patients
be confined in the ground-floor wards that are farthest from the center
building, the best patients in the top-floor wards, closer to the center. "A
classification that admits of no greater mingling of patients than this,"
Kirkbride concluded, "is quite rigid for all practical purposes."[28]

PLATE IV.

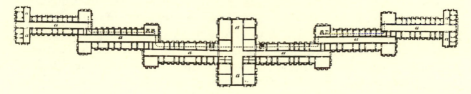

PLAN OF CELLAR.

PLATE V.

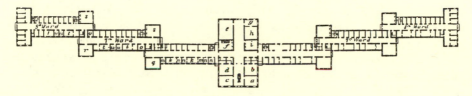

PLAN OF BASEMENT OR FIRST STORY.

PLATE VI.

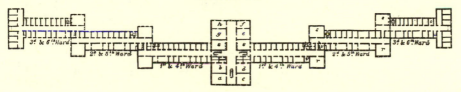

PLAN OF SECOND AND THIRD STORIES OF WINGS, AND
SECOND STORY OF CENTRE BUILDING.

PLATE VII.

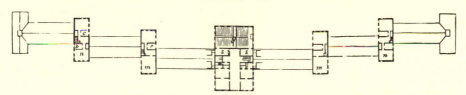

PLAN OF THIRD STORY OF CENTRE BUILDING AND
PROJECTIONS OF WINGS.

Figure 1. The "linear" or "Kirkbride" plan, as it first appeared in Kirkbride's work, *On the Construction, Organization and General Arrangements of Hospitals for the Insane,* 2d ed. (Philadelphia: Lippincott, 1880), pp. 155, 157.

Careful construction of the building's interior might minimize other potentially disruptive events in the hospital. Many of Kirkbride's detailed discussions of ward fixtures reveal his underlying concern with the prevention of destruction, violence, suicide, and escape. While providing the maximum security against these damaging incidents, Kirkbride's designs also had to avoid giving the wards a forbidding appearance. He directed considerable energy to effecting a balance between these two essential yet contradictory aspects of hospital design.

Kirkbride's directions for doors and windows reflect these concerns. He advised that doors always be made to open into the hallway, "as great annoyance and no little danger frequently results from patients barricading their doors from the inside, so as to render it almost impossible to get access to them." "Wickets" should be put in the doors, so patients can be observed or given food "when it might not be prudent for a single individual to enter the room." In the construction of windows, the lower sash should be protected by a wrought-iron window guard, so that it might be opened to admit air without allowing the patient to escape. This guard, "if properly made, and painted of a white color, will not prove unsightly," unlike a cast-iron sash, which when raised, gives the appearance of "two sets of iron bars." The window guard, if "of tasteful pattern and neatly made," appeared no more forbidding than the devices used in the front windows "of some of the best houses in our large cities," Kirkbride claimed.[29]

Kirkbride's attention to doors and windows also reflected his fear of suicide, an event which inevitably contradicted the impression of constant watchfulness and protection he wished to project. For example, he gave explicit instructions for the construction of inside window screens, which prevented the patients from breaking the windows and using the glass for violent purposes. At the same time, the screen's frame had to be fastened carefully or it, too, would be used by patients determined to hang themselves. Other details had to be considered in order to make the hospital as safe as possible. Kirkbride advised buying furniture that had no projections, sharp corners, or "other facilities for self-injury." In his directions for bathing facilities, he directed that the water handles be inaccessible to the patient, so that "improper use," presumably suicide by drowning, could not be made of the tub.[30]

If security was Kirkbride's primary concern in designing hospital fixtures, the general appearance of the building ranked as his next priority. "The process of wear and tear, and even of decay," he noted, occurred more quickly in a hospital for the insane than an ordinary building. In order to "patient-proof" the building against the most destructive patients, he suggested a few simple expedients. Plastering should be given a "hard finish . . . calculated for being scrubbed," in rooms "likely to be much abused by patients." When the floors or patients' rooms might be expected to need frequent washing, he suggested they incline slightly toward the door.[31]

In the section of the building designed for less destructive patients, Kirkbride concentrated on making their wards attractive and comfortable. In order to convince patients and their families that hospital treatment involved no hardships, the wards had to be as homelike as possible. The inevitable smells of an institution formed one of his biggest obstacles in this respect. His concern with ventilation originated in this practical problem. A good system of forced air ventilation was "indispensable to give purity to the air of a hospital for the insane," he felt. A large section of his book contained directions for the most effective form of heating and ventilation; he advocated using steam to heat outside air, and circulating it through an extensive system of flues. In his directions for locating the flues, Kirkbride anticipated certain problems that might have spoiled their good effect. He advised that the hot air flues be placed near the ceilings in the ward rooms, to prevent patients from "congregating around the hot air openings and using the flue as a spitoon." This plan, he noted, also "effectually secures the wards from all the offensive odors with which [they are] frequently filled from articles thrown through the registers."[32]

The toilets also posed a threat to the hospital's appearance of good order. Kirkbride characterized water closets as the most unsatisfactory arrangement in most hospitals; their primitive design made them "a constant source of complaint, and a perfect nuisance in every part of the building where they are found." Yet a proper design might eliminate the unsavory aspects of this indispensable facility. Kirkbride explained that toilets constructed to provide a strong downward ventilation made "unpleasant odors in the wards . . . scarcely possible." All the fixtures of bathrooms, water closets, and sink rooms should be "left open and exposed to view" so that they provided "no harbour for vermin of any kind, no confined spot for foul air, or the deposit of filth." Another frequent nuisance "familiar to all who [spent] much time in the wards" was the "annoyance and unpleasant odors" coming from the wet cloths and brushes constantly used by the attendants. Along with his designs for the toilet facilities, Kirkbride included a detailed plan for a ward drying room, which would eliminate this problem.[33]

These are just selected examples of Kirkbride's use of design and construction details to sustain the image of the asylum he projected in the *Annual Reports.* In a properly constructed hospital, he hoped, no escapes, no suicides, no offensive smells would disturb either the patients or their families. But the building itself was only the foundation of the proper institutional discipline. It had to be maintained by a cooperative staff, who would help manage the asylum pleasantly and efficiently. Thus, along with his suggestion for hospital construction, Kirkbride included an organizational plan that he felt would effectively complement his building design.

The essential prerequisite for proper hospital management was the complete authority of the chief physician. To divide his responsibility with any other officer, Kirkbride felt, would make as little sense as to expect a "proper discipline" and "good order" from a ship with two captains, or an army with two generals. Every fixture of the hospital, "its farms and garden, its pleasure grounds and its means of amusement, no less than its varied internal arrangements, its furniture, its table service and the food, the mode in which its domestic concerns are carried on," he wrote, "everything connected with it, indeed, are parts of the great whole; and in order to secure harmony, economy and successful results, every one of them must be under the same control." This control, he argued, had to exist in a hospital for the insane because all its arrangements had an "influence [on the patients] not readily appreciated by a careless observer."[34]

In order to ensure the proper order of the "great whole," the asylum superintendent had to have complete authority over his staff, for in a mental hospital, divisions among employees had potentially disastrous results. Personnel conflicts might destroy the "active and unceasing vigilance, joined with gentleness and firmness" needed to care properly for the patients. The superintendent prevented disruption of discipline not by constantly exercising his absolute power, but simply by possessing it. He wrote, "The simple possession of adequate authority . . . often prevents the necessity for its being exercised." His authority might be "unseen and unfelt and yet a knowledge of its existence, will often alone prevent wrangling and difficulties in the household, and secure regularity, good order, and an efficient discipline about the whole establishment."[35]

Kirkbride's insistence on "one-man rule" in the asylum represented a departure from the usual practice in general hospitals, as he well knew from his own service at the old Pennsylvania Hospital. He justified the unusual amount of power given to asylum superintendents on the grounds that the asylum had to maintain a higher level of discipline and cleanliness than did the general hospital. Unlike some contemporary observers, who believe that psychiatry's development as a "managerial specialty" was a sign of its weakness, Kirkbride thought this fusion of medical and administrative authority highly desirable. Any asylum superintendent who voluntarily confined himself to the "mere medical direction" of his patients had a "very imperfect appreciation of his true position, or of the important trust confided in him," he wrote. Such an officer would be regarded by all concerned with the hospital as secondary or subordinate. Under such an arrangement, Kirkbride warned, no institution could obtain a "permanently high character."[36]

Effective management depended upon a carefully devised organizational plan, which would ensure that the rest of the staff reinforced rather than countermanded the superintendent's authority. To this end, Kirkbride outlined a suitably hierarchical scheme of management for the asylum. In this plan, the assistant physician served as a less powerful version of the chief physician, that is, he had the same responsibility but limited authority. Kirkbride specified that assistants had to be men of "such character and general qualifications as will render them respected by the patients and their friends." Assistants also had to "perform efficiently" in the superintendent's absence. The steward and matron had a less critical role in the asylum; they attended to the practical necessities that preserved the cleanliness and good order of the institution. If their duties were "precisely defined" and their "subordination to the principal . . . well-understood," their contribution to hospital discipline would be assured. The attendants in many ways had the most critical functions in the asylum. As Kirkbride noted, their "presence and watchfulness" in the wards had to be the superintendent's "grand reliance." To assure proper performance, he advised that attendants be selected carefully and constantly supervised.[37]

The Board of Managers played a particularly delicate role in Kirkbride's scheme of hospital organization. They had to possess sufficient authority to act as an ultimate check on the asylum superintendent without actually interfering with his power within the asylum. Kirkbride realized that the community would need some assurance that the absolute power held by the asylum head was not misused. Therefore, the managers had to be men who "possess[ed] the public confidence" with reputations for their "liberality, intelligence . . . active benevolence," and "business habits," so that they could properly attend to the hospital's financial affairs and enhance its public reputation. He believed that a weekly visit from two managers would furnish enough supervision to convince the public that no abuses or neglect could occur. At the same time, the managers had to maintain an attitude of disinterest in the hospital. For example, they could not have any contracts for its supplies, or show a "personal interest" in any of its subordinates; otherwise people might question the institution's non-profit nature. They also had to be careful not to "weaken the authority of the principal of the institution." Kirkbride warned that the managers should "most carefully avoid any interference with what is delegated to others, or [meddling] with the direction of details for which others are responsible."[38]

Thus from the choice of a site to the proper management of managers, Thomas Story Kirkbride's writings provided the blueprint for the ideal asylum. Despite their varied nature, his directions for every aspect of asylum design and organization had one underlying principle which unified them: the superintendent's absolute control of the hospital environment. In construction as well as management, Kirkbride argued that the ideal superintendent must have complete authority to shape the asylum in his image. Kindly but at the same time firmly, he should rule like a benevolent despot over a hospital kingdom in which every fixture and every inmate was part of his domain.

Yet Kirkbride did not seek power for its sake alone. His asylum philosophy was intimately related to his efforts to win the "generous confidence" of his patrons. As his *Annual Reports* reveal, he strove to furnish his patrons with an easily comprehended and reassuring set of beliefs about insanity and its treatment. Kirkbride's comforting discussions about the causes of insanity, the necessity for asylum treatment, and the nature of hospital care addressed the fears and reservations he so frequently encountered in the family and friends of the insane. To ensure their support for his institution, he created an almost idyllic picture of hospital life, in which their unfortunate loved ones would receive the best medical treatment in a pastoral setting. Sheltered from the less attractive inmates by proper classification, the insane would benefit by friendships with patients of their own social and mental condition. Their days would be a ceaseless round of care and amusements provided by superior attendants. Anxious relatives could contemplate such a fate for the insane members of their family without guilt, secure in the knowledge that the asylum was indeed the best place for the mentally afflicted.

Having raised these expectations as the basis for his patrons' support, Kirkbride had to maintain the hospital as a visible confirmation of their hopes. To this end he devoted his attention to the principles of asylum construction and management. Without the proper site, the impressive but comfortable building, the wards necessary for classification by class and condition, and the measures to prevent suicides and escapes, the patrons' confidence would be shaken. And the maintenance of the ideal asylum, he believed, depended entirely upon the "one-man rule" of the superintendent. Without his vigilance and authority, the "great whole" would inevitably disintegrate.[39]

The grandness of Kirkbride's vision of the ideal asylum did not ensure its success, however. All too often historians have assumed a close correspondence between the asylum superintendents' ideals and the realities of hospital life. But Thomas Story Kirkbride's philosophy of asylum construction and management posited an absolute control of the hospital environment that could never be maintained in practice. Despite his diligence and ability, Kirkbride's own hospital, the Pennsylvania Hospital for the Insane, never fulfilled his ideals. Although he enjoyed great authority, he encountered certain restraints on his power which no effort could overcome.

Contrary to his principles of order and control in building and management, the tendency of hospital life was ever toward disorder and disintegration. Kirkbride, like all superintendents, fought an endless battle against the physical deterioration of his buildings due to overcrowding and hard usage. Poor ventilation, vermin-infested rooms, noisome toilets remained institutional facts of life. Attendants never lived up to the images presented in the *Annual Reports*. Despite the managers' fundamental goodwill, it took careful, time-consuming efforts to procure their cooperation in Kirkbride's plans. Furthermore, the patients refused to be orderly and content. They grew bored, fought with their ward mates, and complained almost endlessly about hospital life. By suicide, escape, and destruction, they continually expressed their resistance to the therapeutic regimen of the asylum.[40]

In the discrepancy between the ideal and the reality of asylum construction and management, Thomas Kirkbride's experience was shared by all the early asylum superintendents.[41] They shared the same conception of paternal absolutism in hospital administration and the same difficulties in maintaining it. The essential disorder and wretchedness of insanity inevitably defeated the medical men's efforts to domesticate the disease and its treatment. This discontinuity between the theory and practice of asylum management remained the most serious weakness of moral treatment. The profession had invested so heavily in the asylum as their chief claim to expertise that when its flaws became apparent, even in the best private institutions like the Pennsylvania Hospital for the Insane, their authority was seriously undermined. The failures so visible in the very buildings the superintendents inhabited left them continually vulnerable to critics and competitors.

The asylums survived their detractors, however. Although imperfectly realized, asylum treatment continued to command the support of its most important constituency, the family and friends of the insane. With all its faults, the hospital regimen still represented an improvement over the families' efforts to treat the disease. The least successful asylum thus retained an efficacy based on desperation. From the nineteenth century until our own time, the mental hospital as an institution of last resort has never lacked a clientele.

Notes

This article first appeared in somewhat different form as a section in chapter 3 of "The Persuasive Institution: Thomas Story Kirkbride and the Art of Asylum-Keeping, 1841–1883" (Ph.D. diss., University of Pennsylvania, 1978). All manuscript materials cited are in the Institute of the Pennsylvania Hospital Archives unless otherwise noted. By agreement with the Hospital Archivist, patient-related items use only initials and dates for identification, in order to protect the confidentiality of patient records.

1. John Galt, "The Farm of St. Anne," *American Journal of Insanity* 11 (April 1855): 354.
2. Gerald Grob, *Mental Institutions in America* (New York: Free Press, 1973), pp. 170–71, 204–5, spends only a few pages discussing hospital architecture. In his study of the Worcester State Hospital, *The State and the Mentally Ill* (Chapel Hill: University of North Carolina Press, 1966), Grob makes a passing reference to building design. He shows the most interest in Superintendent Merrick Bemis's cottage plan, which was not approved by the Worcester trustees. Grob clearly approved Bemis's desire to discard the architectural philosophy espoused by Kirkbride (see pp. 209–22). In *Concepts of Insanity in the United States, 1789–1865* (New Brunswick, N.J.: Rutgers University Press, 1964), p. 141, Norman Dain uses the asylum superintendents' interest in hospital construction as an example of how "practical problems took precedence over scientific study of theoretical questions" in early American psychiatry. In *The Mentally Ill in America*, 2d ed. (New York: Columbia University Press, 1949), pp. 207–12, Albert Deutsch discusses Kirkbride's propositions at some length, as part of the reform movement which he feels greatly improved the care of the insane. Yet he thinks early nineteenth-century mental hospitals resembled "well-conducted boarding houses" rather than truly therapeutic institutions (p. 189).
3. David Rothman, *Discovery of the Asylum* (Boston: Little, Brown, 1971), pp. 134–35. Rothman actually uses the phrase "moral architecture" when discussing prison design (pp. 83–84), but I think it is equally suitable for the asylum. The *Annual Report* of the Boston Prison Discipline Society, which referred to architecture as one of the "moral sciences," inspired his usage of the term.
4. The term *moral entrepreneurs* is borrowed from Andrew Scull, "From Madness to Mental Illness: Medical Men as Moral Entrepreneurs," *Archives Européenes de Sociologie* 16 (1975): 218–61.
5. See Grob, *Mental Institutions*, esp. chap. 4.
6. The career of Kirkbride's protégé, John Curwen, at the Pennsylvania State Lunatic Asylum in Harrisburg provides an excellent example of this point.

Curwen eventually lost his position there largely because he could not overcome problems in the hospital's construction, finances, and his own relationship with the Board of Trustees. The state- and private-hospital superintendents had similar problems; the private institutions simply had more resources to overcome them. See chap. 6 of "The Persuasive Institution" for a more extended discussion of these issues.

7. Thomas Story Kirkbride, *On the Construction, Organization, and General Arrangements of Hospitals for the Insane* (Philadelphia: Lindsay and Blakiston, 1854), p. 11.

8. I base these observations on my reading of the collection of several thousand letters that were sent to Kirkbride by the family and friends of patients. The letters have been preserved in the hospital archives. In these letters, the asylum's patrons frequently recounted the difficulties that led them to commit a patient, and conveyed the expectations they had of asylum treatment. Their demands had a tremendous influence on Kirkbride's asylum philosophy and practice. See chap. 4 of "The Persuasive Institution" for a more extended discussion of their attitudes.

9. Historians have recognized the *Annual Reports* as a form of propaganda used by the asylum superintendents, but have not considered their audience very closely. Norman Dain, *Concepts*, p. 121, realizes that the private hospitals may have inflated their recovery rates to attract patients. However, he doesn't examine in detail how other parts of the *Reports* were written to attract patients. Deutsch, *The Mentally Ill in America*, pp. 206–7, sees the *Reports* as "mediums of beneficial propaganda, addressed to the public in hopes of creating mass backing behind the cause of the insane." The use of the word *public* does not convey the sense of the particular audience Kirkbride wished to attract. Deutsch does characterize Kirkbride's *Annual Reports* as particularly skillful in their appeal to a lay audience.

10. Letters received from patients' families frequently contained requests for copies of the *Annual Reports*. See, for example, patient-related correspondence, M. C. to T. S. K., 9 March 1848; B. B., Sr., to T. S. K., 16 March 1861; W. B. to T. S. K., 15 February 1858. For other perspectives on Kirkbride's conception of his *Reports*' purpose, see *Annual Report of the Pennsylvania Hospital for the Insane*, 1859, p. 33 (hereafter cited as *AR*); "AMSAII Proceedings," *American Journal of Insanity* 28, no. 2 (1871): 316–17 (hereafter cited as *AJI*). Quotes are taken from *AR*, 1855, p. 7 and 1882, p. 37.

11. *AR*, 1853, p. 30; 1873, p. 39; 1858, p. 41; 1843, p. 29; 1858, p. 37; 1882, p. 38. Kirkbride took the same position on the role of heredity in causing insanity when he discussed the subject with his professional colleagues. See, for example, "AMSAII Proceedings," *AJI* 14, no. 1 (1857): 84; *AJI* 14, no. 1 (1857): 84; *AJI* 28, no. 2 (1871): 264. For the following section, only references will be given to the exact quotes used in the text. There is so much repetition in the *Annual Reports* that it would be pointless to supply similar citations; all the points discussed here reappear frequently in the *Reports*.

12. *AR*, 1849, p. 26; 1858, p. 37; 1852, p. 27.

13. *AR*, 1850, pp. 18–22.

14. *AR*, 1858, p. 38; 1857, p. 27; 1864, p. 29; 1856, p. 7.

15. *AR*, 1867, pp. 26–27; *AR*, 1856, p. 30; 1865, p. 8; 1862, p. 12.

16. *AR*, 1865, p. 28; 1849, p. 25; 1846, pp. 1–12. See also *AR*, 1845, pp. 9–10. This is a good example of Kirkbride's efforts to portray his chronic patients in an attractive fashion. He describes one incurable male patient as possessing "all the courtesy of character, polished manner, and social disposition which eminently characterized him in youth, and which still make him one of the most welcome guests at all our parties and entertainments."

17. *AR*, 1882, pp. 37–38; 1860, p. 9; 1865, p. 28. See also 1867, p. 33.

18. *AR*, 1876, p. 27 (see also 1869, pp. 9–10); 1860, p. 9; 1869, pp. 7, 9.

19. *AR*, 1865, p. 24; 1871, p. 40.

20. *AR*, 1844, p. 25; 1844, p. 24.

21. *AR*, 1858, pp. 31–32. See also the list of lectures in *AR*, 1858, pp. 22–31. The slides used in the patient lectures, which were made by William and Frederick Langenheim of Philadelphia, are still part of the institute's archives. Dr. George Layne, a former resident at the institute, has catalogued them and written a paper about their uses, "The Kirkbride-Langenheim Collaboration: Contributions to the Development of Psychiatry and Photography at the Pennsylvania Hospital for the Insane, 1840–1883."

22. *AR*, 1869, p. 26; 1845, p. 38; 1846, pp. 24–25.

23. *AR*, 1844, p. 22; 1843, p. 26.

24. Kirkbride, *On the Construction*, pp. 6–7, 12.

25. Ibid., pp. 11–12.

26. Ibid., p. 11; Institute of the Pennsylvania Hospital Archives, T. S. K. to John Evans, 18 May 1845, Letterpress 1 (1842–1844): 79.

27. Kirkbride, *On the Construction*, pp. 13, 35–36.

28. Ibid., pp. 58, 35–36.

29. Ibid., pp. 16–17.

30. Ibid., pp. 16, 57, 20.

31. *AR*, 1878, p. 15; Kirkbride, *On the Construction*, pp. 15–16.

32. Kirkbride, *On the Construction*, p. 24.

33. Ibid., pp. 20–21.

34. Ibid., pp. 41–42.

35. Ibid., pp. 42–43.

36. Ibid.

37. Ibid., pp. 44–45, 9. Kirkbride opposed the introduction of personnel into the hospital who would not be strictly subordinate to his authority. He thought that consulting physicians were an unnecessary addition to the hospital staff; they would only duplicate duties which properly belonged to the chief physician. He also did not recommend having a chaplain. He felt that religious services should be "as much under the control of the physician as anything else connected with the care of the patients." See ibid., p. 46; *AJI* 26, no. 2 (1869): 158.

38. Kirkbride, *On the Construction*, p. 39.

39. Andrew Scull's discussion of the development of English psychiatry in his two articles, "From Madness to Mental Illness" (see n. 4) and "Mad-doctors and

Magistrates," *Archives Européenes de Sociologie* 17 (1976): 279–305, and more recently in his book *Museums of Madness* (New York: St. Martin's Press, 1979) has many parallels with my argument in this essay and in my thesis, "The Persuasive Institution." While we agree on many points of analysis, we have somewhat different explanations for the importance of asylum construction and design to the emerging psychiatric specialty. My work on a private American asylum has led me to place more emphasis on the doctor/patron/patient interaction as a factor in shaping psychiatric ideology. Scull's contention in "Mad-Doctors," pp. 287–88, 299, that clients and patients formed in essence a captive audience, with little influence on the medical men's conception of professional issues, clearly does not hold for my case. Thus Scull presents the asylum "philosophy" as a response, in the face of therapeutic failure, to those outside the institution (primarily lay critics and state authorities) who threatened to interfere with the asylum doctors' monopolistic claims to expertise. The emphasis on "one-man rule" became a protective device to ensure the specialty the autonomy and integrity that were necessary for a true professional status. While the same forces were certainly at work in American psychiatry, I see the pressure from patrons and to a lesser extent, patients, as an equally important factor in shaping the superintendents' strategies. Whether my disagreement with Scull's argument represents a question of interpretation or a definite difference between the profession's situation in England and America remains to be seen. I plan to explore these issues in a comparative study of Anglo-American psychiatry.

40. This should by no means imply that the Pennsylvania Hospital for the Insane was completely disrupted by such events. Despite his difficulties, Kirkbride did manage to realize many of his therapeutic goals. I would characterize him as the most successful practitioner of asylum medicine in his generation. Nevertheless, he articulated an ideal of asylum management which was impossible to maintain, primarily because it rested on a therapeutic consensus which did not include the patients. Patients were usually committed against their will and did not accept the interpretation of their behavior that was shared by the doctor and family members. Throughout their hospital stay, they formed a constant source of challenges to Kirkbride's authority. The most articulate patients, such as Kirkbride's *bête noire*, Ebenezer Haskell, managed to win enough public support of their protests to help bring about legal measures like the Pennsylvania Lunacy Law of 1883, which circumscribed the power of asylum superintendents. See chap. 5 of "The Persuasive Institution" for a full discussion of these points.

41. I base these observations on research I have done in the papers of other superintendents and hospitals, notably the Pliny Earle Papers, American Antiquarian Society, Worcester, Massachusetts; the Isaac Ray Papers at Butler Hospital, Providence, Rhode Island; the Dorothea Dix collection, Houghton Library, Cambridge, Massachusetts; and the St. Elizabeth Hospital Papers, National Archives, Washington, D.C.; as well as the superintendents' correspondence with Kirkbride, located in the institute archives.

A N D R E W   S C U L L

6 The Discovery of the Asylum Revisited: Lunacy Reform in the New American Republic

During the past fifteen years, with the possible exception of Michel Foucault's work, David Rothman's *Discovery of the Asylum* has attracted more attention than any other book on the history of our responses to insanity.[1] Like Foucault, Rothman has succeeded in reaching an audience far beyond the limited circle of historians who ordinarily concern themselves with social reform and administrative history. Indeed, he has even been widely read among sociologists, despite the well-known aversion of many of them to studying anything but contemporary America.

It is not difficult to suggest reasons for his success. At the very least, they include the following: the belated and welcome rupture with lingering Whiggish tendencies—still evident in many histories of psychiatry, though long since formally renounced in other areas of historical inquiry; the boldness and sweep of his argument, as well as his willingness (deriving in part from his acquaintance with the work of Goffman and others on "total institutions")[2] to seek similarities and connections between the rise of the lunatic asylum and the adoption of segregative responses to other forms of deviance; the intrinsic appeal of his subject matter given the newly fashionable interest in the poor and the powerless, in "history from below"—bolstered in this instance by Rothman's claim that attention to these apparently peripheral concerns could shed new light upon so central an issue as the bases of social order and cohesion; and the resonance of his implicitly antiinstitutional, antibureaucratic, antiexpert analysis, not just with the general intellectual climate of the 1970s, but (ironically enough) with the more particular ideology of a contemporary "reform" movement seeking the deinstitutionalization of the deviant.[3]

One further source of the book's popularity, I think, lies in its subliminal appeal to a certain sophisticated variant of cultural chauvinism. English historians have long treasured and nurtured the myth of "the peculiarities of the English";[4] their American counterparts have been equally enamored of the image of "the city on the hill," the unique and special destiny of the American Republic. And, of course, the central element in Rothman's fundamentally idealist account of the rise of the asylum is his emphasis upon the uniquely *American* properties of the new institutions, and their origins in a peculiarly Jacksonian mixture of angst about the stability of the social order and utopianism about the solutions that are available to meet the difficulty. As I have pointed out elsewhere, such an account is vulnerable to the overwhelming evidence that, so far from being a uniquely American phenomenon, the "discovery of the asylum" was well under way in Europe long before the Jacksonian era began. Furthermore, while Rothman's account persuasively *describes* the anxiety and the vision of perfectibility, it neither explains the emergence of these ideas nor analyzes the social location of those who espoused them.[5]

In this essay, however, I want to take this criticism a step further. For it is not just a comparative perspective on parallel developments in England, France, and elsewhere which undermines Rothman's argument. Rather, in his insistence upon the domestic character of the changes he describes, he gives scant attention to evidence that the lines of influence were precisely the *reverse* of those he implies, to intimations that the first critical stages of the American lunacy reform movement involved a heavy dependence upon ideas and examples that were borrowed from abroad.[6]

In what follows, I shall examine the developments that led, between 1810 and 1824, to the construction of a number of lunatic asylums on the eastern seaboard of the United States. I shall suggest that while each of these so-called corporate asylums[7] had its idiosyncrasies, they all also exhibited striking similarities. I shall also suggest that these "family resemblances" mark them as a distinct departure in the history of American responses to insanity. I shall show that, taken together, these institutions had a profound impact upon the movement to "reform" the treatment of lunatics in the United States, notwithstanding their eventual fate as asylums for the rich, precursors of the dual, class-based system that is still characteristic of our approach to mental disorder. And I shall demonstrate that the early history of these corporate asylums is marked at every turn by evidence of European inspiration and influence.

The new corporate asylums were not, of course, the first institutional provision made for lunatics in the United States. From its foundation in 1751, the Pennsylvania Hospital had made some provision for the distracted, first in the basement of the original building, and later in a separate structure adjacent to the rest of the hospital.[8] Prompted largely by the urgings of two successive provincial governors, the Virginia burgesses had set up a "madhouse," modeled to some extent on London's Bethlem, in 1773.[9] And when a hospital for New York was first canvassed in 1769, its

projectors urged that provision be made for maniacs, as well as for medical
and surgical cases. Following its long-delayed opening in 1791, the maniacs
were assigned to the basement; by 1803, a third story had to be added to
accommodate them; and in 1808, they were moved to a separate building
on the hospital grounds.[10] But each of these early institutions was little
more than a "place of safe-keeping" where the inmates could be "disabled
from injuring themselves and others."[11] At best, those in charge hoped that
"the wretched maniac, sequestered from society, might be made subject to
such regimen and regulations, which if not always the means of recovery,
would at least ensure safety, decency and order."[12] As this implies, these
institutions were intended "to secure" rather than "cure,"[13] and the treatment that was given was dispensed haphazardly, consisting of the application of such standard medical therapies of the period as bleedings, purges,
and emetics.

   If these eighteenth-century institutions had looked to contemporary
English developments for their models—to the growing number of voluntary hospitals of the period and to idealized accounts of the success of the
regime at Bethlem—their nineteenth-century counterparts equally looked
across the Atlantic for inspiration, though with rather different results.
Both England and France were by now in the throes of their own movements to reform the treatment of the insane, and it was to the work of Pinel
and (to a much greater extent) Tuke that the founders of the new corporate
asylums looked for guidance. The means by which they obtained that
guidance were sometimes more, sometimes less, direct, but the impact in
each case was marked, and the outcome was an influential group of asylums that exemplified a radically different approach to the insane,[14] even
while giving that approach some peculiarly American overtones.

   The most direct lines of influence are to be found in the cases of the
Friends' Asylum at Frankford, and in the Bloomingdale Asylum in New
York. The Friends' Asylum, as its name suggests, was, like its inspiration,
a Quaker foundation. The prime mover in the enterprise was Thomas
Scattergood, who had visited the York Retreat during an extended religious visit to England between 1794 and 1800. Beginning at their meeting
in the spring of 1811, the Philadelphia Friends began to debate the question
of making "provision for such of our members as may be deprived of the
use of their reason." Even from three thousand miles away, Tuke's grandson Samuel played a direct role in the process, contributing an anonymous
article, "Hints on the Treatment of Insane Persons," to the October 1811
issue of the Philadelphia *Eclectic Repertory and Analytic Review*. The Philadelphia Friends subsequently sponsored an American edition of Tuke's
Description of the Retreat, which appeared only a matter of months after the
original English printing. The latter "was circulated among Friends in
Philadelphia and the adjoining districts of the Yearly Meeting and served

to stimulate the interest of Friends in collecting funds and in pushing forward the work to completion."[15] By 4 June 1813, the management committee had raised $24,092.50, having met with "extensive approbation of the proposed institution" and contributions from a large number of individual subscribers, as well as from more than twenty district Quaker Meetings.[16] The site selection and construction now proceeded alongside further fundraising efforts, and in 1817 the asylum finally opened its doors to an exclusively Quaker clientele.[17]

The direct lines of communication between English and American Quakers played a similarly important role in the founding of the Bloomingdale Asylum in New York. Unlike Frankford, this was not a completely new foundation, but it resulted from a sharp change in the arrangements for dealing with the insane at an existing institution. As we have seen, the New York Hospital had begun by placing its lunatics in basement cells, but subsequently, it had moved them to a separate building on the hospital grounds, in an effort to diminish the deleterious impact upon the remaining patients of the noise and confusion which they created. This expedient proved to be little more than a palliative measure, as the accumulation of chronic cases, the lack of any systematic plan of treatment or management, the limited interest of the hospital's physicians in dealing with lunacy, and the absence of any unified authority over the insane department combined to create recurring difficulties for the hospital's governors.[18] It was in this largely favorable context that, in April 1815, Thomas Eddy set about converting his fellow members of the hospital board to the advantages of "a course of *moral* treatment for the lunatic patients, more extensive than had hitherto been practiced in this country, and similar to that pursued at 'The Retreat' near York, in England."[19] Highly active in many of the Quaker-inspired reforms of the period (he has been called "the American Howard" for his role in prison reform), Eddy had almost certainly learned of the new approach through the publications and appeals of his fellow Quakers who were on the asylum committee in Philadelphia. However, he also corresponded regularly with Lindsay Murray, a member of the York Quaker Meeting and a close friend of the Tuke family. Mention of his project to Murray brought forth a swift and detailed response from Samuel Tuke himself concerning the principles which should guide "the erection of an asylum for lunatics." Tuke's suggestions were published as a pamphlet in New York in 1815.[20] Eddy proposed a new asylum on a separate site, a farm in the northern part of Manhattan Island, and also proposed an immediate attempt to apply the principles of moral treatment in the existing building[21]—proposals whose realization was made easier when the New York legislature voted an annual subvention of $10,000 to support the erection of more extensive accommodations for the insane.

The new Bloomingdale Asylum opened in 1821.[22] Like the Friends' Asylum at Frankford, it bore a pronounced physical resemblance to the York Retreat, which is perhaps not surprising in view of Tuke's emphasis on the contribution architecture could make to the patients' recovery.[23] All three institutions concurred on the primary qualification of a successful asylum superintendent: he should, in the words of the Bloomingdale committee, be "reasonable, humane, moral and religious, possessing stability and dignity of character, mild and gentle, . . . resolute, . . . compassionate . . . of just and sagacious observation."[24] The omission of medical qualifications was neither accidental nor insignificant. Moral treatment, as I have pointed out elsewhere, had been developed at the York Retreat by laymen.[25] Following this precedent, both the Friends' and Bloomingdale Asylums placed this position in lay hands.[26] At the New York Hospital, William Handy announced that medicine was "rarely given" and that "we do not believe in the specific power of any drug in curing madness." Reiterating Tuke's own conclusions in an American context, he denounced bloodletting, emetics, violent cathartics, setons, and blisters as generally useless, and asserted that with the addition of warm baths, recovery "will be the most certainly accomplished by strict attention to a moral regimen."[27] The superintendent at Friends' Asylum made similar efforts to insist upon the primacy of moral treatment, though here this was in the face of some opposition, for the resident physician continued to insist upon the frequent use of medicine.[28]

Boston had neglected to build a general hospital in the eighteenth century, possibly, as Leonard Eaton suggests, because the homogeneity of the elite there and the consequent lack of religious and social competition hampered the kind of competitive philanthropy that aided the establishment of the Pennsylvania and New York hospitals.[29] By 1810, however, some of the more ambitious young Boston physicians, perhaps resenting the provincial status to which the lack of such a hospital consigned them, were urging the establishment of a hospital and lunatic asylum.[30] The campaign quickly attracted the support of some of "the wealthiest and most respectable men of Boston." However, delayed somewhat by unsettled political conditions, the construction of the two institutions was not completed until 1818.[31] Having learned from the experiences of New York and Philadelphia, the trustees of the new Massachusetts General Hospital from the beginning had planned to keep the hospital and lunatic asylum physically and administratively separate. Now they also sought to imitate the novel and supposedly more curative system of moral treatment. Accordingly, before taking up his appointment as the first superintendent of the asylum, Dr. Morrill Wyman was dispatched by the trustees to view and report back to them on conditions at the Philadelphia, New York, and Frankford asylums.[32] At New York, he was conducted round by Thomas

Eddy, who then presented him with a copy of Tuke's *Description of the Retreat.*[33] His subsequent practice indicates that he became a convinced disciple. In his only separately published writing, a lecture delivered in 1830, Wyman suggested a very restricted role for conventional medical therapeutics because they were "seldom useful in relieving mental disease . . . usually injurious and frequently fatal." The contrast with the value of Tuke's approach was stark: obviously, "without symptoms of organic disease, a judicious moral management is more successful." However, he went on, "moral treatment is indispensable even in cases arising from organic disease."[34]

The evidence of Wyman's practice at the McLean Hospital reinforces this portrait. Chains and straitjackets were absent; high qualifications were demanded of the attendants; patients ate at the superintendent's table, rowed on the Charles River, took country rides, and in some instances were allowed to visit the newly founded Boston Atheneum. In the words of an English visitor, "To gain his confidence and imperceptibly lead him to the exercise of his disused energies and faculties . . . is all that the physician studies in the management of his patient."[35]

In their early years of operation, then, these three asylums tended to play down the importance of the medical armamentarium, and to urge that moral treatment be employed very widely in its place. In this respect, they differed sharply from the fourth corporate lunatic asylum that was built in this era, the Hartford Retreat. For here, from the outset, medicine was accorded the central place in treatment that came to characterize American approaches to the treatment of insanity during the remainder of the nineteenth century.[36]

This inversion of emphasis is scarcely surprising in view of the central place that was occupied by medical men in creating and running the Hartford Retreat. An asylum for the state had first been proposed before the Connecticut State Medical Society in 1812. At that time, little action was taken. But the project was revived again in 1820 by a group of Hartford physicians, led by Eli Todd. In a speech before the local Hartford County Medical Society in December 1820, Todd articulated his conviction that "mental disorder is as definitely a manifestation of disease as is a fever or fracture. It is our duty as civilized men to attack this disease. Let us make diligent inquiry, find out how prevalent this disease is, and then establish an institution for its treatment and cure." Within a year, the state medical society had supported the asylum proposal, and thereafter played a major role in bringing the plan to fruition. Society funds were made available to publicize the project and to print appeals for contributions; with the aid of local clergy, committees were formed throughout the state to collect donations; the public was repeatedly informed of the benefits and advantages of asylum treatment; and a state subvention was successfully sought.

Lacking the concentrations of wealth that were present in New York, Pennsylvania, and Massachusetts, fund raising proved to be far more difficult in Connecticut than it had been elsewhere,[37] and one may reasonably doubt that the Retreat would have been built at this time without the sustained initiative of the medical society—the more so since the state's wealthy inhabitants could clearly avail themselves of the new asylums in New York and Boston. The society's leaders were convinced that "no-one conversant with the records of our profession, can hesitate for a moment to believe that its interests would be greatly promoted by adopting the plan which we have suggested."[38] And in setting up the new institution, the society went to great lengths to ensure the dominance of the profession's interests.[39] The state charter that was passed in 1822 provided that at least a quarter of the committee of trustees were to be physicians, as were all six of the official asylum visitors. Perhaps even more significantly, the power of appointing the superintendent rested with the state medical society, thereby cementing the profession's dominance.[40]

As the very name of the institution indicates, those setting up the Hartford Retreat were heavily influenced by the recent developments in England and France. In his declining years, looking back on his role on the planning committee for the asylum, George Sumner commented, "We had no other guides than 'Pinel on Insanity' and 'Tuke's History of the Retreat,' near York, in England."[41] The English institution was the most frequently mentioned in the fund-raising literature, the public being assured that, in accordance with Tuke's approach, "the inmates of this asylum will in all cases be treated with humanity, subjected to no unnecessary rigour of discipline, and controlled by no force unless their safety requires it. The chains and the scourge, which have too often been the implements of correction, must be abolished, and every attendant dismissed from the institution who resorts to violence in the performance of his ordinary duties."[42]

Shortly after the Retreat opened its doors in 1824, its new superintendent, Eli Todd, informed the public of the principles that guided his practice:

> These are to treat [the insane], in all cases, as far as possible, as rational beings. To allow them all the liberty and indulgence compatible with their own safety and that of others. To cherish in them sentiments of self-respect. To excite an ambition for the good will and esteem of others. To draw out the latent sparks of natural and social affection. To occupy their attention, exercise their judgement and ingenuity, and to administer to their self-complacency by engaging them in useful employments, alternated with amusements. To withdraw, in most instances, their minds as much as possible from every former scene and every former companion, setting before them a new

world and giving an entire change to the current of their recollections and ideas.[43]

The techniques, even the very wording, come directly from the *Description of the Retreat*.

But the Hartford Retreat was no mere copy of its namesake. Breaking sharply with his model, and criticizing the other American corporate asylums for failing to do so, Todd placed great stress on the value of medical treatment. The York Retreat had marked a distinct advance in the treatment of insanity: "Its managers appear, however, to have placed too little reliance upon the efficacy of medicine in the treatment of insanity, and hence their success is not equal to that of other asylums in which medicines are more freely employed."[44] And the managers of the McLean, Bloomingdale, and Friends' asylums had perpetuated the error, with the result that "their treatment is feeble [as] compared to the lofty conceptions of truly combined medical and moral management."[45] "The aid of medicine" was essential, since

> the mind and body are so connected that there can scarcely be a disease of either in which the other is not involved, and in which medical and moral treatment may not be advantageously combined. When mental derangement originates entirely in a diseased state of the body— medication constitutes the paramount, and moral treatment the subsidiary means of cure. On the other hand, when bodily disease is merely the effect of mental derangement, then there is a complete inversion of the relative importance of these curative means. In most states of insanity, therefore, a judicious combination of both promises the most successful results.[46]

Gradually, practice at the other corporate asylums began to resemble that at Hartford. Stress was placed on the traditional medical therapeutics and was soon accompanied by the growing reliance upon opium and morphine that became characteristic of American asylum practice. The McLean from the outset had had a medical superintendent, albeit one skeptical of the value of medical as opposed to moral treatment of insanity.[47] But at Bloomingdale and the Friends' Asylum, the administrative structure was more fragmented and confused, and here the realignment in treatment philosophies was signaled and in large part produced by changes in the asylums' internal organization.

As we have seen, the latter asylums had initially opted for lay superintendents; but they also had a resident physician, a young man who practiced under the supervision of two or more visiting physicians.[48] The superintendent was "entrusted with the general controll of the concerns of the Institution" and the supervision of the moral regimen; the medical men dealt with the strictly medical treatment.[49] At Bloomingdale, this system was abruptly abandoned in 1831, "the position of attending physician being dispensed with and the resident physician given immediate control of the moral and medical treatment of the patients." The lay superintendent, meanwhile, was reduced to the status of a steward.[50] At the Friends' Asylum, the changes were more gradual and subtle: perhaps the Quaker managers here were less willing to abandon Tuke's original vision.

Symptomatic of growing medical ambition, the attending physicians' contribution to the *Annual Report* for 1830 for the first time moved beyond the compilation of routine statistics to a more elaborate discussion of the medical role in patient care. Two years later, the superintendent and his wife resigned, and the appointment of their replacements was accompanied by upheavals in the medical department, with "Dr. Robert Morton and Dr. Charles Evans, appointed attending physicians to the House."[51]

Like Eli Todd, Evans and Morton were convinced that moral and medical treatment were inextricably linked:

> Where a judicious system of medical treatment is steadily pursued [they commented] it exerts a strong influence on the other departments, which would not at first sight be obvious. . . . A course of moral treatment is almost a necessary consequence of a proper sense of the value of medical remedies. They, in fact, are parts of the same system. After what have been called medical means have been successfully resorted to, to remove obvious physical disease, moral treatment will then be found very efficient in restoring and strengthening the functions of the diseased organ.—And we believe that it is only by thus uniting them that full benefit can be derived from either.[52]

Subsequently, they sought a steadily larger role than the superintendent in the dispensing of the "moral" side of the treatment, a campaign bolstered by an insistence upon insanity's somatic basis. In a complaint seemingly intended as much for internal as for external consumption, they commented that "instead of regarding it, as it really is, strictly a morbid state of some of the physical organs, and the deranged manifestations of the mind merely the symptoms of that state, it has been too common to look upon it as an unintelligible malady of the immaterial existence itself; and the unhappy lunatic has been left . . . a victim to the idle and ignorant belief that his disease was immedicable."[53]

The success of their efforts can be measured in a series of changes in the asylum's rules. A new codification in 1840 for the first time included the provision that "it shall be their [the attending physicians'] duty to act in concert with the Superintendent in the moral treatment of the patients and promote their restoration with all the means in their power."[54] A decade later, this uneasy joint authority came to an end. In a further revision of the rules, it was laid down that "the Superintendent shall be a well-qualified Physician, and shall be the official head of the Institution. . . . He shall . . . direct such medical, moral and dietetic treatment, as may be best adapted to [the patients'] relief or comfort."[55]

Important as they were, administrative turbulence and realignments were not confined to these changes or, indeed, to these asylums. At none of the four corporate asylums were the founders familiar with the administrative problems that were associated with the organization and running of large institutions. It is thus not surprising that their first efforts in this sphere usually created unwieldy administrative structures. Thus the McLean was originally seriously understaffed[56] and placed trivial administrative tasks on the superintendent's shoulders—a situation only mitigated somewhat by the appointment in 1823 of a steward who was to assume some of these burdens.[57] Even the Hartford Retreat did not entirely escape these problems. Here, the superintendent from the outset had the aid of a steward, but even during Eli Todd's tenure (1824–1833), there were squabbles occasioned by the absence of clear lines of authority.[58] After his death, the problem became more acute, for his successor as superintendent, Silas Fuller, gave much of his attention to outside activities that were designed to augment his income. The lay steward and matron, who had previously served for four years under Todd and who claimed (correctly) to know more than Fuller about asylum treatment, sought to exploit this situation in order to expand their own roles. Ultimately, the managers only succeeded in restoring the *status quo ante* by obtaining the resignations of all three in 1840. Thereafter, Brigham (Fuller's replacement) quickly destroyed all remnants of divided authority and regained undisputed medical control of the institution.[59]

Thus after a period of experiment, all four institutions converged upon a standard system of authority relationships, one which gave all-embracing hegemony to the medical superintendent. Moreover, in every institution, moral treatment came to be defined as the physician's responsibility, and its administration as inextricably bound up with the employment of conventional medical therapeutics. Consequently, in these matters, as in so many others, these new institutions established the basic framework and ground rules within which subsequent asylums were to operate.

To an important extent, the rapid spread of the asylum idea in mid-century America rested upon the well-publicized success of these early institutions. In their first fund-raising efforts, the asylums' founders had perforce to conduct an extensive campaign to convince the public of the superior merits of their chosen solution. Subsequently, in their printed annual reports and in more occasional addresses (often distributed in editions of two thousand or more)[60] the asylums' officers initiated increasingly complex and extensive discussions of the nature of insanity and its proper treatment, all explicitly aimed at modifying public opinion on these matters.

The public was warned of the inconvenience and danger associated with leaving the madman at large. The threats to life and property, and the distress and hardship visited upon families forced to cope with an insane member, meant that "the whole community is indirectly disturbed by the malady of the one."[61] There were more subtle and perhaps more serious dangers, including those of contagion: "When an individual becomes insane, unless he is removed from his family and associates, it is probable that some of them will become the subjects of the same disorder."[62] Families and physicians alike should recognize that

> in private practice no disorder is more unmanageable. The patient suffers for the want of that steady course of discipline, which is equally remote from cruelty and indulgence—for the want of attendants, qualified for their task and faithful in its performance, and for want of that medical skill which is rarely possessed, by those whose attention is chiefly directed to other diseases. . . . A madman in his own house, has of all situations the worst. The same causes which produced his disorder continue to operate with their original force, and oppose every exertion which is made to mitigate its symptoms or arrest its progress.[63]

The obverse was true, of course, of the controlled environment of the asylum. The evil reputation the madhouse had long possessed in England was not unfamiliar to Americans, even if they possessed scarcely any domestic examples of the phenomenon.[64] The asylum authorities sought energetically to supplant it with the image of a humane institution that was carefully designed as a curative apparatus.[65] And they insisted repeatedly that "it is only in Lunatic Hospitals that the course of treatment indicated by an intelligent consideration of the different phases of insanity can be applied."[66]

Even before their asylums opened, committees announced confidently that, based upon European experience, the new structures would markedly *diminish the number of the insane.*[67] Subsequent experience seemed to suggest that such claims had been overly modest. As little as three years after opening its doors, the superintendent of the Hartford Retreat informed the public that "during the last year there has been admitted twenty-three recent cases, of which twenty-one have recovered, a number equivalent to $91 \frac{3}{10}$ per cent. The whole number of recent cases in the Institution during the year was twenty-eight, of which twenty-five have recovered—equal to $89 \frac{2}{10}$ per cent"[68]—a result he attributed to the judicious combination of medical and moral treatment. Following the announcements of similar successes in 1830 and 1831,[69] he underlined the moral: "It is not an extravagant calculation that three fourths of these would have continued under the influence of mental derangement if no institution like the Retreat had been prepared for their reception."[70] As the "attending physician" at the Friends' Asylum, Charles Evans, had pointed out, the joint experience of the new asylums had demonstrated that, given early treatment, "this deplorable malady is equally with other diseases of the human system under the control of proper medical treatment, the proportion of cures being as great."[71]

There can be little doubt that the superintendents successfully communicated their message to "informed" opinion; or that the optimism which they did so much to foster had much to do with the rapidity with which the asylum solution was to spread. Captain Basil Hall was only the first of a number of English travelers touring the United States to comment favorably on conditions in the new asylums, and to extol their superintendents' extraordinary therapeutic success. That the praise was an isolated moment in the midst of a parade of sour and scornful comments on American manners and mores only increased the attention it received.[72] The result, as Pliny Earle pointed out, was that "the newspapers took it up and sent it throughout the land, and in this way, whatever a few physicians might have learned from the report itself, the people at large received the impression that insanity is largely curable."[73] By the mid-1830s, the *North American Review* could inform its readers, with no little satisfaction, that "no fact relating to insanity appears better established, than the general *certainty* of curing it in its early stage. . . ." The *Review* was able to cite in support of this claim not just such foreign authorities as Tuke and Dr. Willis, Dr. Burrows, and Dr. Ellis, but also the "uniform testimony" provided by the experience of Bloomingdale and McLean Asylums and the Hartford Retreat. Following a review of that experience, the *Review* sounded a theme that was to be the leitmotiv of the American reform movement in the following decade: "We doubt not but that every State in the Union will, within a very few years, be supplied with at least one [asylum]. Interest will prompt the States to this, if feelings of benevolence do not; for it requires but slight observation to see, that the expense of supporting the insane poor will be much lessened by providing them with a good Asylum."[74] In the succinct words of the Pennsylvania Prison Discipline Society, *"The expense incurred in making a proper provision for this class of paupers is a very profitable investment."*[75]

Again and again in her crusade across the American continent in behalf of state asylums, Dorothea Dix was to draw upon such claims, coupling them with her own vivid (and sometimes imaginary) recital of the abuses to which the insane were exposed in the community. Repeatedly she informed state legislatures that "all experience shows that insanity reasonably treated is as certainly curable as a cold or a fever." She drew upon the elaborate statistics provided by her allies among the asylum superintendents (most notably Luther Bell of the McLean) to provide estimates to the penny of the money to be saved by "a combination of medical and moral treatment" in an asylum.[76] And always she succeeded in loosening the states' purse strings.

In the early years at least, the new asylums continued to be indebted in a variety of ways to the earlier generation of corporate asylums. This was true even of new *corporate* asylums built in the 1840s. For example, prior to his appointment in 1841 as the superintendent of the Pennsylvania Hospital's newly separate branch for the insane, Thomas Kirkbride had served a year in 1833 as resident physician at the Friends' Asylum at Frankford; and before entering upon his new duties, he supplemented that experience with a tour of the Bloomingdale and McLean asylums and the Hartford Retreat, as well as the recently opened Worcester State Hospital.[77] And during the construction and organization of the Butler Hospital for the Insane in Rhode Island, the committee utilized Luther Bell of the McLean as its consultant.[78]

The two most influential state hospitals of this period, which set the pattern for similar institutions elsewhere, were the Worcester State Hospital in Massachusetts,[79] and the Utica Asylum in New York. Again, both had close links to the corporate asylums. When Horace Mann sought, in the late 1820s, to secure a state asylum for Massachusetts, he frequently sought advice and support for his project from Eli Todd of the Hartford Retreat, and often visited the Retreat himself to observe the new regime at first hand. Later, when the Worcester asylum was about to open, he tried unsuccessfully to induce Todd to become its first superintendent. When Todd refused, Mann accepted his suggestion that he appoint Samuel Woodward instead. (Woodward was an old friend of Todd's, who had played one of the most active parts in securing the establishment of the Hartford Retreat, and he was intimately familiar with that asylum's operation.)[80]

Even the external appearance of the Worcester asylum—widely copied by other states—was modeled on an existing corporate asylum, this time the McLean.[81] There were important differences, however, emblematic of which was the use of brick in place of stone. As a consequence, Worcester's "cheap and flimsy style of construction presented a striking contrast to the finished massive features of the other. Being intended for the poorer classes, it was the first considerable example of very cheap construction, and one, unfortunately, which building committees have been too ready to imitate."[82]

Todd was at least as influential in New York. "When the New York Assembly first began to debate the advisability of a state hospital for the insane, several of its members visited the Connecticut Asylum."[83] Subsequently, both Todd and Amariah Brigham (who became superintendent at Hartford in 1840) were consulted on the construction of the Utica Asylum. And in 1843, Brigham resigned his post at the Retreat to take over the new state institution.[84]

The spread of state hospitals was to have important consequences for the corporate asylums as a whole, strengthening and intensifying some preexisting tendencies and increasing the homogeneity of their patient populations. In their early years, as virtually the only specialized institutional provision for the insane, the private asylums (with the exception of the Friends' Asylum at Frankford)[85] had been under considerable pressure to make some space available for the poor. They responded with varying degrees of reluctance. At the McLean, in return for a contribution from the state to the initial fund raising, the trustees had not only given the state the power to nominate four of their number, but had agreed to set aside thirty beds for the indigent insane. Two years before the asylum even opened, however, discreet lobbying had secured the repeal of this provision. In the short run, this created problems, especially since the poorer classes were, if anything, more anxious than the wealthy to obtain an asylum.[86] Accordingly, the trustees felt impelled to publish signed notices in the *Columbian Sentinel,* the *Commercial Gazette,* and the *Independent Chronicle* refuting the widespread belief that the asylum would accept only monied patients. This was followed up, in 1817, with "an address to the public [designed] to obviate an impression that the Insane Hospital was designed exclusively for the wealthy."[87] Notwithstanding the repeated denials, the suspicions proved well founded. Two sizable bequests within the first few years of operation rendered the asylum independent of state support; and in response, the McLean became the first of the corporate institutions systematically to exclude the poor and thus to avoid "the odor of pauperism."[88]

At Bloomingdale and Hartford, the situation was somewhat different, and the exclusion of the poor came more slowly. With a much less generous endowment than the McLean, the Retreat perforce had to continue to rely upon state subsidies. And in 1817, the governors of the New York Hospital had accepted an annual subsidy of $10,000 from the New York legislature, to remain in effect for thirty years.[89] Hence both, with some misgivings, took substantial numbers of poor patients. At Bloomingdale, the proportion of publicly supported patients grew from 17 percent in 1828 to 40 percent a decade later; while at Hartford, their share of the total population jumped still more abruptly in 1842 and 1843, when the state legislature granted both capital funds and an annual maintenance sum provided that the asylum would make provision for pauper lunatics.

Eli Todd's fears that any such moves "would lower the character of

the Institution" were amply borne out.[90] Complaints were quickly voiced
of "filthy, noisy or dangerous pauper lunatics" filling the asylum;[91] reported cure rates declined; and the quality of the physical plant began to
deteriorate. Bloomingdale experienced a similar decline. By 1847, the superintendent reported that "the House is filled with a mass of chronic and
incurable cases," and the trustees conceded that most "were listless and
indifferent and wholly unoccupied."[92]

There was obviously an acute danger that both asylums would lose
their well-to-do clientele. Bloomingdale was able to respond to the situation more quickly. Taking advantage of the opening of the Utica State
Hospital in 1843, and the Kings County Lunatic Asylum in Flatbush in 1856,
it no longer offered space for the pauper insane, and ceased to accept state
support in 1857.[93] Henceforth, it concentrated upon "the wealthy" and
"indigent persons of superior respectability and personal refinement"—
"families of clergymen, and other professional persons, . . . teachers and
businessmen who have experienced reverses, . . . [and] dependent unmarried females."[94]

At Hartford, however, the managers of the Retreat remained ham-
strung for a decade more by the failure of the Connecticut legislature to
build a state facility. Their situation grew more desperate as the decline
of state hospitals into warehouses for the unwanted intensified upper-class
objections to any association with paupers. It was therefore with scarcely
disguised relief that they greeted the legislature's decision in 1866 to build
a state hospital at Middletown:

> It is evident [said John Butler, the superintendent] that different
> classes will require different styles of accommodation. The State
> should provide for its indigent insane, liberally and abundantly, all
> the needful means of treatment, but in a plain and rigidly economical
> way. Other classes of more abundant means will require, with an
> increased expenditure, a corresponding increase of conveniences and
> comforts, it may be of luxuries, that use has made essential. This
> common sense rule is adopted in other arrangements of our social life
> —our hotels, watering places, private dwellings and various personal
> expenditures.[95]

To compete successfully for a monied clientele required a substantial
immediate expenditure to upgrade the physical facilities. Renovations
began within weeks of the removal of the state patients, and at a cost of
about $133,500, the managers secured a "beautiful homelike structure,
resembling a country residence of a private gentleman more than a public
building or a hospital."[96]

Ultimately, therefore, all the corporate asylums came to adhere to
Luther Bell's dictum that "to the polished and cultivated it is due as much

to separate them from the coarse and degraded, as to administer to them in other respects."[97] The asylums resembled one another in still another respect: their decline from curative to custodial institutions. For all the extravagant expenditure of money—the opulent surroundings, the provision of French lessons, drawing classes, singing classes, theaters, and the like—they faced the same decline in curability as the "plain and rigidly economical" state asylums. No matter that "its scale of expenditure is from six to eight times as costly" as the pauper institution; that "its sane population (physicians, attendants, nurses, etc.) is about half as numerous as the insane patients, while at [the state asylum] the sane are but one in thirty as compared with the insane. . . ." Inescapably, "like the State hospitals, and almost to the same extent, it has become the resort of incurable lunacy, and its noble endowments are bestowed, not so much for the cure or prevention as for the alleviation of this disease."[98]

In this study, I have shown that the influence of the corporate asylums upon American lunacy reform was pervasive. They played an important role in the conversion of the public to the merits of institutionalization as a response to the problems posed by the mentally disordered. It was through these institutions that Tuke's and Pinel's new "moral treatment of the insane" was most dramatically made known to an American audience. It was here that moral treatment was absorbed and became part of the therapeutic armamentarium of the medical profession. It was the apparent and widely publicized "success" of their programs which encouraged large-scale emulation and expansion of the asylum system. And even if they ultimately became resorts for the upper classes, distinctively different and self-consciously as remote as possible from the harsh realities of the state hospital system, this should not lead us to slight their part in creating, and to some degree shaping, that system. For the earliest state hospitals, the corporate asylums provided not only a model to be copied, but a source of professional staff and advice once they opened. Lastly, given the extent to which the corporate asylums in turn drew upon European antecedents, parochial theories about the American discovery of the asylum must surely collapse.

Notes

1. Michel Foucault, *Madness and Civilization* (New York: Mentor Books, 1965); David Rothman, *The Discovery of the Asylum: Social Order and Disorder in the New Republic* (Boston: Little, Brown, 1971).
2. Erving Goffman, *Asylums* (Garden City, N.Y.: Doubleday, 1961).
3. On this last point, see A. Scull, *Decarceration: Community Treatment and the Deviant: A Radical View* (Englewood Cliffs, N.J.: Prentice-Hall, 1977).
4. The latest, and perhaps oddest, example of this school is the anthropologist turned historian, and former specialist on Nepal, Alan Macfarlane. See his *Origins of English Individualism* (Oxford: Basil Blackwell, 1978).
5. See Andrew Scull, "Madness and Segregative Control: The Rise of the Insane Asylum," *Social Problems* 24 (1977): 338–51.
6. Though I shall not do so here, a similar case could be made about the origins of the penitentiary. Cf. in this regard Michael Ignatieff, *A Just Measure of Pain: The Penitentiary in the Industrial Revolution* (New York: Pantheon, 1978); and R. Evans, "A Rational Plan for Softening the Mind" (Ph.D. diss., Essex University, 1974).
7. So-called because they were built primarily with funds raised by private appeals to the public.
8. See Nancy J. Tomes, "The Persuasive Institution: Thomas Story Kirkbride and the Art of Asylum Keeping, 1841–1883" (Ph.D. diss., University of Pennsylvania, 1978).
9. Norman Dain, *Disordered Minds* (Williamsburg, Va.: Colonial Williamsburg Foundation, 1971), esp. pp. 7–9.
10. S. I. Pomerantz, *New York—An American City 1783–1803* (New York: Columbia University Press, 1938).
11. *Bloomingdale Asylum,* 1818, p. 11.
12. Pennsylvania Hospital Archives, Board of Managers' Minutes, 6:390–92.
13. William Malin, clerk at the Pennsylvania Hospital, 1828, cited in Tomes, "Persuasive Institution," p. 67.
14. See chaps. 2 and 4 of this volume.
15. *A History of Friends' Asylum* (Typescript, Friends' Hospital Archives, Philadelphia, Pa.), p. 16.
16. *Friends' Asylum Contributors' Book,* vol. 1. Both the fund-raising procedures and the organization of the Contributors' Association were borrowed directly from those used by the founders of the York Retreat.
17. These included the publication of reports, in editions of a thousand and more, designed to stimulate further interest in the project. To the 1814 version, "An abridged account of the proceedings of Friends relative to the Retreat near

York, in England, is added, in order to convey correct information of the nature of the proposed establishment, the views of both institutions being nearly the same." *An Account of the Rise and Progress of the Asylum, Proposed to Be Established Near Philadelphia for the Relief of Persons Deprived of the Use of Their Reason* (Philadelphia: Kimber and Conrad, 1814), p. 18. Quaker clientele: Again, it followed here the example of the York Retreat. But unlike the English establishment, the Frankford Asylum was unable to generate sufficient inmates to fill the available space, a situation which persisted until the rule restricting admissions to Quakers was abandoned in 1834.

18. For an insightful discussion of the emergence of similar problems at another "mixed" institution, the Pennsylvania Hospital, see Tomes, "The Persuasive Institution," chap. 1. Tomes astutely suggests that these administrative difficulties may have contributed to the managers' receptivity to moral treatment. But I feel she pushes her case too far when she argues that "moral treatment must be looked at as a product of institutional experience at least as much as emulation of foreign precedents" (p. 69). In this connection, one may note that the Pennsylvania Hospital did not adopt the new approach until 1841, long after the administrative difficulties to which she refers had become apparent.

19. Quoted in Henry Hurd, *The Institutional Care of the Insane in the United States and Canada* (Baltimore: Johns Hopkins University Press, 1916), 3:137.

20. Samuel Tuke, *A Letter to Thomas Eddy of New York on Pauper Lunatic Asylums* (New York: Samuel Wood, 1815).

21. See Thomas Eddy, *Hints for Introducing an Improved Mode of Treating the Insane in Asylums* (New York: Samuel Wood, 1815).

22. Significantly, it is referred to in some early hospital sources as "the Rural Retreat." Cf. William L. Russell, *The New York Hospital: A History of the Psychiatric Service, 1771–1936* (New York: Columbia University Press, 1945), p. 178.

23. See Andrew Scull, "The Architecture of the Victorian Lunatic Asylum," in *Buildings and Society: Essays on the Social Development of the Built Environment*, ed. A. D. King (London and Boston: Routledge and Kegan Paul, 1980). The Friends' Asylum was particularly reminiscent of the York Retreat, incorporating only some minor modifications that had been suggested by Tuke himself, based on his experiences at the Retreat. The most important of these was building patients' rooms on only one side of the corridors in the wings, to make the structure more light and airy. In other respects, the Frankford institution's indebtedness is evident even to the untrained eye, and extended to even so fine a detail as the use of Tuke's design for iron-window sashes. The use of sashes would obviate the need for bars and thus make the building more nearly resemble an ordinary residence.

24. *Bloomingdale Asylum*, 1818, p. 13.

25. See Andrew Scull, *Museums of Madness: The Social Organization of Insanity in Nineteenth-Century England* (London and New York: Allen Lane, St. Martin's Press, 1979).

26. Isaac Bonsall and his wife at Frankford; and Laban Gardner and his wife at Bloomingdale. Both institutions differed from the Retreat, however, in having

from the outset a *resident* as well as a visiting physician. I shall discuss the significance of this fact further on in this essay.

27. *Bloomingdale Asylum*, 1818, pp. 7–10; see also Russell, *New York Hospital*, pp. 178–79.

28. Cf. Norman Dain and Eric T. Carlson, "Milieu Therapy in the Nineteenth Century: Patient Care at the Friends' Asylum, Frankford, Pennsylvania, 1817–1861," *Journal of Nervous and Mental Disease* 131 (1960): 284–85.

29. Leonard K. Eaton, *New England Hospitals 1790–1833* (Ann Arbor: University of Michigan Press, 1957), pp. 11–13.

30. See the 20 August 1810 appeal from Dr. Warren and Dr. Jackson, reprinted in Nathaniel I. Bowditch, *A History of the Massachusetts General Hospital* (Boston: privately printed, 1851), pp. 3–6.

31. Eaton, *New England Hospitals*, pp. 43–46.

32. Nina F. Little, *Early Years of the McLean Hospital* (Boston: Countway Library of Medicine, 1972), p. 63. He made a verbal report to the trustees on 2 June 1818.

33. This copy is still in the McLean Archives.

34. Rufus Wyman, *A Discourse on Mental Philosophy as Connected with Mental Disease, Delivered Before the Massachusetts Medical Society* (Boston: Office of the Daily Advertiser, 1830), p. 24.

35. Edward Sturit Abdy, cited in Helen E. Marshall, *Dorothea Dix: Forgotten Samaritan* (Chapel Hill: University of North Carolina Press, 1937), pp. 78–79. See also Eaton, *New England Hospitals*, pp. 136–37.

36. On this last point, see Gerald Grob, "Samuel B. Woodward and the Practice of Psychiatry in Early Nineteenth-Century America," *Bulletin of the History of Medicine* 36 (1962): 420–43.

37. Cf. Eaton, *New England Hospitals*, p. 72.

38. Connecticut State Medical Society, *Report of a Committee . . . Respecting an Asylum for the Insane, with the Constitution of a Society for Their Relief* (Hartford: Bowles and Francis, 1821), p. 12.

39. Particularly prominent in the asylum movement were Dr. Eli Todd, Dr. Mason Fitch Cogswell, Dr. George Sumner, and Dr. Samuel Woodward (who later, on Todd's recommendation, became superintendent of the new Worcester [Massachusetts] State Hospital).

40. Connecticut State Medical Society, *Report*, 1821, p. 15. This situation contrasted markedly with that at the McLean, where in the early years the state directly appointed four of the trustees; and with that at Frankford, where lay managers were clearly the final authority in the institution's affairs.

41. George Sumner, "Sketches of Physicians in Hartford in 1820 and Reminiscences," Paper read before the Hartford Medical Society, 1 January 1848 (Hartford: Case, Lockwood and Brainard, 1890), pp. 8–9.

42. Connecticut State Medical Society, *Report*, 1821, p. 10.

43. Cited in John Winkler and Adele Norton, "History of the Institute" (i.e., the Hartford Retreat) in typescript at the Institute of Living Library, Hartford, chapters paginated separately, 3:6.

44. Connecticut State Medical Society, *Report*, 1821, p. 10.

45. Eli Todd, speech before the Hartford County Medical Society, December 1820, cited in Winkler and Norton, "Institute," 1:19.

46. Todd, cited in ibid., 3:6.

47. Bulfinch, the asylum architect, had tried to persuade the trustees that appointing a medical man, rather than a lay administrator, to the post of superintendent was "very objectionable." (His report is reprinted in *Isis* 41 (1950): 8–10.) But the board ignored the suggestion, deciding that "it is expedient to unite in one person the offices of Physician and Superintendent of the Asylum" (quoted in Bowditch, *History,* p. 37).

48. The relative status of the two resident officers is clearly indicated by their respective salaries: at Frankford, at its opening, these were $500 per annum for the superintendent (and $250 for his wife, who acted as matron), and only $100 for Dr. Charles Lukens, the resident physician (Friends' Asylum Contributors' Book, vol. 1, 19 March 1817).

49. Ibid.

50. Hurd, *Institutional Care,* 3:140–41. The steward retained some residual power via his control over materials; but clearly this was of minor importance and ultimately, in 1877, even this source of independence was lost.

51. Friends' Asylum, *Annual Report,* 1832, p. 3; 1833, p. 3.

52. Ibid., 1833, p. 3. See also Dain and Carlson, "Milieu Therapy."

53. Ibid., 1836, p. 9.

54. Friends' Asylum, *Rules for the Management of the Asylum, Adopted by the Board of Managers, First Month 20th, 1840* (Philadelphia: Rakestraw, 1840), pp. 11–12.

55. Friends' Asylum, *Rules . . . 1850* (Philadelphia: Rakestraw, 1850), pp. 13–14. Again, the degree to which American developments recapitulated similar events elsewhere is quite striking. In my work on lunacy reform in England, I have demonstrated the extent to which the advent of moral treatment rendered medical control over the treatment of the insane highly problematic for a time, and I have documented the manoeuvering by which medical dominance was reestablished. See Andrew Scull, "From Madness to Mental Illness: Medical Men as Moral Entrepreneurs," *European Journal of Sociology* 16 (1975): 219–61; idem, "Mad-doctors and Magistrates: English Psychiatry's Struggle for Professional Autonomy in the Nineteenth Century," *European Journal of Sociology* 17 (1976): 279–305; and William Bynum, "Rationales for Therapy," chap. 2 of this volume.

56. Eaton, *New England Hospitals,* p. 127.

57. Little, *McLean,* p. 39.

58. Eaton, *New England Hospitals,* pp. 66–67.

59. See Winkler and Norton, *Institute,* chaps. 5 and 6.

60. E.g., Robert Waln, Jr., "An Account of the Asylum for the Insane . . . near Frankford," *Philadelphia Journal of the Medical and Physical Sciences* 11 (1825); Wyman, *Discourse;* Charles Evans, "An Account of the Asylum for the Relief of Persons Deprived of Their Reason Near Frankford, Pennsylvania," *American Journal of the Medical Sciences* n.s. 12 (1846).

61. Connecticut State Medical Society, *Report,* 1821, p. 7.

62. Ibid.

63. Ibid., p. 8.

64. William Ll. Parry-Jones, *The Trade in Lunacy* (London: Routledge and Kegan Paul, 1972).

65. E.g., *Bloomingdale Asylum,* 1818, p. 13; Connecticut State Medical Society, *Report,*

1821; Friends' Asylum, *Account of the Present State of the Asylum for the Relief of Persons Deprived of the Use of Their Reason* (Philadelphia: Brown, 1816).

66. Hartford Retreat, *20th Annual Report,* 1844, p. 17.

67. Connecticut State Medical Society, *Report,* 1821, p. 10, italics in the original. For the actual experience in England, cf. Scull, *Museums of Madness,* esp. chap. 3; and John Walton, chap. 7 of this volume.

68. Hartford Retreat, *3rd Annual Report,* 1827, p. 5.

69. Ibid., *6th Annual Report,* 1830, p. 5; *7th Annual Report,* 1831, p. 5.

70. Ibid., *7th Annual Report,* 1831, p. 7.

71. Friends' Asylum, *Annual Report,* 1835, p. 8. During Wyman's years at the McLean, he refrained from making "the exaggerated claims put forward by most of his fellow superintendents; the highest percentage of recoveries he ever announced was forty-three percent" (Eaton, *New England Hospitals,* pp. 144–45). Perhaps this accounts for the clear preference most visitors showed for the Hartford Retreat. Under Bell, however, the McLean contributed its voice to the chorus.

72. See Basil Hall, *Travels in North America in the Years 1827 and 1828,* 2d ed. (Edinburgh: Cadell, 1830), 2:191–97; see also E. S. Abdy, *Journal of a Residence and Tour in the United States of North America,* 3 vols. (London: Murray, 1835); and Charles Dickens's similarly favorable response to the Hartford Retreat in his otherwise equally jaundiced *American Notes* (London: Penguin, 1972), pp. 122–24.

73. Pliny Earle, *The Curability of Insanity: A Series of Studies* (Philadelphia: Lippincott, 1887), p. 21. The press had earlier given much favorable attention to the founding of the corporate asylums, to the "humane" principles on which they were based, and to the high cure rate they promised to achieve. Cf. Eaton, *New England Hospitals.*

74. "Insanity and Insane Hospitals," *North American Review* 44 (1837): 99, 101, 114.

75. *Pennsylvania Journal of Prison Discipline and Philanthropy* 1 (1845): 60, italics in the original. For similar comments, and for a calculation that the potential savings of asylum treatment on only 150 patients was $179,420 *(sic)* without taking into account that those cured would then return to work, see Connecticut Assembly, *Report of the Committee for Locating a Site for a Hospital for the Insane Poor* (New Haven: Babcock and Wildman, 1840), pp. 12–13.

76. See, among many examples, Dorothea Dix, *Memorial Soliciting a State Hospital for . . . Pennsylvania* (Harrisburg, Pa.: Lescure, 1845), p. 57; idem, *Memorial Soliciting an Appropriation for the State* [of Kentucky] (Lexington: Hodges, 1846), p. 10; idem, *Memorial to the Senate and House of Representatives of the State of Illinois* (Springfield, Ill., 1847), pp. 19, 24–25; idem, *Memorial Soliciting a State Hospital for . . . Alabama* (Montgomery: Office of the Advertizer, 1849), pp. 13–15.

77. Earle D. Bond, *Dr. Kirkbride and His Mental Hospital* (Philadelphia: Lippincott, 1947), p. 39.

78. Isaac Ray, *Description of the Butler Hospital for the Insane* (reprinted from the *American Journal of Insanity* [1848]), pp. 2–3.

79. See Gerald Grob, *The State and the Mentally Ill: A History of Worcester State Hospital* (Chapel Hill: University of North Carolina Press, 1966).

80. See Winkler and Norton, "Institute," chap. 3.

81. Cf. Grob, *The State and the Mentally Ill*, pp. 33–34.
82. Isaac Ray, "American Hospitals for the Insane," *North American Review* 79 (1854): 75.
83. Eaton, *New England Hospitals*, p. 157.
84. Winkler and Norton, "Institute," 6:19–20. Similarly, from its opening in 1836 until 1872, the Vermont Asylum employed William Rockwell, a former assistant at the Retreat, as its superintendent.
85. As a sectarian institution, which had sought no subsidy from the state, and which retained an exclusively or almost exclusively Quaker clientele, the Friends' Asylum was largely spared these pressures.
86. Eaton (*New England Hospitals*, p. 48) shows that, while the poorer wards contributed twice as much for the insane asylum as for the general hospital, the wealthier wards gave the asylum much less preference.
87. Bowditch, *History*, p. 26.
88. Massachusetts State Board of Charities, *Annual Report no.* 8, 1871, p. xli.
89. This was by no means the first such subsidy they had accepted, and as Grob points out, this for a time gave both branches of the hospital a "quasi-public character." Gerald Grob, *Mental Institutions in America: Social Policy to 1875* (New York: Free Press, 1973), pp. 63–64.
90. Hartford Retreat, *6th Annual Report*, 1830, p. 5.
91. Ibid., *19th Annual Report*, 1843, p. 5.
92. Cited in Rothman, *Discovery of the Asylum*, p. 279.
93. Hurd, *Institutional Care*, 3:141.
94. Bloomingdale Asylum, *Annual Report*, 1851, pp. 15–16; 1856, pp. 19–20; 1862, p. 11; 1866, pp. 17–25.
95. Hartford Retreat, *43rd Annual Report*, 1867, p. 33.
96. Hartford Retreat, *44th and 45th Annual Reports*, 1870, p. 21. Modern observers have thought that a more appropriate comparison would be "a luxurious spa hotel." (Winkler and Norton, "Institute," 7:21.)
97. McLean Asylum, *22nd Annual Report*, 1839, in Massachusetts General Hospital, *Annual Report*, 1839, p. 16.
98. Massachusetts State Board of Health, Lunacy, and Charity, *1st Annual Report*, 1879, p. xxxii. The comparison may be extended, of course. The same therapeutic failures characterized the English asylums for the rich. See Scull, *Museums of Madness*, pp. 204–8.

JOHN WALTON

7 The Treatment of Pauper Lunatics in Victorian England: The Case of Lancaster Asylum, 1816–1870

The treatment of the insane poor in England began to undergo two kinds of transformation during the first half of the nineteenth century. Growing numbers of pauper lunatics were removed from the jurisdiction of relatives, neighbors, workhouse masters, and the proprietors of private madhouses, and placed in a new kind of specialized institution, the rate-supported county asylum. Overlapping with this process was the emergence of a new orthodoxy about the proper treatment of what was coming to be seen as mental illness. Evangelical and Benthamite reformers were coming to regard the old coercive methods of dealing with lunatics, the whip, the chain, the straitjacket, and the darkened room, as cruel, degrading, and counter-productive. In their place was to be substituted an orderly and disciplined regime in which socially acceptable behavior would be consistently encouraged, but by moral suasion rather than physical coercion. The aim was "to encourage the individual's own efforts to reassert his powers of self-control," and to provide a stable and comfortable environment in which this transformation could come to pass. "Moral treatment" of this kind originated in subscription asylums that catered mainly to patients of some means, and in small numbers; but it aroused expectations among educated opinion which ensured that its influence would eventually spread to the treatment of pauper lunatics.[1]

These changes took time. The development of the county asylums began before the new orthodoxy of "moral treatment" had really taken hold; and the original motives of the reformers who were responsible for the setting up of the new system seem to have involved a desire to bring pauper lunatics under disinterested medical control, freeing them from the arbitrary cruelties and deprivations of confinement in the workhouse or at home, but without offering any alternative to existing medical practice.[2] Only the earliest of the new institutions originated under these conditions, however, for the County Asylums Act of 1808, which empowered the Justices of the Peace in the counties to set up rate-supported asylums for pauper lunatics, was a permissive measure; and cost-conscious justices were slow to take up the option to pursue such an expensive innovation. The first county asylum was opened at Nottingham in 1811, but by 1827 only eight other counties had followed suit.[3] It was not until the mid-nineteenth century that county and borough asylums began to proliferate, in the aftermath of the Lunatic Asylums Act of 1845, which required local authorities to make adequate provision of this kind for pauper lunatics within three years. Even then, some of the more thinly populated counties continued to drag their feet; but by the early 1850s most pauper lunatics were confined in purpose-built asylums that were maintained at public expense, although many were still kept in workhouses and a significant minority remained in private asylums or under the care of relatives, friends, or neighbors.[4]

The rapid expansion of the county asylum system was encouraged by a mounting conviction among reformers, which was steadily communicated to the educated public at large, that asylums could do more than merely provide a safe refuge for lunatics; they could also cure them, especially in the early stages of the illness, if careful management and kindly treatment were provided. This belief appealed to both the major strands of contemporary reforming thought, for it seemed to combine humanity with cost-effectiveness.[5]

Shortly after the passage of the 1808 Act, the idea of the therapeutic asylum had been given a considerable impetus by the wide circulation given to the ideas of Samuel Tuke, whose *Description of the Retreat* was published in 1813 and received enthusiastic reviews in strategic places.[6] Even before this, the director of the new Nottingham Asylum had studied the operation of the York Retreat, and the Tuke influence was reflected in the classification of patients, the use only of mild physical restraint under strict medical supervision, and the concern to provide adequate exercise space and occupation for the patients.[7] The same influence was brought to bear in the earliest years of the county asylum at Wakefield. Here, Tuke himself was requested to prepare instructions for the architects, and the first medical director, Dr. Ellis, sought from the opening of the asylum in 1818 to exclude "those coercive measures, formerly used in other asylums," and to secure "the employment in some way or other, of every patient."[8] But these seem to have been exceptional cases, and at Wakefield, Ellis's successor, Dr. Corsellis, reverted to a more traditional coercive regime in 1831.[9]

The developing vogue for "moral treatment" was given further encouragement in the late 1830s by the discovery that even pauper lunatics could be managed without mechanical restraint. The "nonrestraint system" was pioneered at Lincoln Asylum, and achieved widespread recognition when John Conolly showed that it could be made to work even in the largest of the pauper asylums, Hanwell in Middlesex, which already housed nearly a thousand patients.[10] This further refinement of "moral treatment" made it all the more necessary that asylums should be well staffed and patients satisfactorily occupied, and its success provided further ammunition for the growing band of believers in the curative power of a well-managed asylum system. The legislation of 1845 furthered the spread of "moral treatment" and "nonrestraint" all the more effectively in the long run by setting up a national asylums inspectorate, the Commissioners in Lunacy, whose views naturally reflected a reforming perspective, although they were at first suspicious of the "nonrestraint" system.[11] They soon decided, however, that even this most controversial extension of "moral treatment" was "really deserving of encouragement," and promoted it vigorously. In the mid-1840s, only five county asylums in England and Wales had abandoned mechanical restraint, and it was the norm in most other English asylums; but by 1854 twenty-seven of the thirty "county or public asylums" had fallen into line, as had nine of the fourteen subscription asylums.[12] Two years later, only one county asylum still employed mechanical restraint, and Conolly himself felt able to praise "the cordial interest taken by Mr. Hill, the superintendent, in the general happiness of the patients" even there.[13]

The great expansion of the county asylum system in the 1840s thus took place at a time when the principles of "moral treatment" were in the ascendant, and the "nonrestraint" system was making rapid headway. The transformation of the treatment of pauper lunatics had made slow progress until the forties; but by the early fifties it was far advanced, despite the persistence of older patterns of treatment in workhouses and private asylums.

How did the new system work out in practice? Recent studies of this question in Britain and the United States have been pessimistic about the extent to which the ideal of the therapeutic asylum survived the constraints and limitations that proved unavoidable in dealing with the insane poor on a large scale. In the United States, attempts have been made to explain the "apparently early transformation in policy, from one emphasizing regenerative therapy to a later preoccupation with regimentation and custody"; and the same issues are now coming to the fore in a British setting.[14] Some, indeed, would argue that the very conception of an asylum "premised on the curative value of confinement" was bound to bring out the "latent repressive features" which ensured that "in the guise of reform and human improvement, new forms of regulation replaced older ones."[15] Without adopting quite so determinist a view, it is possible to point to practical problems which, in the absence of unlimited or even adequate funding and staffing resources, were bound to undermine the principle of a therapeutic asylum and push the new institutions toward a custodial holding operation. In the first place, the tendency for county asylums to increase in size, which was already marked before the spate of new foundations in the forties, was not matched by proportionate increases in staffing, especially medical staffing; and the environment provided for the patients also deteriorated in some respects, especially as new extensions were added one at a time in a manner which often precluded rational planning. All this made treatment and even control more difficult, and ensured a drift toward impersonality, regimentation, and the institutionalization of routine which seriously undermined pretensions to "moral treatment." Secondly, the demand for increased accommodation was fueled by the very Poor-Law authorities who were eager, as guardians of the taxpayers, to cut the cost of patient care; and these local administrators generally sent the patients who were most troublesome and expensive to maintain in the workhouse or in the community, rather than those who seemed most likely to be curable. Instead of the recent cases for whom they held out the highest hopes, the asylum authorities found their institutions swamped by old and chronic patients; and this limited the scope for therapy, diverted resources away from patients with a happier prognosis, and enforced a rigid system of patient classification. Asylum doctors were busily carving out a professional niche for themselves in the forties and fifties, but they were unable to secure effective influence over the size and funding of county asylums, and even the basic criteria of admission generally remained out of their hands.[16]

Under these circumstances, a great deal of responsibility devolved on attendants and nurses, whose character had long been recognized as vitally important to the successful pursuit of "moral treatment." But the long hours and personal restrictions imposed by this often dirty and unpleasant work made the recruitment and retention of suitable staff extremely difficult, and complaints on this score persisted throughout the nineteenth century. As Conolly pointed out,

> The character of particular patients, and of all the patients of a ward, takes its colour from the character of the attendants placed in it. On their being proper or improper instruments—well- or ill-trained—well- or ill-disciplined—well- or ill-cared for,—it depends whether many of (the) patients shall be cured or not cured; whether some shall live or die; whether frightful accidents, an increased mortality, incalculable uneasiness and suffering, and occasional suicides, shall take place or not.[17]

The quality of attendants was recognized to be particularly important in the largest asylums, where they necessarily had a good deal of effective autonomy in the wards; but nothing systematic was being done about training or recruitment in the mid-Victorian period.[18]

These problems were exacerbated by the increasing remoteness of superintendents and medical staff in the larger asylums. The failure of convincing medical therapies to emerge, and the consequent refusal of superintendents to relinquish the administrative responsibilities that were basic to the operation of "moral treatment," but which provided an insecure basis for professional autonomy, led to the decline of the superintendent to a remote supervisory role. Submerged in paperwork, he and his deputies were unable to keep in touch with the needs and problems of their patients, or to maintain effective personal relationships with them; and this made it even more likely that the reality of "moral treatment" would prove to be an empty shell of routine backed up by thinly veiled coercion.[19]

These defects were already becoming apparent in the larger asylums in the 1840s and even the 1830s. Two caveats must be made, however. In the first place, we should remember that conditions in the new asylums remained physically much better than in the alternative places of confinement where many pauper lunatics still languished; and an awareness of this fact helped to worsen the asylums' problems, since superintendents were unwilling to return chronic patients to greater discomfort in the outside world.[20] Secondly, the actual substantiation of the failings of the county asylums has rested on parliamentary reports and contemporary polemics, rather than on any systematic investigation of how particular asylums worked. The allegation that the new asylums soon degenerated into merely custodial institutions with a veneer of humanitarian aspiration has been convincingly supported at the national level; but to probe more deeply into the *how* and the *why*, we need to look more closely at particular examples. In the remainder of this paper, I shall examine the development of an individual asylum during the thirty years after the adoption of a thoroughgoing commitment to "moral treatment" and the introduction of "nonrestraint"; and I shall try to establish the extent to which "moral treatment" degenerated into mere custodial care, and to isolate the most important influences for change and continuity in this respect.

Lancaster Asylum was opened in 1816. It was the fourth of the county asylums to be established under the 1808 Act, and in its early years it reflected the practices of older establishments rather than responding to the new currents of thought which emanated from the York Retreat.[21] The first superintendent, Paul Slade Knight, paid lip service to ideals of humanity and moderation, stressing in particular the need for keepers to be of "good moral and religious characters, minutely clean, mild, firm and intelligent;"[22] but in reality his approach to treatment was firmly grounded in physical coercion and mechanical restraint, and he became widely known for his invention of new kinds of wrist and leg locks.[23]

Knight was summarily dismissed by the Justices in 1824 after the reports of referees failed to clear him of malpractices in the supply of clothing to the patients;[24] but his successors continued to operate along similar lines. We are hampered in our attempts to assess the unreformed regime by the fact that much of our information comes retrospectively from the reports of Dr. Gaskell and Dr. De Vitré, who introduced "moral treatment" and the "nonrestraint" system in 1840; but some aspects of asylum policy can be discerned quite clearly. Physical restraint was in general use; Gaskell and De Vitré found twenty-nine people wearing handcuffs, leg-irons, or straitjackets, and a further thirty or forty patients who were chained up during the day in specially heated rooms "on seats so constructed as to answer all the purposes of water-closets." All new arrivals were chained up at night until it was felt to be safe not to do so.[25] The patients in general were at least kept warm; indeed, one of the visiting justices complained in 1836 that "the fires are too large," and in 1840 the departing superintendent was criticized for having kept "eleven fires . . . burning day and night."[26] This perhaps helped to counterbalance the coldness and dampness of the ground floor rooms, but the deficient ventilation ensured unpleasant consequences, as evil smells resulted from "hot air acting upon the wet of the dirty patients."[27] This indication of neglect is reinforced by evidence that the patients slept on straw;[28] and Gaskell and De Vitré found it necessary to provide "warm cloth boots" for barefoot patients, and to improve the asylum dietary in order to alleviate "the evident feeble condition of the patients."[29]

The physical circumstances of the patients thus left much to be desired in the eyes of the reformers, although the visiting justices who oversaw the working of the asylum had found little to complain of. The most common comments of the 1830s described conditions as "satisfactory," and praised the "order and cleanliness" of the premises. There were occasional complaints about the ventilation, but the patients' conditions and surroundings clearly matched the justices' expectations for most of this period.[30] High windows with "strong iron bars," "massive iron gates," gloomy rooms, chains, and leg-locks were accepted as part of the natural order of asylum management.[31]

Under these circumstances, and given the prevailing high level of overcrowding (which the justices did perceive),[32] it is hardly surprising that the patients' physical health suffered. Between 1819 and 1840, the annual death rate, calculated on the average number resident, rose above one in six for ten of the twenty-one years, and only in 1820–21 did it fall below 10 percent of a population mainly composed of people in their thirties, forties, and fifties. In 1832–33 a cholera epidemic boosted the mortality level to 48.9 percent, and in 1836–37 diarrhea and sickness brought the death rate up to 26.8 percent.[33] In February 1837 the superintendent was asked to keep a book recording deaths and their causes, and to produce it at the quarterly meeting of the visiting justices; however, nothing seems to have come of this.[34]

These high death rates were sharply reduced when Gaskell and De Vitré took over in 1840, and they are all the more remarkable when we bear in mind that surviving case notes exhibit a greater concern for patients' physical conditions than for their mental health. Under the Knight regime, most comments concentrated on the state of the tongue, bowel movements, and general bodily health, with some attention being paid to fits in the case of epileptic patients.[35] By the late 1830s more attention was being paid to the patients' state of mind, but only a minority of the cases seem to have been written up in any detail, and treatment apart from the inevitable recourse to restraint was mainly a matter of bleeding, usually to counteract excitement, and the provision of sherry or brandy and water for those in failing physical health.[36] During Knight's term of office, refractory patients were punished by the use of cold plunge baths and seclusion in dark rooms, and these practices seem to have continued.[37] The uncertainty of the medical officers in dealing with insanity was brought into sharp relief by their eager and inventive response to the appearance of cholera in the asylum in 1832. In September the superintendent and the asylum physician reported on their experiments in treating the disease, advocating the use of bleeding and the ingestion of large quantities of cold water, and pointing out that "brandy, opium by the mouth, and the mustard emetics have been found to be productive of much mischief."[38] Perhaps fortunately, this experimental energy seems not to have been reproduced in new approaches to the treatment of insanity itself. Indeed, the construction of the asylum seems to have been such that it was hardly possible even to classify the patients, although some attempt was made to find useful work in gardens and galleries for those deemed capable of sustaining it.[39]

Comparative material is in short supply, but it seems likely that Lancaster was not untypical of county asylums in the years before the ascendancy of "moral treatment" and "nonrestraint."[40] It will be clear that conditions differed from those in existing asylums, and even from those in workhouses, more in degree than in kind, although the ever-present likelihood of a justice's visitation was some safeguard against the worst abuses. Lancaster was one of the first generation of county asylums, whose buildings, as Conolly remarked, "resemble prisons rather than hospitals for the cure of insanity."[41] Its deficiencies, tolerated as they were by the justices, offer a reminder that until the 1840s the county asylums offered little practical comfort to those who pursued the ideal of the therapeutic asylum.

At the beginning of 1840, the posts of superintendent and consulting physician to the Lancaster Asylum fell vacant almost simultaneously; and at the end of February a well-attended meeting of the county magistrates in Preston elected two replacements. Samuel Gaskell, who had been house surgeon at Manchester Infirmary, polled an absolute majority of the votes on the first ballot, and was duly appointed superintendent; and Edward De Vitré, a local physician who had been one of Lancaster's first Poor-Law guardians, and had worked for the town's dispensary for several years, was elected to the second post by a similarly decisive margin.[42] In only a few months, this partnership brought about a remarkable transformation in the whole working of the asylum; and they seem to have done so with the full backing of visiting magistrates who had offered very little criticism of the previous arrangements. The magistrates must have known what they were getting, for Gaskell was already based within the county, and he probably came armed with an excellent reference from John Conolly, whose adoption of "nonrestraint" at Hanwell was already well known; but the reasons for their espousal of the new principles of asylum management are not at all clear.[43]

Whatever the reasons for their appointment, Gaskell and De Vitré achieved a great deal at Lancaster in a very short time; and although they were spared the internecine conflicts between superintendents, consulting surgeons, and visiting magistrates which hampered innovation elsewhere, their successes were achieved in the teeth of some serious obstacles.[44] Despite the confusion attendant on the extension and rebuilding of the asylum, which began within a few months of their appointment; despite the overcrowded state of the asylum during this period; and despite their subsequent complaint that "the efforts of the superior officers [were] not cheerfully seconded by those placed under them," the new medical officers immediately introduced a full program of "moral treatment," and in little more than a year the last vestiges of mechanical restraint had been abandoned.[45] Lancaster was among the first handful of county asylums to follow Hanwell's lead in this respect.

In their Annual Report for 1845, Gaskell and De Vitré were able to look back on their first five years in office. They had begun by abandoning "all obstacles to freedom of motion . . . then extensively in use . . . obnoxious mechanical contrivances. . . ." In the summer of 1842, the seal had been set on all this by the removal of over nineteen tons of iron bars and gates. The windows had been lowered, the grounds landscaped, and the patients' living standards improved. The most difficult innovation, however, was the inculcation of "a different system of moral discipline," without which physical amelioration would have been unavailing. The patients were classified for the first time, and new rules prescribed that "convalescent and quiet" patients were to be separated from "those who are refractory, noisy or dirty," and the clean kept separate from the dirty. A program of regular occupations and amusements was inaugurated, including battledore, chess, and backgammon, while every effort was made to encourage patients to "follow their particular calling or to learn shoe-making, tailoring or other common and useful trades." Workshops were built, and skilled artisans were employed, working alongside the patients rather than merely supervising them. Exercise in the open air was encouraged, and books and newspapers were provided. There were daily excursions into the surrounding countryside, and a weekly party was held on each ward, while six hundred plants and three hundred engravings had been introduced and placed under the care of the patients. Most important of all, the medical officers emphasized the cultivation of regular, friendly, personal relationships with and between the patients; the rules enjoined that "all the attendants be instructed to treat their patients kindly and indulgently, and never to strike or speak harshly to them." Even visitors were encouraged. All this freedom of action was to be balanced by "the exercise of a regulating and controlling power," but this overriding domination was to be concealed or disguised as far as possible. All this took place without any increase in medication; indeed, expenditure on drugs and medicines halved under the new regime.[46]

At the very least, this was an impressive transformation of the ideology and external appearance of an institution. It echoed Conolly's work at Hanwell, and in some ways it even went beyond it.[47] In the light of recent skepticism about the possibility of translating the ideals of "moral treatment" into reality in the large pauper asylums of early and mid-Victorian England, however, two questions must be asked. Did the high aims put forward by Gaskell and De Vitré really penetrate the inner life of the asylum, or was their acceptance only skin deep? Secondly, was this burst of activity in the early forties a flash in the pan, or was it sustained and built upon in the longer term? In particular, did it survive the departure of Gaskell when he was promoted to the ranks of the Commissioners in Lunacy in 1849?

The sources do not allow us to probe very deeply into the inner workings of the asylum during Gaskell's term of office. It is clear, however, that Gaskell and De Vitré made every effort to build up personal relationships with the patients as individuals, and that they persisted in this aim in spite of considerable difficulties that occurred in the later 1840s.

Gaskell's efforts to get to know his patients emerge most clearly from the transformation of the casebooks under the new regime. His first report indicated that he planned to introduce a standard questionnaire in order to obtain more satisfactory evidence on individual case histories;[48] and the resulting case notes show that what might have been a mere bureaucratic formalization of procedure was actually used as a way of compiling a searching but sympathetic dossier on each patient, which could only have been achieved by painstaking questioning of patients.

The case notes in the 1839 admissions bring out the contrast in proce-dure most clearly.[49] The original entries are brief, and some simply record that no information on the patient's antecedents was available. Often, no comment was made on a patient's progress between admission and dis-charge or death. Where patients remained into the Gaskell era, however, their entries became much fuller, although in many cases it took the new regime until well into 1843 or even 1844 to get around to this. New bio-graphical material appeared, transferring faceless ciphers into well-rounded personalities. Cecilia Bole, for instance, remained just a name in the case notes from her admission in April 1839 until February 1844, after which regular entries chronicled her efforts to learn to read and to learn to live with her lifelong hemiplegia. Robert Butterworth, a tinplate worker, came to life in remarkable fashion, as new entries revealed him to be an earnest Nonconformist who played the bass violin, and who had sup-posedly been driven insane by "study," eventually accusing a neighbor of using ventriloquism against him. In case after case, corrections, amplifica-tions, and completely new material were added in a neat, practiced hand, and patients began to emerge as people, no doubt, to contemporaries as much as to the historian. For admissions under the new regime, the even-tual introduction of Gaskell's questionnaire made little difference, for it was written up in the first instance in a mechanical way by an underling, and it was the subsequent amendments and further comments that brought the material to life.[50] It seems safe to assume that Gaskell himself was responsible for this new approach to record keeping, an approach which expressed the efforts of the superintendent to breathe a new kind of life into an established institution.

These efforts were maintained throughout Gaskell's tenure of office, in spite of serious problems which began to emerge in the mid-1840s, and which were shared by other county asylums to such an extent that they have been given a significant share of the blame for the alleged general decline from therapy into custodialism. In the first place, the size of the asylum continued to increase, putting severe pressure on attempts to treat patients as individuals and to avoid the necessity of a deadening routine.[51] By the time of Gaskell's arrival, the average number of patients resident had already increased more than threefold over the previous twenty years, from 153 in 1819–20 to 523 in 1839–40; and the extensions that were added in the early forties enabled the number to rise still more rapidly in absolute terms during the next decade, to reach 767 in 1848–49.[52] From 1844 on, there were renewed complaints that the asylum was overcrowded, and these persisted until the pressure on space was reduced by the opening of addi-tional county asylums at Prestwich and Rainhill in 1851.[53] By this time, Lancaster was firmly established as England's second largest asylum, yield-ing pride of place only to Hanwell; and it was already several times larger than the optimum size envisaged by the reformers.[54]

Not only was the asylum becoming unduly large and overcrowded; it also passed through a difficult phase when its inability to control admissions allowed the overseers of the poor in the localities to unload large numbers of long-standing chronic and congenital patients, most of whom were felt to be incurable and many of whom were described as "idiots and imbeciles." This was becoming a serious problem by 1846, when it was blamed for the proportion of patients discharged as "cured" falling below 10 percent of the average number resident for the first time; but by the end of the decade, matters had returned to normal, at least as far as the congenital cases were concerned, for only 4 of the 629 patients admitted during 1848–50 were recorded as having been insane "from birth" or "from childhood."[55] With the opening of the new asylums at Prestwich and Rainhill, a new superintendent was able to express satisfaction in 1852 that "patients are now sent at an earlier period of the disease" from the workhouses; but the complaints had died down some years earlier.[56]

The influx of chronic and congenital patients was a passing problem at this stage, then, although it altered the balance of the asylum population for a longer period.[57] In any case, Gaskell met the challenge constructively. He conducted research on the incidence of congenital idiocy and imbecility in the county, and he studied the characteristics of such patients who were in residence, urging the development of special institutions in which those who were able to follow simple occupations could realize their limited but definite potential. He stressed their unsuitability for asylums, especially when their imitative propensities were considered, and he warned of the danger to the curative role of the asylum if the influx were to continue.[58]

Gaskell and De Vitré were able to use their continuing good relationship with the visiting justices to ensure that the asylum never became completely swamped with incurable patients. In 1845 they had agreed "to reserve a certain amount of accommodation at all times for the reception of recent and active cases."[59] In striking contrast with Conolly's experience at Hanwell, indeed, the available evidence suggests that the Committee of Visitors collaborated cordially with the medical officers, allowing Gaskell a degree of autonomy which was often sought in vain by his colleagues elsewhere.[60] In May 1840 there was immediate praise for "the great diminution of severity towards the patients, and the wish to afford recreation and amusement to all,"[61] and the magistrates seem to have readily allowed Gaskell the extra employees that were necessary to make the new treatment system work. In 1842–43, too, they were quick to respond to requests for additional exercise space. As J. T. Arlidge cynically remarked in 1859, visiting committees tended to be particularly impressed by "well-kept wards, well-clothed and well-fed patients, well-filled workrooms, and a well-stocked and worked farm; and, above all, a good balance from the patients' earnings, as a set-off to the cost of their maintenance."[62] Lancaster Asylum offered all these desiderata under Gaskell, and the magistrates responded accordingly. Soon after his departure, their report praised the asylum's "high character for efficiency," sustained over a number of years, and this reputation can hardly have been harmed by the fact that the patients had grown enough potatoes to feed the whole institution for fourteen weeks, or that the female patients had made, among many other things, 1355 sheets and 796 shirts.[63] This was news to gladden even the hardest-hearted ratepayer, and R. Hindle, who published an attack on county rates in 1843 which made much of extravagant spending by the magistrates, could find little fault with the asylum apart from its high building costs and the £300 salary paid to the chaplain when, it was alleged, "some needy curate in the neighbourhood" would have done the job for £50.[64] Even the town of Lancaster itself seems to have tolerated the strange institution on its outskirts remarkably well, for there seems to have been no significant criticism of Gaskell's methods there even when a string of escapes took place during the mid-1840s through windows, from working parties, and even from a cricket match.[65] No doubt the citizens were mindful of the "many thousands a year" which the asylum was said to have fed into the local economy, although this was not contingent on the adoption of a policy of "nonrestraint."[66]

Gaskell and De Vitré satisfied their paymasters, then; but it should be clear that they achieved much more than this. Even in the difficult years of 1846–47, when serious overcrowding was exacerbated by an influx of incurable patients, further innovations were still being introduced. Again following Conolly's lead, the teaching of basic literacy was begun, "under the superintendence of the Matron and Chief Attendant, with such assistance as the ordinary attendant can bestow." These activities were continuing in the evenings two years later.[67] The overall impression is of a genuine attempt by the medical officers to introduce a system of "moral treatment" in the fullest sense, and to change the whole spirit in which the asylum was conducted. There is sufficient evidence to suggest that, up to a point, they succeeded.

Even in these years of enthusiastic innovation, however, there is a darker side to the picture. As Scull has pointed out, "moral treatment" was not just a more humane way of managing patients; that is, through classification and the ward system, the manipulation of status gradations, and little privileges, it placed "a far more effective and thoroughgoing means of control in the hands of the custodians, while simultaneously, by removing the necessity for the asylum's crudest features, it made the reality of that imprisonment and control more difficult to perceive."[68] The limitations of the sources do not allow us to examine this process in action at Lancaster during these years; but what is clear is that alongside the subtle manipulative controls that were inseparable from "moral treatment," the Gaskell regime was still having recourse to measures of direct physical coercion, although these almost always stopped short of the use of mechanical restraint.

On one occasion, however, locks and chains did have to be brought back into use with the superintendent's consent; and the circumstances are revealing. In 1841, a group of epileptic patients misread the temper of the new regime, and attempted "forcibly to demand their discharge." They were duly rebuffed, in a manner which does not emerge from the sources; but in spite of the medical officers' hopes, resentment clearly lingered. Two years later, mechanical restraint was used for the only time during Gaskell's term of office, to coerce "a very violent and uncontrollable epileptic patient, who had got an impression that the Medical Officers durst not have recourse to any coercive measures, such as were formerly in constant use, no matter how outrageous his conduct."[69] This episode may tell us something about the frustrations of epileptic patients who believed themselves to be wrongfully confined; but it reminds us much more convincingly of the ever-present latent threat of punishment and degradation, without which the facade of "nonrestraint" could never have been sustained. There are other hints in this direction in the records. In 1842 it was remarked that some patients still had to be forced to have showers;[70] and a few patients were regularly placed in solitary confinement during periods of excitement; this, indeed, was a standard feature of "moral treatment."[71] Plunge baths were also used for patients who were felt to be in need of "moral reformation."[72]

This was not a heavy use of physical coercion; it was just sufficient to cope with the occasional otherwise uncontrollable outburst, and to remind "refractory" patients that the benign face of "moral treatment" concealed powerful sanctions which could be brought to bear if necessary. Seclusion was probably conducted under the system described subsequently by Conolly, which was expressly designed to minimize the amount of physical force involved;[73] and the evidence of the reports and case notes suggests that the repressive face of "moral treatment" seldom obtruded in an asylum which ran surprisingly smoothly for a large institution which dealt with an often rough working-class clientele.

This impression may be dangerously misleading. As we have seen, and as contemporaries were well aware, the success or failure of "moral treatment" depended in large measure on the personal characteristics of the attendants, who exercised constant surveillance over the patients, and who enjoyed a considerable degree of effective autonomy between the occasional visits of overworked medical officers.[74] Even the most enthusiastic superintendent could not hope to operate a genuinely humani-

tarian and therapeutic asylum without the wholehearted support of able
and experienced attendants, for there was infinite scope, and often prov-
ocation, for innumerable acts of petty cruelty and physical coercion as
soon as the attendants were left alone with the patients. As a result, the
day-to-day reality of life on the wards could be very different from the
picture painted in the medical officers' reports and minutes, based as
they were on occasional inspections and observations. Contemporaries
alleged that attendants were recruited from the lower reaches of the laboring poor, "persons unsuccessful or dissatisfied with their previous
calling, or otherwise tempted by the higher wages obtainable in asylums."[75] Conolly remarked on the average attendant's lack of education,
intelligence, training, and, all too often, benevolence, and complained
that "attendants are generally persons of small intelligence, and easily
inflated by authority; they love to command rather than to persuade, and
are too prone to consider their patients as poor lost creatures, whom they
may drive about like sheep."[76] Comments of this kind flowed particularly
readily from the large London asylums, whose often disillusioned medical officers tend to dominate the literature. How far was Gaskell's regime
at Lancaster similarly threatened by an inability to secure, retain, and
control an adequate nursing staff?

The problem was perceived at the outset. Until the advent of Gaskell
and De Vitré, the attendants had been known as "keepers," and had worn
a "police-like garb." It was tartly remarked that they "had been in the habit
of considering their duty finished when they had chained down the patients," and they were clearly unwilling to adjust to an apparently dangerous and more demanding redefinition of their role, and to cultivate the
necessary "watchfulness, care and ingenuity." For the new system to work
properly, something more than grudging acceptance was necessary, and in
1841 the medical officers were already reflecting sadly on the paradoxical
nature of the attendant's role: "The office is essentially a menial one; but
although the required duties partake of a routine character, something
more than a mere servant is required."[77]

Attempts were soon being made to reconstruct this unpromising material in the desired image. The staff was encouraged to set a good example
to the patients in their general behavior; "coarseness of manner" and
"impropriety of conduct" were checked whenever possible, and the medical officers sought to "elevate and improve the demeanour and general tone
of the servants."[78] To some extent, no doubt, this involved an attempt to
force the behavior of the attendants into an alien cultural mode of refinement and respectability, which was more likely to be assumed on appropriate occasions than to be effectively internalized.[79] Alongside these attempts
at general cultural amelioration, at any rate, Gaskell and De Vitré constructed a new disciplinary system. The supervisory post of chief atten-

dant was created, and new rules were introduced. We have seen that kind
and indulgent treatment was enjoined, and the rules prescribed that any
attendant who was caught striking a patient was to be dismissed. Drunkenness carried the same penalty, and attendants were forbidden to receive
perquisites or to "traffic" on the patients' behalf. The mechanical restraint
or seclusion of patients was permitted only by medical authority. Vigilance was encouraged by the standard provision that attendants were to
bear the cost of recapturing patients who escaped from their custody.[80]

We have no way of knowing how effective these rules were, as no staff
records for these years seem to have survived, and the asylum's Day Book
is unhelpful in this respect. The Commissioners in Lunacy were certainly
impressed by the public face displayed by the attendants. Their skill in the
successful operation of "nonrestraint" was praised as early as 1842, and in
1848 special mention was made of their "gentleness and patience."[81] These,
of course, were attendants on their best behavior, and we must set other
kinds of evidence alongside these transitory impressions.

The asylum authorities were apparently able to recruit staff in sufficient numbers during these years. The rules issued in 1846 prescribed
ward ratios of one attendant to every twenty-five "tranquil or convalescent" patients, and one to every fifteen dirty, violent, refractory, or dangerous patients; and these staffing levels seem to have been maintained.[82]
They almost matched the ideal ratios proposed by Conolly in his subsequent textbook on asylum management.[83] Moreover, the demand for jobs
at the asylum seems to have been strong at this time, for the superintendent was required to keep lists of applicants, giving details of age, place
of residence, previous occupation, and qualifications.[84] The stagnant or
depressed state of Lancaster's economy probably helped to ensure a
healthy flow of recruits of both sexes, especially as pay and conditions
were quite competitive.[85] Admittedly, the hours were long and the work
demanding, dirty, and potentially dangerous. Attendants worked a thir-
teen-hour day which began at 6 A.M., and they were tied to the asylum
except for specified periods of leave, which ran to three hours on alternate evenings (although married attendants were allowed to stay out all
night), with alternate Sundays free and one day off in every four weeks.[86]
On the credit side, most of the work was indoors, and generally in warm
surroundings. Above all, it was secure, at a time of recurrent trade depression in most sectors of the local economy. Work at the asylum paid
quite well, too; certainly much better than domestic service, and at least
as well as most kinds of outside manual work. In 1841 the chief male
attendant received £50 per year, his second-in-command, £35, and the pay
of thirteen attendants ranged from £25 to £31–10s. On the female side,
thirteen nurses earned between £13 and £15–15s. The laundress received
£16, but even the cook only commanded £14, and the other domestic servants obtained less than the nurses, while on the male side the two porters

earned £28 and £25.[87] All of these wages included board and lodging, and it was this that lifted the asylum to a strong competitive position in the local labor market, especially as the employees were well fed. The earliest information we have about the attendants' and nurses' dietary comes from 1857, and it offers an impressive array of basic fare. As well as fourteen pounds of potatoes per week for both sexes, it included seven pounds of bread, at least a pint a day of milk and beer, 5.25 pounds of butcher's meat for the men and 4.25 for the women, and allowances of butter, cheese, sugar, coffee, and tea.[88] This was luxury indeed for a mid-Victorian manual worker.[89] Moreover, money wages increased steadily during the 1840s. By 1852 twenty male attendants received between £27–12s. and £37–12s. per year, according to the length of service. Most were paid £34–2s. or more, which suggests a strong leavening of experience and continuity in the labor force. On the female side, rates had risen to between £15–12s. and £19–8s. per year for nurses.[90]

All this suggests that asylum work was quite attractive to working-class Lancastrians. There is some evidence for rapid staff turnover in the early 1840s, when the Day Book shows ten attendants and nurses leaving and being replaced in a single year. This was about one-third of the labor force, and it may have reflected the dislike of the existing staff for Gaskell's innovations.[91] Subsequently, however, things settled down, although marriage and motherhood must always have been a drain on the female nursing staff; but the development of greater stability in this respect was bound to make for the better working of a system in which experience and continuity of service were important virtues.

Although the power of hiring and firing attendants was officially vested in the Committee of Visitors, the superintendent had a right of recommendation on the filling of each vacancy, and he had full authority within the asylum to suspend attendants, advising the committee subsequently on the appropriate disciplinary action.[92] This relationship does not seem to have generated any significant conflict between Gaskell and the visiting magistrates, and he probably had effective autonomy in this respect.[93] He proceeded with some caution. Attendants and nurses had to serve a three-month probationary period, and on several occasions women were promoted from the ranks of the kitchen maids and laundry maids after showing suitable attributes.[94] We know nothing more of the occupational background of recruits, but the 1851 census provides more general information. The male attendants were almost all in their twenties and thirties, with a median age of thirty, and two-thirds of them had been born in Lancaster and the surrounding villages. Two-thirds were unmarried. The median age of the nurses was twenty-five, the youngest being nineteen, and they were all single. Almost all were of local origin.[95] The age structure of the nursing staff strongly suggests that the medical officers' advice carried great weight in the appointment of recruits, for it is remarkably consistent with Conolly's views on the subject: "As a general rule, the attendants, when entering on their duties, should not be more than thirty years of age, or rather, five and twenty. . . . I have scarcely ever known a female attendant prove efficient who commenced her duties after thirty."[96] It is difficult to imagine an age structure of this kind emerging spontaneously from the local labor market, and it seems much more likely that the influence of Conolly's ideas, which can be detected in so many other aspects of the asylum's operation, was also at work here. The tendency to recruit from the locally born also suggests a concern to obtain a stable labor force whose references and personal antecedents could readily be checked; and at the outset the medical officers had stressed that attendants' "principles and moral character should stand the test of the closest investigation."[97] It is clear that Lancaster Asylum was able to pick and choose in its appointment of attendants and nurses, and that the medical officers' advice was a major influence in decision-making on matters of staffing. Conolly's advice, as published in 1856, was already being put into practice: "The physician who justly understands the non-restraint system well knows that the attendants are his most essential instruments; that all his plans, all his care, all his personal labour, must be counteracted, if he has not attendants who will observe his rules, when he is not in the wards, as conscientiously as when he is present."[98]

This is not to argue that Gaskell's subordinates were actually converted into paragons of virtue and wholehearted enthusiasts for "moral treatment" during the 1840s; but it is suggested that considerable pains were taken in the selecting, molding, and controlling of personnel who were drawn from strata well above the dregs of the labor market. We cannot know how these policies affected the day-to-day life of the wards, but we can show that the importance of the attendant problem was recognized early, and tackled in a positive way.

In spite of these endeavors, however, the Gaskell regime failed in its ultimate goal. It improved the lot of the patients, whether we compare it with the previous state of the county asylum, or with the conditions that still prevailed in workhouses and private asylums; but it did not reap the anticipated rich harvest of cures. Indeed, in cold figures Gaskell's record was much worse than that of his precursors. Between 1831 and 1840, those discharged as "recovered" amounted to about 20 percent of the average number resident in most years; but in 1844, after a few years in the mid-teens, the rate fell to 11.2 percent, and thereafter it hovered close to the 10 percent mark.[99] This fall in the success rate was common to most large asylums, and Gaskell and De Vitré fell into line with their contemporaries by attributing it to the failure of workhouse masters to send patients at a curable stage of the disease, and by pointing to the swamping of asylum facilities by a flood of incurable patients who survived longer in the more benign environment of "nonrestraint."[100] Gaskell may well have been less generous than previous superintendents in his definition of "recovery," too, for his registers show that many patients discharged after a short time were labeled "relieved" or "not improved."[101] Even so, the figures were disappointing, and it was fortunate for the asylum's reputation that criteria of humanity and, perhaps, convenience carried more weight with its paymasters than apparent efficiency as measured in "cures."

Gaskell departed from Lancaster early in 1849. He had presided over the introduction of "nonrestraint" and "moral treatment" under unusually favorable circumstances, with the active help of his consulting physician and the full support of the visiting magistrates. He and De Vitré had made a thorough and sustained effort to change the spirit of an established and growing institution, and in large measure they had succeeded. But there was little scope for further initiative within the framework of "moral treatment." The machine was running, and all it needed was the occasional minor adjustment and refinement. This, indeed, was the key problem left behind by Gaskell. How could a system that depended on freshness, enthusiasm, and the cultivation of personal contact maintain its vigor in a large and growing institution, with a shortage of medical staff, a high proportion of chronic and congenital patients who might be maintained but not cured, and little scope for further innovation? In the short run, and in the first flush of experiment, Gaskell and De Vitré had managed to make "moral treatment" work unusually well, as far as can be judged. At worst, they had greatly improved the quality of the patients' lives. But the perils of mechanical routine, of the reduction of patients and attendants to the status of cogs in an almost self-regulating machine presided over by a remote superintendent, had to be faced at the mid-century. How far did Gaskell's attempt to realize the ideal of the therapeutic asylum survive the departure of its main moving spirit?

Gaskell was succeeded by his assistant, John Broadhurst, who had participated in the introduction of the new system in the early 1840s.[102] A further measure of continuity was provided by the persistence in office of De Vitré until 1858, although the role of the consulting physician was steadily declining in importance by this time, and he was not replaced.[103] He maintained his connection with the asylum for some years as a member of the Committee of Visitors; but by this time he seems to have admitted the primacy of the asylum's custodial and protective function, as opposed to the therapeutic vision of earlier days. In 1858 he expressed retrospective pleasure at his contribution to promoting "the triumph of humane principles in the treatment of the insane"; but two years later he moved a proposal for the expansion of the asylum by a further three hundred patients, overcoming an amendment based on the ideal of the asylum as a small, intimate, therapeutic community, which urged that further growth was not in the institution's best interests.[104] Broadhurst, for his part, held office for over twenty years, but he, too, seems to have come to accept a humane but essentially custodial role for the asylum. During the fifties and sixties the stream of innovation dried up, and a pattern of asylum routine became established in which a growing measure of control and autonomy became vested in attendants who received little supervision from their harassed superiors. It was during these years, despite the continuity of direction from the Gaskell era, that the asylum degenerated into a custodial institution in which the forms of "moral treatment" were still observed, but the main aims of the officials were directed toward restraint and control rather than cure.

Attention to the material comfort, recreation, and occupation of the patients was maintained, but it seems to have been increasingly selective in its operation, and the initiative began to pass from the asylum authorities to the visiting Commissioners in Lunacy. In 1854, the successful band that was formed "under the auspices of the Steward and Chief Attendant" demonstrated a continuing vein of liveliness, but it took another five years before Lancaster came into line with other asylums of more recent construction by acquiring a purpose-built recreation hall.[105] Here, the band was able to play for regular dances, and "theatrical performances" were held, as well as "coffee parties" for "social games and talk."[106] The regular program of reading and elementary education on the wards continued, and the chapel was well attended. The chaplain was pleased with his influence on his captive audience, many of whom "before entering the Asylum, appear[ed] to have had little or no religious training, nor [had] they been accustomed to attend public worship." But they "often" remembered and repeated the substance of his sermons, and in 1863 he felt able to assert that, "the beneficial effect of religious instruction has been manifested by the way in which it has influenced the mind for good, improved the habits, and controlled and restrained the passions."[107] The chaplain thus saw himself as an important component of the "moral treatment" system, and his high salary and new chapel (opened in December 1866) might seem to endorse this view.[108] In practice, however, he was firmly subordinated to medical control, to such an extent that he had to obtain the superintendent's permission before a patient could receive Holy Communion, and by the mid-sixties his reports were not deemed worthy of being forwarded to the Clerks of the Peace for printing.[109]

In practice, the medical superintendent had little more to offer than the chaplain. By the mid-fifties, a regular asylum routine was firmly established, and the patients' work and recreational activities fitted into this. In summer, especially, a few variations were encouraged, as bathing parties visited Morecambe Bay, walks were taken in the surrounding countryside, and cricket, croquet, and skittles could be enjoyed in the asylum grounds.[110] But the completion of the new recreation hall in 1859 called forth the ominous comment that, in winter especially, "asylum life is apt to become monotonous and wearisome to both servants and patients."[111] In spite of this, the inadequacy of the asylum's grounds for exercise and enjoyment was frequently alluded to, and it took several adverse comments from the Commissioners to bring about an extension on land which was already available.[112]

The patients' immediate surroundings and material conditions continued to be improved. In 1857 bookcases and improved looking glasses were provided, and birch bedsteads replaced "many of the old and unsightly cribs"; and by 1865 many patients had acquired chairs, bedside carpets, and doormats. Some of the dayrooms were wallpapered, and the floors covered with carpet or fiber matting.[113] But the Commissioners in Lunacy showed increasing dissatisfaction during the sixties, as they urged the provision of additional dayrooms for the women, and complained of a shortage of washbasins. In 1868, although new facilities enabled the men's shirts to be changed twice weekly, each ration of bath water was still having to be shared between at least three women.[114] Funds were no longer sufficient to keep amenities in line with rising expectations.

The general tone of the Commissioners' reports, however, remained decidedly favorable. The patients were still quiet, orderly, well dressed, and comfortable, and these were becoming the main desiderata of the well-run asylum.[115] Although the patients were being looked after, however, only a minority of them were actually being treated in the sense envisaged by the advocates of "moral treatment." The standard procedures were well established by 1853: "It is unnecessary to burden each successive report with the general details of treatment or management. In these respects there is little or no deviation from the principles which have been acted upon for many years. . . ."[116]

Eight years later, the limited relevance of medical expertise and the persistence of routine were both clearly indicated by the superintendent:

> As regards the medical treatment of the patients, it has not differed from that pursued in former years. Insanity is accompanied in most cases with symptoms of debility, and has to be treated with an abundant allowance of nutritious food, together with the use of wine and porter where indicated. When the patient is restless and excited, active and prolonged exercise out of doors is found to be very beneficial when combined with the use of sedatives; the good effects of the latter remedy however in many cases appear to be transient and uncertain, and when continued for any length of time, an increased quantity does not succeed in producing the desired result.[117]

Broadhurst's skepticism about the value of sedatives was reflected in expenses for "surgery and dispensary" which continued to run at less than one penny per patient per week as against, in 1853, sixpence for clothing and more than fourpence for furniture and bedding.[118] Only a small proportion of the patients received even this limited and negative form of medical "treatment" for insanity. The same could be said of the residual commitment to "moral treatment," for the proliferation of long-lived chronic patients seems to have led to a concentration of effort and resources into a limited number of wards. The Commissioners in Lunacy commented in 1861 that "the patients in some of the wards struck us as being in an apathetic state, and efforts should be made to excite and keep up their attention."[119] Five years later, they were more explicit: "The wards occupied by the more intelligent patients were well supplied with books and games, but in those where the imbeciles were placed we thought that there was not enough effort made to rouse and interest them."[120] By 1868 the men's wards in general were being criticized as "deficient in ordinary means of amusement."[121] The suggestion of a double standard of care, with the chronic patients being allowed increasingly to vegetate, is borne out by the case notes and by the pattern of "recoveries." The case notes, although generally kept up with increasing thoroughness, show a tendency to ignore those chronic patients who showed no physical symptoms;[122] while as early as 1855 it could be regarded as "a gratification" that a patient recovered after spending six years in the asylum, most of those discharged as "recovered" seem to have been patients of less than one year's standing.[123]

The ideal of "moral treatment" was also undermined by an increasing resort to the seclusion of excited or difficult patients as a matter of routine, as Broadhurst and De Vitré had feared in their annual report for 1854.[124] The Commissioners in Lunacy were remarking on the more frequent use of solitary confinement by the early sixties, and in 1870 it was used on 155 patients at a time when the average number resident was 1026.[125] This was seen as a high incidence of seclusion, and its routine character was made generally apparent when a court case revealed that the superintending attendants were empowered to consign patients to padded cells on their own initiative, with a duty to report to the chief attendant but not, apparently, to a medical officer.[126]

The case in question involved the prosecution of two attendants, who in March 1870 were found guilty of manslaughter for beating and kicking a patient to death. The evidence brought the collapse of the asylum's "moral treatment" regime into sharp relief, revealing the inability of overworked medical staff to supervise the wards adequately, still less to get to know the patients as individuals, in what was now a vast and overcrowded institution containing over a thousand patients. The attendants were convicted on the evidence of a patient, James Dutton, who convinced the jury after intensive cross-examination. He alleged that attendants often used violence toward patients, and explained that he did not report assaults to the medical staff "because it is a common occurrence. . . . I have seen him (the victim) and others ill-used before . . . by striking heavy with the fists and kicking." Broadhurst himself admitted, "on being closely pressed," that Dutton had been moved to another ward for fear that "there might be some anger felt" toward him for giving evidence. John Dobson, the ward supervisor, added further information about the hidden workings of the asylum, revealing that "fights frequently [took] place between the patients"; that despite the abandonment of full mechanical restraint, patients were often obliged to wear "lock collars" at the behest of the attendants; and that Dutton suffered from delusions that had not been reported to the doctors or the chief attendant, "because they are very common among the patients." It becomes clear that behind the bland facade of the official reports, the asylum was effectively ruled by the cunning of the attendants, supplemented by force when necessary, and sometimes giving way to unpleasant teasing and gratuitous violence. Medical supervision was effectively nonexistent. The high ideals of "moral treatment" were reduced to John Dobson's perception of what made an effective attendant: "The success of the attendants with the patients depends on their humouring their peculiarities."[127]

These revelations of violence and petty tyranny on their wards shocked the visiting justices. Their distress was exacerbated by the discovery that some of the other attendants had subscribed toward the defense of their colleagues, thereby tending to confirm the prosecuting counsel's belief in a malign esprit de corps among the "warders," as he chose to call them. The possibility of dismissing the organizer of the fund was discussed, but the idea was abandoned on a narrow vote.[128] Subsequently, a subcommittee reported on the causes of the disaster. It recommended closer supervision of the wards by the chief attendant and the assistant medical officers, but its most important paragraph showed a revealing awareness of the root of the trouble:

> But no machinery, no arrangements however minute or perfect are half so important as a constant *personal* intercourse—free and friendly between the superior officers and *all* the patients—this *alone* will enable the responsible Heads of the Establishment to check off the reports and judge of the conduct of the attendants—the regularity essential in all large institutions naturally degenerates into a lifeless routine. We would therefore strongly urge upon the superior officers frequent and irregular visits to the wards, at various and unexpected hours.[129]

The tragic events of 1870 were subsequently glossed over, even by the Commissioners in Lunacy;[130] but they were the outcome of a deep-seated malaise that had been visible in the long-term degeneration of "moral treatment" into custodial care over the past twenty years. Why did it happen? Three malign influences must dominate an explanation. In the first place, the asylum was becoming too large for a system based on personal contact to work effectively; and this problem was exacerbated by attempts to cut costs which led to a shortage of qualified medical staff. Secondly, too many of the patients were incurable, making it difficult to maintain staff morale in what was becoming a holding operation rather than a curative enterprise. These areas of explanation have already been given prominence in the existing literature.[131] Beyond this, however, the paradox of the position of the attendant in a system of "moral treatment" also emerges as vitally important, and at Lancaster the lack of supervision from above seems to have been compounded by problems of recruitment and morale during the sixties. We must explore these points further.

The asylum continued to grow steadily through the fifties and sixties. The average number of patients had fallen to 650 in 1852, but by 1863 it had crept up again to 745, and subsequent enlargements lifted it to 1026 by 1870, at which time the older buildings had been seriously overcrowded for some years.[132] In 1867, the Commissioners in Lunacy noted the signs of strain, observing that the asylum had now "reached the limits which admit of due supervision, and the individual treatment of the patients."[133] Only three years earlier, Broadhurst had at last acquired a second assistant medical officer; and in 1858 he had lost the services of De Vitré, who had clearly taken an active part in the work of the asylum well into the 1850s.[134] Hanwell and Colney Hatch were showing even worse staffing ratios at about this time, but this can have been small consolation.[135] To make matters worse, a steady process of cheeseparing was being operated to bring down the average weekly cost per patient.[136] It would have been impossible, even under the most favorable circumstances, to maintain the original spirit of "moral treatment" under these constraints; but additional pressures were also being felt.

Complaints about the subversion of the ideal of the curative asylum by the poor-law authorities' tendency to send incurable chronic or congenitally deficient cases, leaving recent and possibly curable patients behind in the hope that they would make an inexpensive spontaneous recovery in the workhouse, were as old as the county asylum system. In fact, it is hard to demonstrate from the available evidence that matters worsened in this respect at Lancaster after 1850. There was a slight tendency for patients to be admitted at a greater age, but it was hardly sufficient to justify the allegations some have made that asylums were being used as dumping-grounds for workhouse geriatrics.[137] The median age for new admissions on the male side was thirty-seven in 1816, the first year of the asylum's operation; it was still in the high thirties in 1848–50, and in 1871 it stood at forty. On the female side, the three periods examined all showed median ages in the mid-thirties. Although the proportion of admissions over sixty years of age in 1871 was more than twice that for 1848–50, it still amounted to only 10 percent. Nor was there a marked increase in the proportion of patients admitted in a chronic and incurable state, if the recorded previous duration of their illness is any guide. In 1848, when matters were back to normal after the spurt of chronic admissions in the mid-forties, 50 percent of the admissions were reported to have been insane for two months or more, 18 percent for six months or more, and 9 percent for a year or more. In 1871, the figures were 56, 19, and 13 percent.[138] If we look more generally at the proposition that the asylum became a dumping-ground for derelicts and deviants of all kinds, the occupational data on admissions offer little support. The proportion of admissions in the largest low-status occupational categories, laborers and domestic servants, was smaller in 1871 than in 1848–50; and, as in the earlier years, the handful of hawkers and the occasional fringe occupation, like the solitary "singer in a concert room," who might be tentatively consigned to a subculture of the dissolute, must be balanced against such respectable-looking categories as a schoolmistress, a bookkeeper, and several shopkeepers.[139] Further research on case notes will be needed before these superficial labels can be properly explored, and we cannot yet be sure that the years analyzed are typical of the periods they represent; but it seems likely that the pattern of new admissions did not change significantly in measurable ways between the late forties and the early seventies.

Nevertheless, there was a significant increase in the proportion of long-term chronic patients in the asylum. It was brought about by the low rate of "recoveries," which never rose above 9.8 percent of the average number resident between 1851 and 1870, and sometimes dipped below 5 percent.[140] This, coupled with the persistence of the reduced death rates associated with the Gaskell regime, meant a low level of patient discharges, and ensured that long-stay patients would increasingly predominate. This was reflected in the age structure of the inmates, as opposed to that of the new admissions. The median age of resident patients increased slightly, but not spectacularly, from forty for men and forty-two for women in 1851, to forty-three and forty-five twenty years later. But the really noticeable change came in the proportion of patients who were over sixty years old. On the male side, this rose from 6 percent to 13 percent during this period, and on the female side the figures were 10 percent and 18 percent.[141] Even this was not a high figure; and the rise took place in spite of anxious attempts by the asylum authorities to return chronic patients of quiet demeanor to the workhouses, and replace them with cases with a more hopeful prognosis. Fourteen patients were removed in this way in 1855, and such transfers became a regular practice; but by 1861 increasing caution was

being exercised, as experience showed that many patients lost their tranquillity after transfer, and had to be returned to the asylum in a worse state
than before.[142] Soon afterward, new legislation led the Commissioners in
Lunacy to prescribe minimum standards for workhouses that were receiving old chronic cases in this way, requiring separate wards, "a liberal
dietary analogous to that of an asylum," plenty of exercise space, adequate
medical attention, and "properly qualified paid attendants" as opposed to
inmates working for pocket money or tobacco.[143] At first, this must have
slowed the rate of transfer; but in 1866 the Boards of Guardians were
reminded that even under the new regulations, workhouse accommodation would be much cheaper than the asylum. By the end of the decade,
a growing number of large workhouses were becoming acceptable as
receptacles for old chronic cases, and new optimism was being expressed
about the possibility of the asylum reasserting its role as a curative institution.[144]

This optimism was misplaced, although the problem of chronic and
congenital cases was probably less serious and more soluble than the problems associated with size, organization, and the tyranny of monotonous
routine. Here, the role of the nursing staff was particularly important; and
increasing deficiencies of the staff during the 1860s form the third main
element in the asylum's decline.

In 1859, the Commissioners in Lunacy were full of praise for the "very
respectable and efficient class" of attendants at Lancaster; but a year later
the superintendent pointed to the first serious evidence of difficulty in
attracting and keeping "active and intelligent" staff, especially on the
female side.[145] Subsequently, symptoms of strain began to appear in a
decade which saw renewed industrial growth in Lancaster, for competition for labor was certain to have a significant effect on recruitment and
behavior.[146] The wage scales for ordinary attendants and nurses, moreover, actually fell slightly during the generally inflationary years between
1852 and 1870, and dissatisfaction was expressed in a series of deputations
to the visiting justices in search of higher wages, only one of which resulted in even minimal concessions.[147] To make matters worse, the attendants' beer allowance seems to have been withdrawn in 1864, in spite of
their protests.[148] It was still not difficult to recruit sufficient numbers of
male staff, and a three-man deputation of complaint about the reinstate-
ment of a colleague "over their heads" found the visiting justices perfectly
willing to accept their resignations.[149] Women were becoming harder to
recruit, and in the spring of 1870 a nurse had to be sought by advertisement
in five consecutive issues of the local newspaper, even though the only
criteria, much as in 1816, were that she should be tall, strong, active, and
not under twenty years of age.[150] On the male side, attendants in 1870 still
exhibited dramatic, photographic, and musical talents, but the most pro-

mising-looking recruit, Samuel Wood, who was being considered as an organist for the chapel in August 1869, was languishing in jail a year later as one of the villains in the manslaughter case.[151] This followed two unsubstantiated allegations of cruelty to patients within a short time, and although Broadhurst remarked that the attendants were being severely tried by "violent and troublesome" patients, this merely reinforces the impression of a breakdown of morale among an untrained and undersupervised group whose living standards had been eroded, and whose conditions of work had suffered from the increasing size and anonymity of an asylum that was coming to be dominated by the tyranny of routine.[152]

What can we learn from this case study? It is clear that even the most carefully nurtured and firmly established of "moral treatment" regimes was vulnerable, in the long run, to the combined pressures of increased scale, cheeseparing economies, overworked medical superintendence, aging patient populations, and untrained, undersupervised nursing staff which afflicted all the county asylums following the euphoric confidence of their initial establishment. At Lancaster, despite important continuities of personnel and outlook from the Gaskell era, "moral treatment" for most patients was becoming a mere facade by the 1860s. Even so, Lancaster's record compares favorably with other large asylums, especially the London ones. Despite all the pressures, Broadhurst did not bring back the full paraphernalia of mechanical restraint, although the use even of the lock collar was a significant retreat from the "nonrestraint" ideal. Elsewhere, it was sometimes a different story. At Wakefield, mechanical restraint was reintroduced in the late sixties, and the same was true of Colney Hatch.[153] Lancaster's degeneration seems to have come later and less spectacularly than was the case at other asylums, and its relatively good performance probably owed much to the legacy of Gaskell, assisted by the willingness of the justices in a prosperous county to spend relatively freely on the insane poor, and by a local labor market which eased the recruitment and retention of an adequate nursing staff for many years. But inherent in the "nonrestraint" system was the danger of routinization, and the likelihood of frustration when the expected cures failed to materialize; and it is doubtful whether even Gaskell could have kept the flame of enthusiasm burning through the encroaching darkness of the fifties and sixties. We need to know more about the experiences of other county asylums in the English provinces; but it seems likely that if the pressures of routine and impersonality overwhelmed even the relatively successful regime at Lancaster, they must have proved generally disastrous elsewhere. The details may vary, but the trend is strongly marked.

We can end on a positive note, however. The "mammoth asylums" of the mid-Victorian years may have come to represent a sad departure from the ideals expressed by the apostles of "moral treatment" and "nonrestraint"; but at least they represented a much less uncomfortable alternative to the workhouses in which so many of the congenitally inept, socially incompetent, and derelicts were still being confined in 1870. Horror stories lived on, and although they were deployed as exemplary admonitions by advocates of the asylum system, such as Gaskell himself, we need not doubt the truth of the graphic descriptions of neglected and maltreated patients that were brought before the Select Committee on Lunatics in 1859.[154] Despite widespread improvements during the sixties, which owed much to the efforts of the Commissioners in Lunacy, plenty of black spots remained. We need to know much more about the treatment of pauper lunatics outside the public asylums during this period.[155] The county asylum was only one of several available institutions of confinement and control for this anomalous sector of the dependent pauper population; and the Lancaster evidence drives home the point that, whatever its failings when measured against an unattainable ideal, at a more practical level it provided a relatively humane alternative to the other methods of coping with the most vulnerable fringe elements in Victorian society. With all their faults, we must remember that the county asylums could be refuges as well as places of incarceration; and with all its deficiencies, the record of Lancaster Asylum is particularly significant in this context.

Notes

1. Andrew Scull, *Museums of Madness: The Social Organization of Insanity in Nine-teenth-Century England* (London: Allen Lane, 1979), esp. pp. 54–70; K. Jones, *Lunacy, Law and Conscience 1744–1845* (London: Routledge and Kegan Paul, 1955), pp. 49–65; W. L. Parry-Jones, *The Trade in Lunacy: A Study of Private Madhouses in England in the Eighteenth and Nineteenth Centuries* (London: Routledge and Kegan Paul, 1972), pp. 170–84.
2. Scull, *Museums of Madness*, pp. 61–62.
3. Jones, *Lunacy*, pp. 70–78, 116.
4. Scull, *Museums of Madness*, pp. 186–88; R. Hodgkinson, "Provision for Pauper Lunatics 1834–71," *Medical History* 10 (1966): 146; *Parliamentary Papers*, 1859, p. iii, Select Committee on Lunatics, evidence of S. Gaskell, Q. 1391–92 (hereafter cited as *PP*).
5. Scull, *Museums of Madness*, pp. 102–12.
6. Ibid., pp. 67–70; Jones, *Lunacy*, p. 79.
7. Jones, *Lunacy*, pp. 99–100.
8. J. S. Bolton, "The Evolution of a Mental Hospital—Wakefield, 1818–1928," *Journal of Mental Science* 74 (1928): 588, 596–97; A. Walk, "The History of Mental Nursing," *Journal of Mental Science* 107 (1961): 1–17.
9. Bolton, "Wakefield," pp. 604–5.
10. Jones, *Lunacy*, pp. 149–56.
11. Scull, *Museums of Madness*, pp. 110–13; J. Conolly, *Treatment of the Insane without Mechanical Restraints* (1856; reprint ed., Folkestone: Dawsons, 1973), p. 300.
12. J. Conolly, *The Construction and Government of Lunatic Asylums* (1847; reprint ed., London: Dawsons, 1968), p. 175.
13. Conolly, *Treatment*, pp. 300–302.
14. J. S. Zainaldin and P. L. Tyor, "Asylum and Society: An Approach to Indus-trial Change," *Journal of Social History* 13 (1979–80): 23–25; Scull, *Museums of Madness*, pass.
15. Zainaldin and Tyor, "Asylum and Society," pp. 24–25.
16. Scull, *Museums of Madness*, pp. 113–24, 164–204.
17. Conolly, *Construction*, p. 84.
18. Walk, "Mental Nursing," pp. 6–9; J. T. Arlidge, *On the State of Lunacy and the Legal Provision for the Insane* (London: Churchill, 1859), pp. 105–9.
19. Scull, *Museums of Madness*, chaps. 4–6.
20. Ibid., p. 123; Jones, *Lunacy*, pp. 160–68; *PP* 1859, p. iii, Select Committee on Lunatics, Q. 1498–1548.
21. Jones, *Lunacy*, pp. 116–17, 122–23.
22. Lancaster Public Library (hereafter cited as LPL), Moor Hospital file, extract from *Lonsdale Magazine*, 1821.

23. Jones, *Lunacy*, pp. 121, 151.
24. *Lancaster Gazette*, 3 July 1824.
25. LPL, Medical Officers' Report for 1841, p. 4; Lancashire Record Office, Preston (hereafter cited as LRO), QAM/5/3, pp. 18–20.
26. LRO, QAM/1/33/11, 23 November 1836, 20 January 1839; *Preston Pilot*, 29 February 1840.
27. LRO, QAM/1/33/11, 17 January 1838.
28. Jones, *Lunacy*, p. 122.
29. LRO, QAM/5/39, p. 6.
30. LRO, QAM/1/33/11, pass.
31. LRO, QAM/5/39, p. 4.
32. LRO, QAM/1/33/11, 16 August 1839.
33. LRO, QAM/5/19, table 4.
34. LRO, QAM/1/33/11, 9 February 1837.
35. LRO, HRL/1/1.
36. LRO, QAM/1/30/15; HRL/1/10.
37. LRO, HRL/1/1, cases of Sarah Goodier, John Aspinall.
38. *Lancaster Gazette*, 22 October 1832.
39. LRO, QAM/1/33/11, 1 September 1839; *Lancaster Guardian*, 8 August 1840; Jones, *Lunacy*, p. 123.
40. Jones, *Lunacy*, pp. 116–26; Andrew Scull, "Museums of Madness: The Social Organization of Insanity in Nineteenth-Century England" (Ph.D. diss., Princeton University, 1974), p. 110; Bolton, "Wakefield," pp. 596–600, 604–5, 613–22.
41. Conolly, *Construction*, p. 7.
42. *Lancaster Guardian*, 29 February 1840; *Lancaster Gazette*, 11 December 1839.
43. Conolly, *Construction*, introduction to 1968 edition by R. Hunter and I. MacAlpine, p. 26.
44. Ibid., pp. 25–29, and text pp. 129–30; Scull, *Museums of Madness*, pp. 173–77; Bolton, "Wakefield," pp. 590–96.
45. LRO, QAM/5/39, p. 8.
46. LRO, QAM/5/39; QAM/5/38, 1846 Rules; LPL, 1841 Report, p. 11; R. Hindle, *An Account of the Expenditure of the County Palatine of Lancaster* (1843), p. 239.
47. Conolly, *Construction*, pass.
48. LPL, 1841 Report, p. 9.
49. LRO, HRL/1/10.
50. LRO, HRL/1/11.
51. Note the flexibility of the 1846 Rules, LRO, QAM/5/38, with regard to the use of airing grounds (General mangement, 8: airing grounds to be accessible for at least three hours, morning and evening, weather permitting), and visits (General management, 13).
52. LRO, QAM/5/19, table 4.
53. LPL, 1844 Report, p. 6; LRO, QAM/1/33/11, 17 September 1850; QAM/5/1, p. 6.
54. Scull, *Museums of Madness*, pp. 116–17.

55. LRO, QAM/5/40, pp. 6–7; QAM/1/29/4.

56. LRO, QAM/5/1.

57. Cf. Scull, *Museums of Madness*, pp. 123–24. Lancaster may have been unusually fortunate in this respect.

58. LRO, QAM/5/42; LPL, pt. 688, Gaskell to the chairman of visiting justices.

59. LRO, QAM/5/39, pp. 19–20; QAM/5/38, Resident Medical Officer, Rule 10.

60. Conolly, *Treatment*, introduction to 1973 edition by R. Hunter and I. MacAlpine, pp. xxx–xxxv; Scull, *Museums of Madness*, chap. 5.

61. LRO, QAM/1/33/11, 25 May 1840.

62. Hindle, *Expenditure*, pp. 156–59; Arlidge, *On the State of Lunacy*, p. 105, quoted in Scull, *Museums of Madness*, pp. 176–77.

63. LRO, QAM/5/1, pp. 5, 14, 20.

64. Hindle, *Expenditure*, pp. 238–39.

65. LRO, QAM/1/33/8, 1844–46.

66. *Lancaster Guardian*, 11 July 1840.

67. LRO, QAM/5/40, pp. 3–4; QAM/5/42, p. 6; Conolly, *Construction*, pp. 129–30. Conolly specifically mentions the work of De Vitré in this context, and it is clear that he played an active part alongside Gaskell in the introduction of the new regime.

68. Scull, *Museums of Madness*, p. 121.

69. LPL, 1842 Report, p. 5; 1844 Report, p. 8.

70. LPL, 1842 Report, p. 8; but 1841 Report stresses that showers were not to be used as a punishment.

71. LRO, QAM/1/33/11, 13 September 1847, 29 August 1848; HRL/1/10, case of Joseph Singleton.

72. LRO, HRL/1/16, case of Jane Cane.

73. Conolly, *Treatment*, pp. 44–47; cf. LPL, 1841 Report.

74. Conolly, *Construction*, pp. 83–86; Arlidge, *On the State of Lunacy*, pp. 104–9.

75. Arlidge, *On the State of Lunacy*, p. 105.

76. Conolly, *Treatment*, p. 95.

77. LRO, QAM/5/39, p. 14; LPL, 1841 Report, pp. 7, 12.

78. LRO, QAM/5/39, p. 10.

79. P. Bailey, "Will the Real Bill Banks Please Stand Up?" *Journal of Social History* 12 (1978–79): 336–53.

80. LPL, 1841 Report, p. 12; LRO, QAM/5/42; QAM/5/38, General Management, Rules 11 and 12.

81. LRO, QAM/1/33/11, 25 October 1842, 29 August 1848.

82. LRO, QAM/5/38, General Management, Rule 3.

83. Conolly, *Construction*, p. 83.

84. LRO, QAM/5/38, Committee of Visitors, Rule 15.

85. P. J. Gooderson, "The Social and Economic History of Lancaster, 1780–1914" (Ph.D. diss., Lancaster University, 1975), pp. 160–91.

86. LRO, QAM/5/42.

87. Hindle, *Expenditure*, p. 161.

88. LRO, QAM/1/38, 3 March 1857.

89. J. Burnett, *Plenty and Want* (London: Nelson, 1968), chaps. 3 and 8.

90. LRO, QAM/5/1, p. 22. R. Hunter and I. MacAlpine, *Psychiatry for the Poor* (London: Dawsons, 1974), p. 93, provide similar figures for Colney Hatch.
91. LRO, QAM/1/33/8, year beginning 19 August 1843.
92. LRO, QAM/5/38, Committee of Visitors, Rule 15; Resident Medical Officer, Rules 2–3.
93. Cf. Conolly, *Treatment*, p. xxxii, for Conolly's difficulties at Hanwell.
94. LRO, QAM/1/33/8.
95. Public Record Office (hereafter cited as PRO) HO.107/2272.
96. Conolly, *Construction*, p. 85.
97. LPL, 1841 Report, p. 11.
98. Conolly, *Treatment*, p. 98. The problem of the recruitment of suitable attendants runs parallel to the similar difficulties experienced in obtaining turnkeys and constables for the reformed prison and police services. The asylum attendant was clearly a cut above the police constable in the Lancashire of the 1840s, but the position of the prison service is more obscure. See E. C. Midwinter, *Social Administration in Lancashire 1830–60* (Manchester: Manchester University Press, 1971), pp. 158–60; M. Ignatieff, *A Just Measure of Pain: The Penitentiary in the Industrial Revolution 1750–1850* (New York: Pantheon, 1978), pp. 191–92; Frances Finnegan, *Poverty and Prostitution* (Cambridge: Cambridge University Press, 1979), pp. 63–65, 122, 147–49.
99. Calculated from LRO, QAM/5/19, table 4.
100. Scull, *Museums of Madness*, pp. 188–94; LRO, QAM/5/39, pp. 19–20; QAM/5/40, pp. 6–7.
101. LRO, QAM/1/29/4.
102. Hindle, *Expenditure*, p. 238.
103. LRO, QAM/5/7, p. 9.
104. LRO, QAM/1/38, 5 January 1858, 20 November 1860.
105. LRO, QAM/5/3, p. 20; QAM/5/8, p. 17.
106. LRO, QAM/5/17, pp. 12–13; QAM/5/12, p. 21.
107. LRO, QAM/5/8, p. 9; QAM/5/7, p. 9; QAM/1/38, 26 December 1863.
108. LRO, QAM/5/15, p. 8.
109. LRO, QAM/5/7, pp. 9–10; QAM/1/38, 19 December 1868.
110. LRO, QAM/5/8, pp. 17–18; QAM/5/12, p. 21.
111. LRO, QAM/5/8, p. 17.
112. LRO, QAM/5/7, p. 11.
113. LRO, QAM/5/6, p. 17; QAM/5/14, p. 14; QAM/5/12, pp. 18–19.
114. LRO, QAM/5/15, p. 15; QAM/5/17, p. 11; QAM/5/18, p. 14.
115. LRO, QAM/5/15, p. 12; QAM/5/17, pp. 10–11.
116. LRO, QAM/5/2, p. 15.
117. LRO, QAM/5/10, pp. 17–18.
118. LRO, QAM/5/2, p. 31.
119. LRO, QAM/5/10, p. 13.
120. LRO, QAM/5/15, p. 12.
121. LRO, QAM/5/17, pp. 10–11.
122. LRO, HRL/2/5, HRL/3/4.
123. LRO, QAM/5/4, p. 16; and cf. QAM/5/15, p. 24, which shows that only 3 of the 68 patients discharged in 1866 had been more than five years in the asylum.
124. LRO, QAM/5/3, pp. 18–20.

125. LRO, QAM/5/10, p. 11; QAM/5/19, pp. 12–13.
126. *Lancaster Guardian,* 5 March 1870.
127. Ibid., and 15 January 1870.
128. Ibid., 15 January 1870; LRO, QAM/1/37, 26 March 1870.
129. LRO, QAM/1/37, 26 March 1870.
130. *PP,* 1871, p. xxvi, Twenty-fifth Report of the Commissioners in Lunacy, pp. 165–66.
131. Scull, *Museums of Madness,* chap. 6.
132. LRO, QAM/5/19, table 4; QAM/5/14, p. 18.
133. LRO, QAM/5/16, p. 13.
134. LRO, QAM/1/38, 4 October 1864.
135. Conolly, *Treatment,* pp. xxxiv–v.
136. LRO, QAM/5/7, p. 9.
137. Cf. Scull, *Museums of Madness,* pp. 250–52.
138. Calculated from the admissions registers. The two-month category includes admissions whose illnesses were said to be of unknown duration.
139. J. K. Walton, "Lunacy and the Industrial Revolution: A Study of Asylum Admissions in Lancashire, 1848–50," *Journal of Social History* 13 (1979–80): 12; LRO, QAM/1/29/5.
140. LRO, QAM/5/19, table 4.
141. Calculated from the census enumerators' books: PRO, HO.107/2272; RG.10/4232.
142. LRO, QAM/5/4, p. 15; QAM/5/10, pp. 16–17.
143. LRO, QAM/1/38, 26 December 1863.
144. LRO, QAM/1/38, 26 December 1866, 2 February 1869; QAM/5/19, p. 18.
145. LRO, QAM/5/8, p. 12; QAM/5/9, p. 63.
146. Gooderson, "Lancaster," p. 196.
147. LRO, QAM/5/19, pp. 32–34; S. G. Checkland, *The Rise of Industrial Society in England 1815–85* (London: Penguin, 1971), p. 229; LRO, QAM/1/38, July and August 1860, August–October 1866; QAM/1/37, August and September 1870.
148. LRO, QAM/1/38, 1 November 1864.
149. LRO, QAM/1/38, 3 May 1864.
150. *Lancaster Guardian,* from 14 May 1870.
151. *Lancaster Guardian,* 8 January 1870, 5 March 1870; LRO, QAM/1/38, 3 August 1869.
152. LRO, QAM/5/15, p. 14; QAM/5/17, p. 18; QAM/5/18, pp. 18–19.
153. Bolton, "Wakefield," p. 617; Hunter and MacAlpine, *Psychiatry for the Poor,* p. 86.
154. *PP,* 1859, p. iii, Select Committee on Lunatics, evidence of S. Gaskell, Q. 1503–27.
155. Cf. Parry-Jones, *Trade in Lunacy,* pass.

PART THREE
Changes in the Profession and Its Orientation

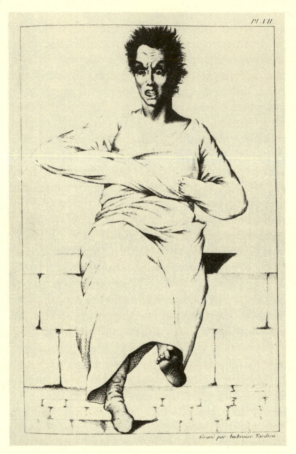

"A Case of Mania"

This woman in her late thirties was one of Esquirol's patients at the Saltpetrière. In his notes on the case, Esquirol commented that "everything in this woman conveys the highest degree of disturbance of the intellect and the affections together with the most violent rage.... Her animated though cross-eyed gaze gives the physiognomy of this maniac a character which perfectly reflects the disorder and exultation of her ideas and emotions." On admission to the Saltpetrière on 29 June 1813, in the throes of her second attack of madness, she "was extremely emaciated, with a very dark complexion, constantly loquacious, her delirium was all-embracing, she had numerous hallucinations, shouted obscenities, uttered threats, was violent; the sick woman broke everything she could lay her hands on, tore off her clothes, remained nude, rolled around on the ground, sang, danced, shouted, rejected whatever food was offered to her." After a long period of confinement, she was eventually discharged as recovered.

(Source: Jean Etienne Dominique Esquirol, *Des Maladies Mentales* [Paris: J. B. Baillière, 1838] 2:160–62 and plate 7.)

William Ll. Parry-Jones

8 The Model of the Geel Lunatic Colony and Its Influence on the Nineteenth-Century Asylum System in Britain

The story of the lunatic colony at Geel begins in the darkness and mists of Ireland in the late sixth century. The king of Ireland had a gentle and beautiful wife, Odilla, who became a Christian through the influence of Gereberne, a priest. The king and queen had a daughter, Dymphna. Her birth was a disappointment to her father, who had her removed and placed by Odilla in Gereberne's care. Later, Odilla died and the king was deeply distressed. Such was his grief that, finally, he ordered a search for another woman exactly resembling his late queen. After much fruitless searching, his men decided to find Dymphna, who, by this time, had the appearance and all the beauty of her mother. When Dymphna met her father, the king denied their relationship and claimed her for his bride. Faced with the prospect of an incestuous union, Dymphna fled with Gereberne. Finally, they settled in the forests near the community of Geel, in the country that is now Belgium, and here she decided to dedicate herself to devotion and celibacy. But the old pagan king followed and discovered the fugitives. Again, Dymphna refused to marry him, and her continued obstinacy made the savage monarch furious. He attacked her, severing her head from her body, and his soldiers decapitated Gereberne. It is reputed that these cruel deeds so greatly frightened several lunatics who witnessed them that they became cured, as if by enchantment. In this way, Dymphna, who had resisted the spirit of evil, was seen ever afterward as the patron of demented victims; later, miraculous cures took place at the scene of her martyrdom.[1]

There are many versions of this legend and, if that recounted here is not the authentic one, it has, at least, the merit of very colorful detail. Some versions simply describe Dymphna's refusal to abandon Christian beliefs as the reason for her flight, but her murder is a common feature and it is an interesting fact that saints martyred by beheading do acquire particular powers over disorders of the head. The belief in the occurrence of miraculous cures at Geel spread far and wide. Dymphna's church was founded in 1349, but it seems likely that the Dymphna cult had been active, even as early as the mid-thirteenth century.[2] Initially, the cure appears to have been for many kinds of afflictions, but from the second half of the fourteenth century on, Geel became a special place of pilgrimage for lunatics, who sought a cure through Dymphna's intercession. At first, pilgrims appear to have been sheltered in chambers adjoining the church or lodged with the local population. However, in 1480 a sick room was built close by the church. In 1532, a college of ten clerics was established in relation to the church, and they were entrusted with the care of the sick. Later, this was enlarged to a chapter of ten canons, who directed the religious services. An elaborate ritual of ceremonial offerings, penances, processions, and prayers was established. In the first instance, these rituals lasted for nine days. Unless the lunatic's condition was improved at the end of this time, the treatment continued for another nine days. If, by this stage, the evil spirits had not been exorcised, the lunatics could remain with a family near the church, to be cared for and allowed to participate in further prayers and invocations at the shrine. Throughout the ceremonies, which took place in the rooms adjoining the tower, the lunatic was closely chained by wrist and ankle and was tied down in a wooden bed at night. In 1687, a new sick room was built on the south side of the church tower. However, this provision proved insufficient for the influx of pilgrims, and accommodation was increased by housing them with local inhabitants. Once having settled in the vicinity, many lunatics began to stay on in Geel indefinitely.

In this way, a large number of lunatics began to congregate in the area, with considerable implications for the town and neighborhood of Geel. Between 1676 and 1754, the local council issued three sets of regulations concerning the supervision of the lunatics and the relationships between the civil and ecclesiastical authorities. In 1797, the Church of St. Dymphna was closed by the French revolutionary armies, and, thereafter, care at Geel became increasingly secular. Major legislative changes also followed in the wake of the Revolution, and, in 1803, legislation that regularized the custody of lunatics was introduced. It is a familiar story, however, to find that such early legislation was not adhered to strictly, and it is recorded that in the opening years of the century lunatics were illegally in residence at Geel.

Little is known about conditions in Geel at the start of the nineteenth century. Some sources suggest that the communal administration simply treated the accommodation of lunatics as a business, extolling the economic advantages that Geel offered. According to Dr. J. Parigot, who later became superintendent of the colony, when inspectors were first appointed in 1803, the lunatics had been treated perhaps even more cruelly than the Negroes he had seen in South America.[3] The legislation of 1803 provided for a regular system of inspection by representatives of the patients' communes, but their interference was opposed fiercely by the council of the commune. Consequently, effective controls were minimal until further legislative reform of 1850 transferred responsibility for the colony from commune authorities to the state government.[4]

Esquirol was the first to draw the attention of the scientific world to Geel in his "Des Maladies Mentales," a book he wrote after visiting the colony in 1821.[5] He found between four hundred and five hundred lunatics, both males and females, who wandered freely in the streets and countryside, without anyone seeming to supervise them. Various means of mechanical restraint were noted to be in use for patients who were furious or those who tried to escape, and it did not appear that any medical means of treatment were employed. In 1828, Sir Andrew Halliday wrote about a visit he had made to "Gheil" and was obviously impressed by the experience. He recorded that

> if the governors of St. Luke's were to form such an establishment, upon some of the heaths or commons that are no great distance from the metropolis, they would more effectually, I imagine, fulfil the intentions of the benevolent supporters and contributors to this institution, than by transferring their supposed incurables, after a twelve months' trial, to the white and red houses at Bethnal Green, as very uniformly has hitherto been their practice for a number of years past. And that such an establishment might be formed at a very small expense, must be apparent to all who will give themselves the trouble to think on the subject.[6]

W. A. F. Browne, of the Crichton Royal Institution, who was well known for his monograph "What Asylums Were, Are, and Ought to Be," visited Geel in 1838, claiming to be the first British doctor to do so. His reports about Geel were dismal.[7] Brierre de Boismont visited Geel in 1846, and, like Browne, he found no evidence of physical and moral treatment of patients.[8] After this time, a stream of visitors began to make their own pilgrimages to Geel, reporting their visits in the scientific journals of the day. The first reports in English journals were made in 1857, by John Webster, in the *Journal of Psychological Medicine*, and in 1858, by Henry Stevens, in the *Journal of Mental Science*.[9] The number of such reports proliferated, and in the first thirty-eight volumes of the *Journal of Mental Science*, 1853–92, there were over twenty indexed references to Geel. More popular accounts also appeared, such as that written by the intrepid traveler, Mrs. William Pitt Byrne.[10] By the end of the century, therefore, Geel had developed a voluminous literature of its own.

It is clear that in the first half of the nineteenth century conditions at

Geel left much to be desired and, as Browne stated in 1861, "The humane impulse which has changed the condition of the lunatic in many lands was late in reaching West Flanders."[11] But, by mid-century, when there were approximately one thousand lunatics at Geel, a slow transition was made from the cult of Dymphna to a more orthodox medical administration and care. In 1851, a royal commission was appointed to inspect asylums in Belgium. In the following year, the colony became a state institution and nonecclesiastical medical directors were officially appointed, the first being Dr. J. Parigot. Further developments and changes continued to be made at Geel, where the family-care system of treating mental patients has remained a vocation to the present day.[12] The number of patients in the town increased steadily, reaching a peak of 3,736 in 1938.[13]

In 1856, Dr. Bulckens took over as superintendent of the colony. At this time, the commune of Geel had approximately eleven thousand inhabitants, of whom four thousand lived in the town itself. The commune covered twenty-seven thousand acres and measured 14 by 8 miles. For the purposes of administering the colony, the commune was divided into four sections, each of which had an assistant physician, an apothecary, and a guard or inspector. There was a medical superintendent for the whole establishment, and he was assisted by a surgeon. The patients were entrusted to householders, the *nourriciers,* each being allocated up to three patients, with males and females being lodged in separate houses. The classification of patients always appears to have been based on pragmatic rather than nosological considerations, and under Bulckens's superintendency the whole organization was further refined.[14] Tranquil patients and many of those who paid the highest fees lived in the center of the village. The others were arranged in four cordons in surrounding hamlets. In the innermost cordon were those who required special care. Next came imbeciles, idiots, the maimed, the demented, and those of dirty habits. Then came the epileptics, who were placed in areas where there was no danger from brooks and pools. In the outermost cordon of remotely situated farms and cottages were the violent and the furious. Here, they would be safe and cause the least amount of annoyance to the rest of the community. A new central infirmary was built in 1858, which could accommodate sixty lunatics, and was used for initial assessment and for more specialized care.

During the period of Bulckens's superintendency, intake to Geel was not intended to be comprehensive, and clear limitations were set on entry. Actively suicidal, homicidal, or mischievously disposed patients were rarely received or allowed to remain long. Instead, they were transferred elsewhere to a more appropriate asylum.[15] Henry Stevens, medical superintendent of St. Luke's Hospital, London, who visited Geel in 1856, found the residents to be, "almost without exception, . . . the subjects of dementia, harmless chronic mania, brooding habitual melancholia, or helpless para-

lytics or epileptics."[16] Not unexpectedly, visitors' reports in the 1850s indicated that Geel was not a curative establishment. Stevens reported that
of the 905 patients who were under treatment in 1856, 29 were cured and
10 relieved. He added, "This is a success hardly to be envied by our asylum
superintendents." This was a somewhat overconfident claim, bearing in
mind the very low percentage of curable patients who were in British
asylums a decade later. In fact, when Webster revisited in 1866, he found
more encouraging evidence, that is, about a quarter of the patients who
were admitted in the preceding ten years were cured.[17] A further significant fact was that nearly 70 percent of the 436 patients deemed curable on
admission were eventually discharged. Similar figures continued to be
reported, and by the 1890s, for example, 21 percent of admissions were
being discharged as recovered.[18] Such statistics are notoriously difficult to
interpret, but they do, at least, indicate a general trend toward a more
clearly therapeutic orientation within the colony.

At the present, the institution is controlled by the Ministry of Public
Health and is known officially as Rijkspsychiatrisch Ziekenhuis-Centrum
voor Gezinsverpleging ("State Psychiatric Hospital-Center for Family
Care"). Information supplied by the Hospital indicates that in 1970 it
catered for about 1,700 patients of whom 60 percent were subnormal, 30
percent psychotic, and 10 percent suffering from organic brain disorders.[19]
Over a thousand patients were boarded out among host families, and the
remainder stayed in the central infirmary. The standard practice is to have
two patients of the same sex and about the same age in a family. Close
supervision is maintained by doctors and nurses, enabling smooth inter-
change between foster families and the central infirmary. It is generally
accepted that the institution functions most successfully in the management of chronically disabled patients, who may find at Geel a supportive
environment for a lifetime.[20]

Since many of the reports of the nineteenth-century visitors to Geel
were lengthy and verbose, it is a difficult task to summarize their findings
usefully and to extract significant conclusions. Moreover, these reports
describe an evolving institution viewed through the eyes of visitors from
many different countries. The visitors were, for the most part, accustomed
to widely discrepant methods of managing the insane. Not unnaturally,
the most critical were the superintendents of established, leading asylums,
who warned that those visitors without experience of asylum management
might be misled by the merits of Geel and believe that they had stumbled
across "the apotheosis of all that modern education and civilization could
produce in the way of psychiatry."[21] William Letchworth, president of the
New York State Board of Charities, concluded that "the Gheel system is
of little practical value to America, except as demonstrating that a great
amount of freedom is possible in the care of certain classes of the insane."[22]

Many of the early visitors reported that they found the accommodations in the cottages and farms to be dirty and squalid. Certainly, there were no baths outside the central infirmary, which led Stevens to record that "the rooms and persons of the patients give evidence to the enquiring nose of anything but freshness and salubrity." However, little attempt was made to evaluate such conditions in the context of the standards of ordinary cottage life elsewhere in that part of Europe or in England. Similarly, the peasant dietary was often commented on adversely, and the use of mechanical restraint in a colony that emphasized liberty was always seen as paradoxical. Stevens found ninety-three patients in restraint and spoke of "the helpless, purposeless, wandering imbecile . . . fettered like the hedge-side vagrant donkey."[23] By the 1860s, however, the number of patients under restraint does not appear to have been abnormally high. The presence of patients who seemed basically unsuitable for the "free-air" treatment was usually remarked upon, often coupled with comments about the risks of offenses being committed against morality and propriety. There were worries about illegitimate births among the patients and fears of assaults by them.[24] But the recurring and fundamental objections were concerned with the lack of medical supervision and systematic, disinterested nursing care, services which would normally be provided in well-run asylums. Numerous examples were cited of deranged or infirm patients who were receiving no active treatment. Medical treatment as such was minimal, and Bulckens acknowledged to Stevens in 1857 that it was not used, "except in so far as the colonial bowels required moving, or the chance exhibition of expectorants or demulcents when fogs prevailed in that uncomfortable looking plain."[25] Using arguments that were well rehearsed against private asylum proprietors, doubts were cast on the possibility of achieving consistently humane care in the households of the *nourriciers* who were paid for the job. Frequent concern was expressed about the excessive importance of religion and superstition in the treatment of the mentally ill, coupled with the persistent significance of the ordeal of Dymphna.

The advantages of the Geel colony were always more difficult to pinpoint than the demonstrable abuses. This is to be expected since the advantages had to do with the absence of what were regarded as the adverse features of contemporary asylums, which Griesinger expressively called "barracking." The merits, therefore, were concerned with the concept of liberty, literally in the "free air," the absence of restraint, and the possibility of living a happier, healthier, and more useful home life than in the traditional asylum. In addition, there were specific benefits such as the greater possibility of employing lunatics in occupations of a kind previously pursued and allowing patients to have a more familiar life-style than that permitted in the asylum which was part palace, part barrack, and part prison. These benefits were especially important during convalescence. A further recommendation was that the regime was much more economical than that followed in conventional asylums. However, significantly, this merit was accorded little praise by many of the visiting county asylum superintendents.

Despite the divergent opinions about the merits and demerits of the regime at Geel, it is indisputable that it provided a prototype for an alternative approach in the care of the chronic insane to that offered traditionally within the asylum system. It was this feature that drew visitors to the colony and continued to capture their imaginations. The approach at Geel was based on the dispersion of chronic lunatics rather than on their sequestration in asylums. It was this clear distinction that polarized opinion sharply and often bitterly. The development of the asylum system in Britain was shaped largely by the dual problems of containing the insane who were poor and managing the insane from the middle and upper classes in private asylums and public-subscription hospitals, a problem which presented very different issues. The ethos and system of care of private asylums were based on an essentially domestic family model.[26] Sibbald, writing in 1861, suggested that "the most complete illustrations of the best form of cottage treatment, are met with in a small and good private asylum for the higher classes."[27] But few contemporary observers were as perceptive in acknowledging the merits of the private system of care.

By the beginning of the second half of the nineteenth century, it was becoming abundantly clear that the problem of pauper lunacy was not being contained by the county asylums. The common experience in most asylums was that, despite careful planning to meet the estimated demands, they became overcrowded rapidly and additional accommodation had to be built every few years. The asylums were literally besieged by previously unheard of applicants for admission, who formed an increasingly heterogeneous group of lunatics, idiots, epileptics, paralytics, the elderly, and the physically infirm, many of whom had spent long periods in workhouses. The proportion of curable pauper lunatics in county asylums declined rapidly, and from 1844 to 1870, for example, the proportion of curable patients fell from 15 percent to 7 percent.[28] Therapeutic optimism was at a low ebb, and the outcome was that asylums settled down as understaffed, overcrowded establishments, in buildings whose very size and appearance spoke of authority and repression. Some contemporary observers sounded the alarm. In a thoughtfully reasoned account of the adverse effects of huge asylums, J. T. Arlidge, formerly of St. Luke's Hospital, observed that

> many asylums have grown to such a magnitude, that their general management is unwieldy, and their due medical and moral care and supervision an impossibility. They have grown into lunatic colonies

of eight or nine hundred, or even of a thousand or more inhabitants, comfortably lodged and clothed, fed by a not illiberal commissariat, watched and waited on by well-paid attendants, disciplined and drilled to a well-ordered routine, gratified by entertainments, and employed where practicable, and, on the whole, considered as paupers, very well off; but in the character of patients, labouring under a malady very amenable to treatment, if not too long neglected, far from receiving due consideration and care.

Further, he cautioned that "in a colossal refuge for the insane, a patient may be said to lose his individuality, and to become a member of a machine. . . . In all cases admitting of recovery, or a material amelioration, a gigantic asylum is a gigantic evil, and, figuratively speaking, a manufactory of chronic insanity."[29] These prophetic words were followed by constructive proposals for remedying the situation, including the distribution of certain patients in cottage homes. But by the 1860s the pace of large-scale institutional confinement was still accelerating. The time was ripe, therefore, in the 1850s and 1860s for a tidal wave of doubt about the efficacy and desirability of the asylum system. Alternative approaches were examined, tried out, and vigorously debated. It was in this context that the Geel colony offered an appealing model.

In England, J. C. Bucknill, superintendent of the Devon County Asylum, experimented with two ways of relieving the pressure on his overcrowded asylum, by opening a temporary branch asylum and by housing patients in cottages in the neighborhood. The removal of forty-two patients from the Devon County Asylum to a seaside house lasted a year, from 1856 to 1857, while a new building was being constructed at the asylum.[30] At the time, this was a bold experiment, which proved that the redundant population of an asylum could be disposed of temporarily under less institutional conditions. The whole enterprise was of great interest, but particularly significant was the alarm voiced by the local residents, who petitioned the secretary of state against the move. Subsequent events would be familiar to anyone who has been involved in new developments within the community involving the mentally ill or deviant members of society. The objections were the following:

> That the existence of the pauper lunatic asylum at Exmouth would prevent invalids and tourists visiting the town as a marine watering place; that the hotels and houses let as lodgings would be unoccupied; that the value of house property would be greatly deteriorated; that the residents would be distressed and terrified by painful scenes, and that in taking their usual walks upon the beach and the sands, they would be in danger from the violence of the patients whom they would meet.[31]

In fact, the fears were groundless. The summer seasons of 1856 and 1857 were unaffected, and later, it was agreed that opposition to the asylum had been mistaken. Bucknill was encouraged by the experiment, and he saw the "free social life, differing little from a large private family," of the Exmouth asylum as an essential ingredient of progress.

Bucknill's innovative work in developing what was called "the English cottage system" was directly associated with the model of Geel. Patients were discharged on trial from the asylum and boarded with neighboring cottagers who were selected as being trustworthy. Many of these householders were attendants, domestics, or artisans at the asylum, and Bucknill felt that this greatly improved their qualifications for the work. Bucknill visited the patients regularly and carefully selected chronically dependent or convalescent patients for this type of care. The underlying reasons for adopting this program were due partly to pressure on the asylum facilities but also because Bucknill felt that patients would be happier and more useful in this setting. He likened the experiments to the work of the Geel colony and called for an impartial trial in this country of the cottage system, which he saw as an adjunct to the asylum system.

Others echoed Bucknill's sentiment, and various plans were put forward. The superintendent of the Gloucester Lunatic Asylum, in 1864, considered that the cottage system was the best means for treating the insane, and he proposed a plan for a colony comprising twenty-nine cottages.[32] Webster, in 1865, reported a plan, at the Inverness District Asylum, that he likened to "the Gheel system." It was proposed that there should be cottages in the grounds for married attendants and their families, in whose charge would be placed patients who would be "treated like ordinary members of such households, taking part also in the customary domestic arrangements."[33] The design of asylum cottages became a new area of interest, and Baron Mundy of Vienna, one of the chief European protagonists of the cottage system, erected a fully equipped model cottage, at his own expense, in the Paris exhibition of 1867. It had two parts, one for the attendant's family, and the other for the patients, with a bedroom, bathroom, and padded room.[34] Some enthusiasts suggested more radical developments. W. Lauder Lindsay, physician to the Murray Royal Hospital, Perth, for example, proposed the construction in Scotland of one or more "National Colonies on the Gheel plan," although his ideas did not find favor with the authorities.[35]

Approaches analogous with the system prevailing in Geel came to be viewed collectively as the "family system," and for a time, developments within this system focused attention on Scotland. The practice that aroused attention was that of boarding out pauper lunatics with strangers. Although this practice was widespread, particular villages in certain parts of the country were more heavily used than others, which led them to be referred to as "Geels of the North." These villages included Kennoway, in Fife; Balfron, in Sterling; Aberfoyle, in Perth; and Loanhead, near Edinburgh. In addition, boarding took place extensively in the Shetlands and on the island of Arran. Visitors trooped through these villages, much as they did at Geel, and, for a time, the pages of the *Journal of Mental Science* and the *Journal of Psychological Medicine* reflected the exceptional interest aroused. It was something of a misconception, in fact, to view the Scottish boarding out regime as a specialized system of family care. After all, the boarding of single lunatics, both private and pauper, had been and remained common practice in England and Wales. The main difference in Scotland was the aggregation of relatively large numbers of lunatics in one locality. Kennoway, which received most of its boarders from Edinburgh, was the best documented "Scottish Geel," and rather stereotyped and often acrimonious debates took place about what was to be found there. When J. B. Tuke, of the Fife and Kinross Asylum, visited Kennoway in 1869, he found some twenty-five lunatics in "hovels" in a decaying village.[36] The patients were mainly dements and idiots. He noted the regular visits of the Deputy Commissioner in Lunacy and the parochial surgeons and inspectors. He also acknowledged that the system was cheaper than conventional asylum care. But he concluded in an outspoken way that all the patients would have been better off in asylums. In fact, this was not the view of Dr. Arthur Mitchell, one of the Deputy Commissioners in Lunacy for Scotland. In 1870, Mitchell reported on the use of houses with special licenses to accommodate patients, and he provided a very detailed account of the group of houses at Kennoway, where thirty-one patients had been boarded since licenses were first issued in 1863. With regard to the principal groups of houses, he concluded,

> Enough indeed has been seen and done at these places to show that it would be quite a possible thing to repeat in this country such an institution as that at Gheel; but in the present state of matters, and without the existence of some favouring circumstances which are not likely to arise, it would be unwise to attempt the creation of such an institution. It is better, in the meantime, to have several small groups than one large one. If the conditions of any particular group favour its development, these should be allowed to operate, but should not be unduly fostered.[37]

Other reports, like that of Professor Jolly of Strasbourg, in 1875, provided an optimistic view of family care of the insane in Scotland and discussed in a balanced way the merits of the system and the supervision of the Board of Lunacy.[38] However, as at Geel, the case against the system was easily made. It rested upon the poor selection of patients; inadequate supervision; the impossibility of obtaining consistently reliable custodians and the difficulties inherent in any training; the insufficiency of proper official inspection; the liability of improper treatment and the misuse of patients; and the fears of "moral injury" to the custodian's family, especially its younger members. Many critics made the point that only the impoverished were willing to accept boarders. When wages were high and employment constant, it did not pay persons of the laboring class to take in boarders. Certainly, it is true that in Fife, the decay of handloom weaving increased the number of cottagers who were eager to supplement their incomes. Clearly, there were abuses and scandals under this system. The colony on Arran was disbanded after the discovery of brutal treatment there, and even the inhabitants of Kennoway were moved to petition the General Board of Lunacy against the use of their village for boarding of the insane.[39] This petition made two particularly salient points. The first was that "the system of boarding out is founded upon a mistaken philanthropy, because the parties boarding them have no more regard for these imbeciles than to look upon them as paying objects"; the second point emphasized "the propriety and reasonable necessity for each parish providing within its own boundary accommodation for its own helpless creatures, and not to oppress with their imbecile men and women neighbouring communities." The last word in this debate perhaps could be left with the patients. In 1872, in the course of reviewing an article that was critical of the "out-door system" as practiced in Kennoway, Dr. T. W. McDowall,[40] of the Inverness District Asylum, remarked, "How astonished the patients in that quiet village would be could they understand the interest taken in them, and how well they would behave could they but believe that some people are anxious to make out that they are not fit for living outside an asylum, in which institution they would be happier, freer, and better cared for!"[41]

Elsewhere in Europe, other variants of the family system were tried out. In Belgium itself, an additional colony, initially regarded as an annex of Geel, was established at Lierneux, in the Ardennes, in 1884.[42] This was an entirely new development, and its very success refuted to some extent the claims that the Geel community had unique characteristics that could not be replicated. Another colony was established at Dun-sur-Auron, in the Département of Cher, France, in 1892.[43] A variety of specifically agricultural colonies for the insane were set up, for example, at Einum, in Germany, associated with the asylum at Hildesheim, and at the Fitz-James and Villers colonies, associated with the Clermont Asylum in France.[44] Similarly, colonies were opened in various parts of the United States and Canada, despite much criticism of the Geel system.[45]

In summary, the family system comprised several different models.[46] The colony proper was typified by those at Geel and at Lierneux, and it is well described by Bulckens's term *L'Asile Patronale*. Annexes to asylums were of two kinds. First, there were cottage asylums, with cottages in the grounds of asylums or in the vicinity, designed for the asylum staff who undertook to supervise chronic or convalescent patients. Second, there were the farm asylums or agricultural colonies like that at Fitz-James. Boarding out or the "Scotch System" involved the placement of single patients as boarders in licensed houses, in relatively small groups, not amounting to planned colonies.

In practice, the concept of a cottage, family, or colony system never gained ground in Britain. Bucknill's experiment only lasted a few years. Opposition from leading asylum psychiatrists was always too great, and even the proposal to set up a committee to consider the principle of the cottage system was rejected at the Annual General Meeting of the Association of the Medical Officers of Asylums and Hospitals for the Insane in 1862; one leading figure, Dr. Harrington Tuke, called the scheme "utopian and absurd."[47] Boarding out continued on a widespread scale, especially in areas remote from asylums and workhouses. In fact, placement in workhouses was considered to an increasing extent, much against the better judgment of the Lunacy Commissioners. In England and Wales, in 1870, 61.8 percent of pauper lunatics were in asylums, 23.5 percent in workhouses, and 14.7 percent boarded out.[48] In the late 1870s, the possibility was discovered, often with some surprise, that quiet, harmless patients, especially those who were "passed the procreative period of life," could be safely discharged home. Interim placements between asylum and home were discussed, and a significant development was the founding of the Mental After-care Association in 1879, with Bucknill as president and Lord Shaftesbury as patron.[49] But this association only had lukewarm support from asylum staff and its influence was trivial. The most durable developments were in the asylums themselves, where efforts were directed toward approximating asylum life to the domestic ideal. The concept of the open-door system, initiated in the Scottish asylums, gained ground, with greater liberty on parole, on trial leave, and a general minimizing of irksome and degrading restraints, coupled with increased useful employment in asylum farms and workshops. Much thought went into the design of new asylum buildings, the emphasis being on detached villas in the grounds. But when faced with the overwhelming problem of chronic insanity, the authorities always sought solutions within the asylum system. The reply to the ever-mounting pressure for accommodation continued to be phrased in bricks and mortar, as may be still seen in the huge, cheaply built, auxiliary asylums for incurable inmates that were built at Leavesden and Caterham in the 1860s.

The story of Geel began with the magic of Dymphna and was sustained by the compassion of the Geeloise peasants and the "free-air" treatment they provided. It is interesting to reflect on the question as to whether the flurry of excitement, the traveling, the enthusiastic support, and the antagonism generated by the Geel colony during the nineteenth century was of any avail. Certainly, by the end of the century, a fairly clear consensus had emerged that a considerable number of the chronic insane, universally housed in asylums, could be provided for outside, in accommodations that more closely resembled everyday life and where there was less restriction of personal liberty and freedom of movement. But the idea of relatively unsupervised management amongst strangers was never really acceptable. Despite their extreme concern about chronic lunatics, the Commissioners in Lunacy made their position quite clear. In 1873, for example, they noted, "The risk of placing such patients to board with strangers is so great that, in the existing state of the law, we think it would be unwise materially to extend the practice."[50] In this context, it is important to recall that the English asylum system was inspired and sustained by the ideology of reform, philanthropy, and nonrestraint. The near-phobia of abuse had a paralyzing effect, and superintendents and their committees believed that only constant vigilance could control violations of duty and abuse of humanity, even in asylums. How much easier it would be for neglect to occur in the cottage system, where the guardian's responsibility was so small, the temptation to fraud and tyranny so high, and the chances of detection, so few.

Many visitors to Geel found a new vision for the management of the chronic insane by combining domestic care in the cottages of the rural population with medical supervision. Was this vision, after all, just a Utopian ideal, just a mirage? Was it perhaps "the last glimpse of a mediaeval condition, incrusted with the stains and decay and corruption of a worn-out organization, where the faith in the supernatural had faded away, and the sun of science had not yet arisen?"[51] Or was the vision real, and still awaiting fulfillment? Contemporary psychiatrists and their colleagues still wrestle with the ambivalence that mental illness has always evoked and, in turn, perpetuate their own versions of the myth of community care. In this context, it is intriguing to note that the Geel Family Care Research Project originated in a decade colored by the antipsychiatry movement and continuing doubts about institutional treatment. As always, the regime at Geel is alluring, holding out the hope that its ancient practices can still serve as a model for an alternative system of psychiatric care in the community.

Notes

1. The insanity of the king is often mentioned, with suggestions that the martyred Dymphna not only forgave her murderous father, because of his madness, but also wished to relieve similar madness in others. See the version reported in William P. Letchworth, *The Insane in Foreign Countries* (New York and London: Putnam, 1889), pp. 242–43.
2. This historical summary is based on information from a variety of sources, including Roland Pierloot, "Belgium," in *World History of Psychiatry*, ed. John G. Howells (London: Baillière Tindall, 1975), pp. 136–49; Eugeen Roosens, *Mental Patients in Town Life: Geel—Europe's First Therapeutic Community* (Beverly Hills: Sage Publications, 1979). These works contain useful references to Belgian sources.
3. Report to the Brussels Society of Medical and Natural Sciences, 1859. See Foreign Psychological Literature, *Journal of Mental Science* 13 (1860): 600–602.
4. For a historical account of Belgian psychiatry, see Pierloot, "Belgium."
5. J. E. D. Esquirol, *Des maladies mentales, considérées sous les rapports médical, hygiénique et médico-légal,* 2 vols. (Paris: Baillière, 1838), 2:715–20, 21.
6. Andrew Halliday, *A General View of the Present State of Lunatics and Lunatic Asylums in Great Britain and Ireland and in Some Other Kingdoms* (London: Thomas and George Underwood, 1828), pp. 53–58.
7. He described dirty cottages and dark sickrooms in which many of the insane were chained in disgusting states of filth and degradation. W. A. F. Browne, "Cottage Asylums," *Medical Critic and Psychological Journal* 1 (1861): 213–37.
8. Ibid., p. 220.
9. John Webster, "Notes on Belgian Lunatic Asylums, Including the Insane Colony of Gheel," *Journal of Psychological Medicine and Mental Pathology* 10 (1857): 50–78, 209–47; Henry Stevens, "Insane Colony of Gheel," *Journal of Mental Science* 4 (1858): 426–37.
10. Mrs. William Pitt Byrne, *Gheel. The City of the Simple* (London: Chapman and Hall, 1869).
11. Browne, "Cottage Asylums," p. 216.
12. The town of Geel is in eastern Belgium, approximately 50 miles from Brussels and 25 miles from Antwerp, set in a plain of heaths and copses. It is a busy town with a population of about 30,000. It has a small museum and there is much of interest to be seen in the church, including a painting of 1639 that purports to depict part of the hospice as it was at that time. This painting has been described in detail by Goldin. The sick rooms on view today are a modern reconstruction of the third version, which, together with the church tower and roof, was demolished during World War II. Grace Goldin, "A Painting in Gheel," *Journal of the History of Medicine* 26 (1971): 400–412.

13. Roosens, *Mental Patients,* p. 31.
14. Dr. Bulckens died in 1876. See "The Late Dr. Bulckens, of Gheel," *Journal of Psychological Medicine and Mental Pathology* n.s. 3 (1877): 326–28.
15. Elsewhere in Belgium, the growth of other institutional provisions had followed a characteristic pattern. The ancient city hospitals, which made very limited provision for the insane, were followed by the rise of private madhouses and then by the foundation of new institutions in the mid-nineteenth century. These were administered almost entirely by religious orders. The standards achieved were never high and nineteenth-century Belgian psychiatry never acquired any special repute.
16. Stevens, "Insane Colony."
17. John Webster, "The Insane Colony of Gheel Revisited," *Journal of Mental Science* 12 (1867): 327–40.
18. John Sibbald, "Gheel and Lierneux, the Asylum-Colonies for the Insane in Belgium," *Journal of Mental Science* 43 (1897): 435–61.
19. See the following pamphlets issued by the hospital: "Colony for Family Care of Mental Patients, Geel"; "Colonie pour le traitement familial de malades mentaux, Geel."
20. There have been few accounts published in English of the organization and therapeutic milieu at Geel, but in the late 1960s, a collaborative Belgian and American research program, the Geel Family Care Research Project, was established. This was an extensive, multidisciplinary project, and recently, Roosens has reported about the social anthropological study of the interaction between Geelians and boarders in public community life. Roosens, *Mental Patients;* M. P. Dumont and C. K. Aldrich, "Family Care after a Thousand Years—A Crisis in the Tradition of St. Dymphna," *American Journal of Psychiatry* 119 (1962): 116–21; M. F. E. V. Doms, "The Geel Family Treatment," *British Journal of Social Psychiatry* 1 (1966): 299–303; Mary Hampson, "The Town That Cares," *World Medicine* 2 (1971): 17–23.
21. Stevens, "Insane Colony," p. 436.
22. Letchworth, *The Insane,* p. 278.
23. Stevens, "Insane Colony," p. 433.
24. Such fears were still being voiced by Letchworth in 1889, when he observed, "Looking at the commune in its moral aspect, one cannot help thinking that the shockingly immodest exhibitions which here and there meet the eye must have a baneful influence on the large number of children of both sexes growing up in their midst." Letchworth, *The Insane,* p. 278.
25. Stevens, "Insane Colony," p. 436.
26. William Ll. Parry-Jones, *The Trade in Lunacy. A Study of Private Madhouses in England in the Eighteenth and Nineteenth Centuries* (London: Routledge and Kegan Paul, 1972), p. 184.
27. John Sibbald, "The Cottage System and Gheel," *Journal of Mental Science* 7 (1861): 31–61. Relevant in this context is a report of outdoor occupations at the madhouse of Francis Willis Senior at Greatford, Lincolnshire: "As the unprepared traveller approached the town, he was astonished to find almost all the surrounding ploughmen, gardeners, threshers, thatchers and other labourers attired in black coats, white waistcoats, black silk breeches and stockings, and the head of each '*bien poudré, frisé, et arrangé.*' These were the doctor's patients,

and dress, neatness of person, and exercise being the principal features of his admirable system, health and cheerfulness conjoined to aid recovery of every person attached to that most valuable asylum." From *Life and Times of Frederick Reynolds*, cited by L. Melville, *Farmer George*, 2 vols. (London: Pitman, 1907), 2: 216–17. Reference is made to the lodging of patients at farms within 4 to 5 miles of this madhouse. *Bibliothèque Britannique (Littérature)* 1 (1796): 762.

28. Report of Metropolitan Commissioners in Lunacy, 1844, pp. 185–87; Twenty-fourth Report of the Commissioners in Lunacy, 1870, p. 97.

29. J. T. Arlidge, *On the State of Lunacy and the Legal Provision for the Insane, with Observations on the Construction and Organization of Asylums* (London: Churchill, 1859), pp. 102, 104.

30. J. C. Bucknill, "Description of the New House at the Devon County Lunatic Asylum, with Remarks upon the Sea Side Residence for the Insane, Which Was for a Time Established at Exmouth," *Journal of Mental Science* 4 (1858): 317–28.

31. Annual Reports of County Lunatic Asylums for 1856, *Journal of Mental Science* 3 (1857): 477–78.

32. E. Toller, "Suggestions for a Cottage Asylum," *Journal of Mental Science* 10 (1865): 342–49.

33. John Webster, "Rural Sites for Lunatic Asylums" (letter to the editor), *Lancet*, 11 November 1865, pp. 548–49.

34. "The Asylum Cottage at the Paris Exhibition," *Journal of Mental Science* 13 (1868): 425–26.

35. W. Lauder Lindsay, "The Family System as Applied to the Treatment of the Chronic Insane," *Journal of Mental Science* 16 (1871): 498.

36. J. B. Tuke, "The Cottage System of Management of Lunatics as Practised in Scotland, with Suggestions for Its Elaboration and Improvement," *Journal of Mental Science* 15 (1870): 524–35.

37. Appendix F., *General Reports on Single Patients by the Deputy Commissioners, 1. Report by Dr. Mitchell*, Twelfth Annual Report of the General Board of Commissioners in Lunacy for Scotland, 1870, pp. 250–68.

38. Friedrich Jolly, "On the Family Care of the Insane in Scotland," *Journal of Mental Science* 21 (1876): 40–60.

39. "Dr. Fraser on the Disadvantages of Boarding Out Certain Harmless Lunatics, and on the Advantages of 'Open Doors' in Asylums," *Journal of Mental Science* 24 (1878): 297–99.

40. T. W. McDowall, "American Psychological Literature: Hospital and Cottage Systems for the Care of the Insane," *Journal of Mental Science* 18 (1872): 132.

41. For a later account of the "Scotch System," see Letchworth, *The Insane*, pp. 130–41.

42. Sibbald, "Gheel and Lierneux," 1897.

43. "Notes and News," *Journal of Mental Science* 45 (1899): 205. See also J. Chantraine, "Evolution actuelle de placement familial psychiatrique des adultes à Lierneux," *Acta Neurologica et Psychiatrica Belgica* 68 (1968): 392–406.

44. For a detailed account of the Fitz-James and Villers colonies, see Letchworth, *The Insane*, pp. 229–38. The author concluded that "the free and natural condi-

tions of life existing at Fitz-James and Villers are marked characteristics of these colonies, nor can one forbear to note the admirable judgement and delicate tact displayed in adjusting the employments to the experience, physical capacity, and mental condition of the patient."

45. Jerome M. Schneck, "United States of America," in John G. Howells, *World History*, p. 447.
46. For a résumé of the family system by an enthusiastic, but disappointed, protagonist, see W. Lauder Lindsay, "Family System," pp. 497–527.
47. Annual Meeting of the Association, "Original Communications: Dr. Mundy on the Cottage Asylum System," *Journal of Mental Science* 8 (1862): 333.
48. Twenty-fourth Report of the Commissioners in Lunacy, 1870, p. 9.
49. "After-care of Convalescents," *Journal of Mental Science* 25 (1879): 453, 601–2.
50. Twenty-seventh Report of the Commissioners in Lunacy, 1873, p. 18.
51. Browne, "Cottage Asylums," p. 221.

BARBARA SICHERMAN

9 The Paradox of Prudence: Mental Health in the Gilded Age

Physicians in the late nineteenth century took the lead in telling the American public what must be done to prevent mental illness and to promote mental health. If the advocates of "mental hygiene"—asylum superintendents and neurologists for the most part—wrote with urgency, it was because they judged insanity difficult if not impossible to cure and their countrymen especially prone to mental and nervous disorders. They also shared with many medical colleagues the optimistic belief that modern science would soon conquer the scourges of mankind, including insanity.[1]

Although mental hygienists believed that their advice conformed to scientific canons, their conception of health reveals more about their own values, and particularly their fears, than about the nature of health.[2] Indeed, it is this subjectivity that is of importance to historians. Since definitions of mental health in the Gilded Age differ not only from those in current use, but also from those in use a generation later, they provide an insight to a particular cultural ethos. The context was distinctly medical. From their clinical observations of patients who had failed to meet life's demands, physicians drew conclusions about the ills of society as well as the personal weaknesses of the victims.

Although they were at times banal and even condescending, mental hygienists grappled with the same problems that troubled many of their contemporaries: ambition, when both the rewards of success and the penalties of failure seemed particularly high; spiritual values, when religious doubt flourished; and ill health, when some men, women, and especially children often died prematurely and debilitating diseases kept others from enjoying life. At a time of declining confidence in religion and growing reverence for science, physicians quite consciously offered guidance on behavioral matters which, as one explained, "the custom of centuries has wrongfully confided exclusively to the profession of theology."[3]

The physicians' advice to their contemporaries was sometimes fash-

This essay was originally published in the *Journal of American History* and is reprinted here by permission.

ioned out of their own lives. George M. Beard and Mary Putnam Jacobi clearly illustrate the continuity between personal experiences of depression, religion, and childhood fears, and an interest in preserving mental health. Beard, a zealous neurologist, popularized neurasthenia (literally, weakness of the nerves) as a medical diagnosis, worked to improve treatment of the mentally ill, and tried to incorporate psychological data into the rather inhospitable framework of late nineteenth-century somatic medicine. Jacobi, a sophisticated physician of broad medical, literary, and philosophical interests, specialized in neurological and children's diseases. For neither Beard nor Jacobi had a sense of purpose come easily. Both had been preoccupied with sickness in childhood and adolescence; both had early encounters with personal tragedy and felt an intense need to find some useful way of serving humanity; and both had acquired an exacting moral scrupulosity from zealous family members, which, if they did not entirely discard, they later channeled into professional pursuits.[4]

Not all mental hygienists responded to similar pressures in precisely the same ways. But there can be little doubt that experiences of this sort shaped their hopes and fears, their conceptions of mental health, and in some cases their choice of profession. Those who had triumphed over such difficulties had reason to pass on whatever wisdom they had acquired. By devoting themselves to healing others, perhaps even as they would have liked to have been cared for as children, they may have discovered the purpose in living that had once eluded them.[5]

Mental hygienists who came to professional maturity in the 1860s and early 1870s were members of possibly the last generation expected to undergo the traditional religious-conversion experience. This generation was also the first to feel the impact of evolutionary theory. *The Origin of Species* was published when Beard was twenty and Jacobi seventeen. And this generation was almost the first to embrace the canons of an international scientific community. Many members of this generation found it difficult to reconcile their childhood imperatives and their adult values. By working for mental hygiene, individuals like Beard and Jacobi reintroduced traditional values—always under the cloak of science—and asserted their right, as physicians, to lead others to the desired goals.[6]

Advice on mental hygiene in the Gilded Age resembled nothing so much as the religious precepts these physicians had assimilated as children. But theirs was a liberalized behavioral ethic, better suited to the more secular and bourgeois world of late nineteenth-century America. They emphatically rejected the idea of excessive restraint—the abstemiousness in food, sex, drink, and, particularly, the obligatory self-scrutiny—once imposed by evangelical parents or grandparents. Unable to free themselves from their own pasts or even to follow their own advice, it is likely that the physicians continued to live between high hopes and aspirations and lingering doubts and fears.

In matters of mental hygiene, the Gilded Age did not call forth heroic virtues. Physicians advanced what has been called a "minimal" conception of health—freedom from incapacitating symptoms and good resistance to stress. Fearful that even the "utmost circumspection" might not guarantee health, they settled for what was prudent rather than energizing.[7] Health was widely perceived as the absence of illness rather than as a quality in its own right. According to Jacobi, "Health is like the silent existence of those happy nations that have no history. But disease represents the commotion, the storm and stress, the drama and the convulsions into which the disturbed history of our race has usually been thrown."[8]

If health was a kind of idealized calm, it was also the "successful adaptation to the conditions of existence." And in the Gilded Age, following Herbert Spencer, adaptation meant the *"continuous adjustment of internal relations to external relations."* The human organism must mold itself to a fixed environment rather than shape that environment to its own ends.[9]

Mental hygienists considered contemporary life particularly ill suited to health, repose, or security of any sort. Beard gave voice to the common belief when he declared that neurasthenia, a disease thought frequently to lead to insanity, was a product of nineteenth-century American civilization. Not every physician agreed that the disease was exclusively American, or accepted Beard's list of causes—he emphasized the printing press, the railroad, the steam engine, the telegraph, and the increased mental activity of women—but most physicians considered the disease distressingly common.[10]

Physicians also agreed that each man and woman possessed a limited amount of nervous energy. Given the seemingly unlimited demands on that supply, the wise individual learned to live within the margins of his endowment. Neurasthenia was the paradigmatic illness for mental hygienists; the exhaustion of its victims provided the perfect object lesson of what might happen to those who attempted too much. Consequently, they viewed the individual as a passive being—"tinder waiting for the spark" —at the mercy of hostile external forces and of dangerous internal ones as well. No wonder, too, that strategies for preserving health were largely defensive.[11]

The mentally healthy person, in theory at least, sought neither individual fulfillment nor daring exploits that might take him far from conventional social norms. On the grounds that eccentricity approached insanity, physicians even warned against any course that departed from average or "normal" behavior and recommended that children be taught to "avoid eccentricity and not to defy the requirements of custom without some very excellent reason."[12]

Mental hygienists agreed that the healthy person had complete control over his emotions. He never allowed his temper to get the better of him, or gave way to "depression of spirits." In the well-conditioned brain there was "strict accordance between thought and will." As one physician put it, "Perfect inhibition is the sign of perfect mental health." Some claimed that every surrender to impulse threatened a person's sanity, was in fact "a qualified sort of insanity," and that "he only is a perfectly sane man whose mind is in due subjection to the God-given authority of the will, whose life is governed by reason."[13]

In their search for stability, mental hygienists also warned against extreme emotions. Even great happiness might damage the nervous system, although presumably not as much as grief. They explained that "every strong emotion, or train of thought, temporarily affects the nutrition of the nerve centers, and if such excitations are frequently repeated, there results an organic physical condition which becomes the basis of habit and character." To care too much about anything also left one prey to disappointment and loss, and thus to considerable nervous strain. Thus Jacobi advised, "Healthy and justly proportioned indifference is essential to healthy equilibrium." While directed primarily to those predisposed to nervousness, such admonitions might speak to anyone who wished to avoid "storm and stress."[14]

If the healthy man lacked passion, he was admirably compensated by an equable disposition. Approximating the golden mean in every respect, he struck a balance between work, celibacy, and abstemiousness on the one hand, and frivolity, licentiousness, and indulgence on the other. Mental hygienists condemned any kind of fanaticism, including, despite the recognized dangers of alcohol, teetotalism. One superintendent explained that "abstemiousness and excess are not prudent living; neither can be commended." Even immoderate concern about health could undermine the constitution: "Regular modes of living carried to excess are the road to invalidism, and irregular habits of living within rational limits the highway to health." Prudence itself might be carried too far.[15]

Physicians urged Americans to moderate their ambition, their love of money, and—a new concern for this generation—their compulsion to work. Although the dangers of a competitive culture had been decried as early as 1830, physicians in the Gilded Age pitted themselves, probably with little effect, against "popular-success" writers like Horatio Alger. Mental hygienists did not believe that every American could attain fame and fortune; asylums housed many patients of aspiring temperaments who lacked the ability to achieve their objectives. More "modest" goals, they claimed, would lead to more certain achievement.[16]

Physicians did not believe that work in itself was harmful—only "intemperance of work." With S. Weir Mitchell, the neurologist who developed the "rest cure" for neurasthenia, they distinguished between wear (normal use) and tear (abuse). To a generation of physicians intrigued by mechanical analogies, the body was a machine that might easily be driven beyond its capacity. Their warnings against ambition and overwork also revealed a distinct class bias. They emphasized these dangers to working-class students who, by studying Latin and algebra, acquired false notions of their opportunities and believed themselves above manual labor; to businessmen engaged in speculation or other ventures of high risk and dubious morality; to self-made men catapulted into positions of responsibility for which they were unprepared; and to the nouveaux riches who became self-indulgent, idle, and perhaps morbidly fanciful. In practice then, physicians stressed the dangers of worry, risk, or anything that might take an individual into dangerous or novel territory.[17]

Whatever their qualms about ambition and success, mental hygienists considered idleness and luxury even more hazardous to the nervous system. These interests inclined individuals to "imagine the most fascinating personal romances. They selfishly dwell upon subjective feelings, developing more and more complete egoism; they modify sensations into symptoms, and symptoms into diseases, until nervous invalids result by the hundred." Like other Victorians, physicians had an ingrained fear of fantasy and introspection (with their implications of sexual indulgence), of eccentricity and lack of control. These were also the traits they daily observed in their own patients.[18]

Mental hygienists agreed that childhood was the best time for instilling the "habits of self-control, self-reliance, devotion to duty, and calmness" that would assure mental health in adult life.[19] They seemed to believe that parents possessed almost unlimited power over the development of their offspring. "It is . . . largely in our power to determine the nature of the ideas of any child who is *thoroughly* guarded from his cradle," Jacobi boldly asserted. She believed that personality was built up by incorporating ideas, feelings, and volitions into the original physical substratum of the mind. Since disease was the "invasion of false ideas," the child's ego must be strengthened to guard against the entrance of delusions. On the grounds that grief, shock, excessive egoism, and introspection might cause mental illness, she recommended that children acquire a sense of their own insignificance in the vast scheme of the universe and a capacity for self-denial, so they could bear misfortune in later years and learn to pass easily from one mood to another. More sophisticated in her outlook than most mental hygienists, Jacobi still reached the familiar conclusion that a strong will was the basis for preserving mental health.[20]

Despite the emphasis on emotional control, children were not to be hurried into adulthood. Mental hygienists condemned precocity, which many of them considered "but the token of an inward defect," and felt it should be repressed by watchful parents and teachers. Some physicians, maintaining that all mental labor should be deferred until a child reached ten, prescribed physical exercise and nature study for the preservation of mental and physical health.[21]

Mental hygienists shared the ambivalence of many Americans toward intellectual endeavor. They feared that intellect might blunt an individual's moral sensibilities but deplored the ignorance of the masses. What probably disturbed them most was the "apparent want of intellectual development of the great majority" of patients in any asylum. Thus, while they condemned intellectual excess, they agreed that education and culture were "strong defenses against disease, insanity included."[22]

Although primarily concerned with intellectual precocity, mental hygienists warned against "excitement or perversion" of the sexual instinct. For many, this meant masturbation. They were less dogmatic about this practice in adults than physicians of the preceding generation and many contemporaries as well. They considered it often a symptom rather than a cause of insanity. But they agreed that the practice was especially harmful to children. Like many Victorians who sentimentalized children as innocent, they sought to protect them from sexual knowledge.[23]

A boy reared with due attention to all these matters would, presumably, acquire the necessary imperturbability of character, "tested, it may be, by the extremity of both joy and sorrow—prosperity and adversity— but never disconcerted by either." Physicians assumed that women, whom they considered more emotional by nature and more subject to the vagaries of their reproductive systems, suffered even more acutely from the familiar burden of limited nervous resources and excessive strain. While physicians sometimes noted the harm caused by woman's "limited sphere of physical and mental occupation, as compared with that of the male sex," they were more apt to stress the dangers of "undertaking, with perhaps insufficient equipment, a career just a little beyond her real mental strength." Women were urged to choose the safest course; this inevitably meant marriage and motherhood.[24]

If mental health were largely a matter of emotional control, then presumably women as well as men should be educated to maximize their rationality. But Victorian physicians were inconsistent on this point. Mitchell, for example, pointedly contrasted the strengthening education given boys, which taught them to control their emotions, with the indulgence granted girls, which only encouraged them to give way to their already heightened sensibilities. But he still urged women not to strive for intellectual attainment and to be content as wives and mothers. Although he hoped women would become less impulsive and more self-controlled, Mitchell opposed "even a very steady use" of the brain before a girl reached seventeen. If she ignored this advice, he believed, a girl would endanger her health and "every probability of future womanly usefulness"; her destiny would be "the shawl and the sofa."[25]

Jacobi was almost alone in challenging the conventional wisdom about women's health. She attributed many of their ills to alcoholic fathers, husbands who had venereal diseases, and enforced celibacy imposed by "bad social arrangements." If women sometimes strained themselves to the breaking point in pursuit of success, it was not because of any native deficiency, but because they had been inadequately prepared for responsibility. She criticized her male colleagues for encouraging women, already too removed from the stoicism of their ancestors, to dwell on their ills. Insisting that weakness could be eliminated only by the cultivation of strength, she hoped to train both sexes to bear responsibility.[26]

The thrust of advice on mental health in the Gilded Age was clearly toward self-restriction—of emotional attachment and expression, aspiration, imagination, creativity, and even individuality. Fears of going too far, having too much or too little, and losing control were not unique to this generation. But they have rarely been elevated into a rationale for designing a way of life.

How did physicians arrive at a conception of health that specialists today regard as limited? The husbanding of resources was a central metaphor in nineteenth-century America, one that dominated the cautionary literature on sexual behavior as well as mental health. Since physicians urged others to lead conventional, safe, productive lives, it may be tempting to interpret their work as an exercise in social control, intended to keep workers and women in prescribed roles and to transform middle-class boys into productive clerical or professional workers.[27] But on closer analysis, it is apparent that the restrictive model of mental health was a metaphor that helped physicians make sense of their own professional and personal experiences.

Like physicians in any era, mental hygienists in the Gilded Age began with the example of those who had already broken down. Since they hoped to provide guidelines by which others might avoid a similar fate, it is not surprising that definitions of mental health read like an inventory of personality traits opposite those observed in their patients. If the mentally ill lacked control over their emotions, were self-absorbed, and suffered from delusions or hallucinations, then it followed that the individual who was emotionally temperate and not unduly introspective or egotistical must be healthy. Physicians believed that these desirable traits provided protection against stress.[28]

Physicians of this generation addressed themselves to human fears rather than hopes, perhaps because deprivation and loss were common experiences to all classes. The death rate was extremely high during the second and third quarters of the century, when most of the mental hygienists had been children. As late as 1880, a male at birth could expect to live only to the age of forty-two, a female slightly longer. Although some illnesses were coming under control by 1870, mortality from tuberculosis and typhoid remained high, and infant mortality was variously estimated at one in four or five live births. The childhood diseases—diphtheria, croup, enteritis, diarrhea, and scarlet fever—yielded to medical control only after 1900.[29]

Many mental hygienists had undoubtedly lost parents or siblings at an early age. Their medical training notwithstanding, they were often powerless to save their own children. Not everyone experienced such losses, but premature death was common enough to remind even the fortunate that loved ones might die suddenly. Perhaps this limited their ability to trust their environment or count on a happy future and made them long for the emotional detachment that experts today consider an unfortunate but probable consequence of early separation from parents.[30]

Certainly mental hygienists in the Gilded Age were often preoccupied with the themes of deprivation, death, and danger. In a speech on childbirth, Jacobi made much of the external dangers threatening the individual: "Looking back over our own careers, we seem to trace a narrow path winding between so many disasters, here skirting a precipice, there barely escaping an impending avalanche,—again, emerging from a black quagmire that threatened to engulph,—so many dangers barely escaped, so many others unescapable;—one may well ask whether it be worthwhile to launch another sentient being upon such a difficult and dangerous course. . . ."[31]

But the dangers also came from within, from the disturbing thoughts that suggested to physicians of this generation that no absolute line separated the normal from the insane. As one of Mitchell's fictional physicians declared, "There are times when I seem to hang awed over the abyss of my own mind, with wonder near akin to terror. That out of this world of thought, feelings, and memories should come, to the most healthy nature, at times inexplicable desires, moments of unreason, impulses which defy analytic research, even brief insanities, is not strange to me. I wonder, indeed, at the permanence of mental health. . . ."[32]

The emphasis on self-restriction may have been primarily a defense against the anxieties aroused by such threats. Mental hygienists in the Gilded Age offered a formula for reducing anxiety. By limiting aspirations, they suggested, one could avoid failure, loss, and disappointment. By stifling imagination, they argued, one could keep out unwanted and terrifying thoughts.[33] Perhaps only those who wanted a great deal out of life needed to construct such defenses. Whether or not mental hygienists actually desired such safe lives for themselves, they were addressing problems that had caused some of them acute discomfort—ambition, troublesome imaginations, morbid self-examination, fierce tempers, a sense of their own willfulness. Those who triumphed over such tendencies, often by tremendous effort, must have believed that others could do the same. Those who had not entirely succeeded may have felt compelled to warn others of the dangers.

Beard struggled with many of the conflicts experienced by Victorians who were reared as Calvinists. Among mental hygienists he probably went furthest in rejecting the constraints of that tradition.[34] Born in 1839 in Montville, Connecticut, he was the youngest of four children. His mother died when he was three, and the evidence suggests that at least some of the Beard children lived with relatives, perhaps even after their father remarried in 1843. It was a highly charged religious household. Beard's father, a Congregational minister of slender means, was ever mindful of the temptations of earthly life. Both of Beard's brothers became ministers, and his stepmother hoped that he would also receive the call.[35]

Between 1856, when he completed his preparatory course at Phillips Andover Academy, and 1862, when he graduated from Yale, Beard suffered many of the symptoms he later incorporated under the rubric of neurasthenia—ringing in the ears, pains in the side, acute dyspepsia, nervousness, lack of vitality, feeling "blue." He questioned the purpose of living and tried to reassure himself that when his health improved he would find enough to enjoy in this world. Beard encountered many fellow sufferers, not only among strangers, but also, most important, in his own family. His sister and both brothers suffered from ill health, nervousness, and "lack of vitality"; the college careers of his father and one brother had been interrupted for reasons of health.[36]

Determined to recover, Beard experimented with every remedy that came to his attention. He dieted—on bread, milk, and crackers—since he considered overeating his besetting vice. He also sought relief, despite his family's ridicule, with electricity, a new and not yet medically respectable therapy that Beard later popularized. In his efforts to systematize a proper regimen—"order is heaven's first law"—Beard at twenty was very much the physician in the making.[37]

During these years Beard also struggled to regain "the humble, trustful faith of my younger days, the zeal, the confiding earnestness." He could "not bear this hanging back," and he tried to revive his flagging piety by attending prayer meetings, conducting a sabbath school, and deploring the worldliness of those who profaned the sabbath by fishing, sailing, or engaging in other " 'sinful pleasures' (ice cream parties and other joyful occasions)."[38]

Beard was especially troubled by the conflict between worldly success and spiritual salvation, an understandable concern for one who at seventeen received the following advice from his father:

> Happy to hear of your health & prosperity. You will I hope be on your guard against the dangers which are found in all cases the attendants of success & prosperity. In no condition while in this state of probation are we exempt from what may be inimical to our best interests, if not avoided. In the day of adversity there is the danger of becomeing thereby unbelieving, unsubmissive & despondent; ... on the other hand in the day of prosperity there is the danger of immoder-

ate elation of too great self dependence or of an over estimate of our powers, attainments and goodness. . . . To the injurious & hateful influence of prosperity here refered to we are all exposed especially so in early life before experience has had time to make us see the folly of the self conceit & pride which ever is the forerunner of a fall. I have refered to this subject not because I have seen any thing special in your case, but only to put you on your watch against a danger to which all are exposed in that part of ocean of life where your bark is now sailing.³⁹

In this situation whenever Beard achieved any personal triumph—even an improvement in health—he felt constrained to ask if he were sufficiently grateful. Advice of this sort must have contributed to Beard's depression, especially because he considered himself "inordinately ambitious," and wanted not only to find a useful purpose in life, but also to outdistance his fellows.⁴⁰

Beard's decision to become a physician finally gave him the long sought sense of purpose: "I wish to make my pen the servant of my profession—to make all my writing ability of practical service in the reformation & progress of medical & Hygienic knowledge. This is my earthly ideal." He embraced medicine with the passion of a true vocation: "I love my studies. I love them for their own sake—I can but love them. I was *born* to be a physician. I should do wrong to study any other profession. . . . I have a genius—a decided taste for the *Theory & Practice* of Medicine." Beard still wished he "had equal zeal in Religion," and even as he looked forward to life and success could not help asking this question: "How long will it be before I shall be humbled & crushed?"⁴¹

By this time Beard had also begun to enjoy the worldly pleasures he had once condemned. He attended champagne parties and smoked Turkish tobacco. He also enjoyed skating and the company of young ladies, and in January 1863 he became engaged. Although he finally joined a church, he did not long remain a member. By the time Beard started practice in New York City, after serving as an assistant surgeon in the navy, he was, according to his partner, "quite positively but unobtrusively agnostic."⁴²

Beard found a profession that permitted him to advance humanity's cause as well as his own. He was eager to do both. If Beard did not entirely avoid the pitfalls of ambition against which his father had warned—his propensity for claiming world-shaking discoveries perturbed more cautious colleagues—his aims were undeniably altruistic. He could even draw on his own early troubles to bring comfort to others. As a physician interested in the functional nervous disorders, he served individuals who, like himself, had temporarily lost their direction in life. He was, in the words of a colleague, "intensely therapeutical" and even tried remedies like "mental therapeutics" that had not yet attained medical respectability. Whatever the specific therapy (he insisted that no two patients should be treated alike), Beard reassured them that they would recover. Since he had once declared that "each day is lost in which I have not conferred happiness on some one," the gratitude of his patients must have been extremely important to him. Certainly his empathy was apparent.[43]

Beard was less enamored of the prudent virtues than most of his contemporaries. He was a rebel who welcomed and, by his own admission, "courted" opposition. Perhaps this quality made him particularly critical of the "repelling . . . distressing, wearisome and saddening" educational methods that had been forced on "children of the past generation"—his own presumably—who learned "that to be happy is to be doing wrong." Beard had struggled too hard against his own "hanging back" to recommend it to others. Thus he preferred speculative German science to the "dull and safe" American university system, which he blamed on Puritan ancestors, and absolutely denied that mental activity in any way compromised health. "A well-trained intellect," he insisted, "is itself medicine and hygiene, enabling its possessor to guard successfully against the appeals of passion and the storms of emotion." This was as true for women as for men, for Beard maintained that intellectual women were rarely nervous.[44]

When Beard recommended moderation in food and drink, he was attacking the vegetarianism that had flourished in his youth, not only among "popular charlatans," but also among physicians, and the teetotalist position still advanced by clergymen. He also reassured his patients about their sexual problems, at a time when quacks and physicians alike still urged the direst remedies for masturbation or spontaneous emissions. Beard proposed a "gospel of rest" to promote calmness, serenity, and repose. But he was no great partisan of the rest cure; he himself had early discovered that he felt best when hard at work. Before his death of pneumonia at forty-three, he published ten books and almost eighty articles. Clearly work, intellectual engagement, and, as a hostile reviewer suggested, his typewriter contributed to Beard's emotional well-being. As a dedicated healer, he would not deny this to others.[45]

Beard's experiences with religion, doubt, and nervousness were not unusual in the Victorian era. His less restrained attitude about mental health probably resulted from the intellectual and emotional liberation that often accompanied the casting off of evangelical faith. The greater caution of many of his contemporaries may have reflected their lingering anxieties as well as personal or familial pressures.[46]

Jacobi best illustrates the paradox between the lives of mental hygienists and the advice they sometimes offered.[47] Born in 1842, she was the eldest of the eleven children of George Palmer Putnam, founder of the publishing house, and Victorine (Haven) Putnam. Despite her cosmopolitan background, she preferred rural Staten Island and Yonkers to Manhattan, where she suffered from "ennui." She had considerable freedom—even her education was "helter-skelter"—but her memories of early childhood were filled with tales of sickness, epidemics, punishment for misdeeds, and a season of nightmares and insomnia. Perhaps her near-death by drowning at the age of eight gave rise to a constant preoccupation with illness and death. She claimed to have been unable to understand her parents' gratitude to the workman who rescued her. This anaesthetizing of experience, in reality or in memory, parallels her later advice to cultivate indifference.[48]

Her paternal grandmother, an austere Baptist, took charge of the girl's spiritual well-being, principally the matter of rigorous self-examination for signs of wrongdoing. At nine, she kept a diary recording her daily vices and virtues. At twelve, she informed her grandmother of her "alarming sins, such as passion, inordinate selfishness, envy and jealousy," of which her "awful passion" was the worst. She attributed her initial success in overcoming these vices to a strong effort of will, "assisted by the Holy Ghost." But the "tranquillity of mind" and "a fancied dangerous security" only preceded her relapse into "careless, sinful habits." In this world, even good feelings could not be trusted. She became a Baptist during a religious revival, when a charismatic young minister converted the entire family. Six years later, at the age of twenty-one and following four years of doubt, she rejected Calvinist doctrine and severed her relationship with the church. She attributed such action to intellectual opposition to the principles of probation and authority, the Trinity, atonement, and eternal punishment. To prove that she was not motivated by worldly desire, she promised to abstain from theater and opera for ten years, a resolution steadfastly maintained despite the temptations of student life in Paris.[49]

Precocious in ambition as well as self-analysis, at the age of ten she wrote, "Vague longings beset me. . . . I would be great." She was even then interested in healing, which she associated with the ministerial role. In a story written by Jacobi when she was nine, the minister-hero declares his superiority to the less noble poet and merchant: "I will not bury myself within myself, or upon mountains. Neither will I spend my life in the acquisition of dull gold; but will devote it to the sick bed, to the cell where dark crime and poverty lurk. I will smooth the pillow of the dying, and call sinners to God. I will snatch infants out of the wiles of sin, and preach the Gospel to all. Thus will I pass my life, and I hope to sink to the grave lamented."[50]

To those who knew her as an adult, Jacobi must have seemed an intrepid and dedicated professional. She was graced as well with a "keen sense of humor . . . a suggestive wit." The first woman admitted to the École de Médecine in Paris, she became one of the most respected physicians of her generation. She impressed her vitality and determination on family and colleagues, which is perhaps the reason her father did not seriously interfere with her ambition, despite his conviction that medicine was not an "agreeable pursuit." She was, by her own account, clear and definite in her views and rarely inclined to ask advice of others. Unlike most professional women of her generation, she combined marriage and motherhood with a career. She produced medical papers of high quality, taught medical school, did dispensary work, wrote about philosophy and education, and worked to improve medical opportunities for women and factory conditions for workers. She also became a fierce champion of Positivism, an optimistic creed that she believed would help humanity triumph over evil, the most terrible of which was death.[51]

Yet there are puzzling contradictions about Jacobi that suggest the continued impact of her early experiences. Her professional aspirations and her interest in feminist causes did not keep her from voicing the wish —should she marry at all—to find a man more eminent than herself and more interested in his work than in her. And when she married in 1873, her husband had already made his mark as a founder of American pediatrics. Although she once thanked her parents for allowing her so much freedom as a child, she supervised her daughter's life to such a degree that the child exclaimed, "You make everything a lesson, Mama." When upbraided for this by her own mother, Jacobi replied, "When she can pick the flower it seems a pity not to have her notice what she lately learned about it." Perhaps she was more ambivalent about her own independence than she cared to admit and had craved more attention than she received from her own young mother, who had been busy with a large brood.[52]

Jacobi rejected what she probably considered the most destructive aspects of her own upbringing, including the "constant gloom" of a "ferocious" religion. She warned against doctrinal training on the grounds that any "uprooting of fundamental religious ideas" was invariably disturbing. On learning of her grandmother's death, she tartly observed that the old woman had been "most rare in her entire ignorance of herself. I think that was really astonishing especially in a person who devoted so much time to self-analysis and introspection." Jacobi found it "highly favorable for peace of mind and effective action, to dwell upon what I am sure of and not to be distressed by what remains uncertain." Yet her advice on child rearing resembles admonitions she must often have heard from her grandmother. The sins she owned up to at twelve—"passion, inordinate selfishness, envy and jealousy"—resemble the traits she thought parents must guard against in their children, traits such as egotism, willfulness, and passionate attachments.[53]

Jacobi's admonition to cultivate "justly proportioned indifference" had less to do with any lack of feeling on her part than with an intense need to avoid pain or loss and to come to terms with her fears. As a young adult she keenly sensed the precariousness of health and happiness: "I do not know any time of my life that I have not been more afraid of losing the present than really sanguine about the future." On her twenty-fifth birthday she wondered why she should "nearly always have what I want, when hardly anybody else has." If she suddenly became an invalid or cripple, she claimed it would be "only fair balance for the uninterrupted happiness that has been granted me." She also feared tidings of death whenever mail arrived. While she attributed this to "living so constantly in the presence of death," her decision to enter medicine may have represented a need to face the enemy squarely.[54]

Jacobi seems to have cultivated qualities she suspected were not natively hers. Noting that "a more miserable creature than a human being in a state of fear,—of terror—can scarcely be imagined," she deplored effeminacy and women's penchant for cultivating weakness. In comparison to heroes who risked their lives, a fearful person could only "feel the bitterest self contempt" for such qualities. Perhaps when she traveled alone to New Orleans to nurse her brother through a bout of malaria (he was a soldier in the Union army), she made clear her intention never to be one of those who "fall asleep at his post."[55]

It is particularly ironic that Jacobi's description of the change in personality accompanying a meningeal tumor that eventually caused her death bore a striking resemblance to her earlier definition of health: "I began to lose the initiative, which had formerly been so active with me. I was not at all depressed or melancholy, but relatively indifferent. It seemed as if a fine gauze veil were thrown over all the objects in which I had formerly been so intensely interested. It was like the life after death as the Greeks understood it when they described Hades."

That Jacobi contrasted this state of indifference with her earlier "vivacity and strength" suggests that she had not attained the "justly proportioned indifference" she recommended to others. Indeed, given her statement elsewhere that "the object of living . . . consists in the development of all faculties to their greatest extent to which the individual organization admits of, and in the satisfaction of all desires to their utmost possible capacity," it is unlikely that she ever really wished to achieve such a state. For to the question "What do you want from Life?" she had once answered, "Everything." To one who alternately emphasized the feasibility of triumphing over evil and the precariousness of life, the admonition to cultivate indifference must have been a self-protective device.[56]

On balance, mental hygienists' views on health represented at once a partial emancipation from traditional religious precepts and a reaffirmation of their essential premises. Jacobi was probably not aware of the similarity between her ideas on child rearing and the religious precepts that she had learned as a child and later consciously rejected. But some hygienists who remained formally religious, among them the superintendent of the Hartford Retreat, who was also director of the Connecticut Bible Society, made the connection explicit: "The laws of health and those of religion go hand in hand; the two fundamentally agree. . . . Temperance, honesty, obedience to parents, truthfulness, chastity, recognition of sacred ties, and brotherly kindness are no less in accordance with the laws of bodily and mental health, than they are with the laws and ordinances of the Christian religion, and when man sins against one he does also against the other."[57]

In the introduction to one of his popular medical works, Mitchell observed that he was tempted to call his essays "lay sermons, so serious did some of their subjects seem to me." He compared the role of the physician who treated nervous patients to that of the priest hearing confession. In later years he also maintained, "So great is my reverence for supreme wholesomeness, that I should almost be tempted to assert that perfect health is virtue."[58]

Mental hygienists in the Gilded Age for the most part disavowed the more repressive aspects of their childhoods. They did not speak of breaking the will, but of training it in the proper direction. While complaining of a breakdown in discipline, they believed that "undue repression dwarfs the faculties when it does not derange them."[59] The abstemiousness, the joyless Sundays, the constant exhortations to search one's conscience—all seemed more likely to promote illness than genuine piety.

In place of such a regimen, mental hygienists hoped to substitute "rational enjoyment" that might bring "warmth and sweetness" into the lives of the sturdy New Englanders who had inherited a "coldness and austerity of manner" from their ancestors. Mitchell noted his fear of men who had no "petty vices," and one physician went so far as to declare that "even syphilis must be acknowledged to be a rarer cause of insanity than the enforced celibacy which our civilization demands or the excesses which marriage sometimes allows." If this proved an unfortunate prediction about the relationship between syphilis and mental illness, the liberalizing intention is still clear.[60]

But the innate caution of physicians of this generation, their fear of loss of control and of inordinate wants that could not be satisfied, prevented them from venturing too far in the direction of freedom. They endorsed the close supervision of children—the careful guarding from the cradle—against signs of morbid introspection, fantasy, or willfulness, just as parents of a preceding generation might have watched for evidences of sin. They recommended outdoor exercise or nature study not for children's enjoyment but for health. Physicians of this generation also preferred gymnastics to more strenuous intercollegiate sports; even roller skating, if indulged in at great speed, might prove too exhilarating.[61]

Mental hygienists offered an outlet for individuals who found the pressures of a demanding society excessive—license to seek rest and repair under the guidance of a sympathetic physician. Ironically, prudence rarely characterized the lives of the mental hygienists. Good Victorians, some of the most ardent advocates of mental health were fiercely ambitious and prodigious workers. Mitchell made as many as fifty-two house calls in a single day, found time for research and clinic duties, and had a consulting practice that brought $70,000 in a good year. He even began writing novels to avoid boredom in his leisure hours. Indeed, Mitchell regularly departed for vacations in a state of exhaustion; and it was while recovering from one such episode that he wrote *Wear and Tear,* a book that eloquently warned others of the dangers of overwork.[62]

Mental hygienists were perhaps no more inconsistent than other moral counselors who urged followers to heed their advice rather than their actions. For those who had experienced the social and personal strains about which they wrote, prescriptions for health may variously have reflected satisfactory personal solutions to their own problems, attempts to remedy the perceived errors of their own upbringing, and perhaps even goals for others that they themselves could not, perhaps did not wish to, achieve. Perhaps some considered themselves special individuals, tried and tested for higher ends.[63]

Whatever the personal dimension of their work, mental hygienists addressed themselves to the cultural discontinuities that troubled many Americans in the late nineteenth century. Life-styles and values had changed drastically since the 1850s and for none more than for physicians like Beard who made the difficult transition from village Congregationalism to science and New York City. A generation of Americans sought new certainty as old truths failed them. Some turned away from religion entirely. Others looked to new faiths like Christian Science, which claimed to be both science and religion, and New Thought; both faiths took root in the late 1870s and 1880s.[64] Bolstered by the growing prestige of science, mental hygienists contributed to this quest by providing a secular rather than a religious context for evaluating the good life.

Physicians were just beginning to offer such advice in the Gilded Age, but by 1917 they were widely accepted as experts on matters of personal happiness and social welfare, once fields that were largely outside their domain. Definitions of health also changed. In Beard's day, human capacity seemed almost tragically limited. But the generation that admired Theodore Roosevelt preferred William James's exhortation that the will could open "deeper and deeper levels of energy" to admonitions of prudence. When James wrote his famous essay, *The Energies of Men,* in 1907, he actually reversed a position he had taken fifteen years earlier. Then he had argued, "We must change ourselves from a race that admires jerk and snap for their own sakes, and looks down upon low voices and quiet ways as dull, to one that, on the contrary, has calm for its ideal, and for their own sakes loves harmony, dignity, and ease." In the intervening years, both James and American culture had changed.[65]

Notes

Research for this essay was supported in part by a grant from the National Institute of Mental Health, U.S. Public Health Service, and by the Radcliffe Institute. The author wishes to thank Yale University and George Beard Walker for permission to cite the George M. Beard Papers, and the Schlesinger Library of Radcliffe College as well as the heirs of Mary Putnam Jacobi for permission to cite the Mary Putnam Jacobi Papers.

1. The term *mental hygienist* is used because *psychiatrists,* as they are now defined, did not exist in the late nineteenth century. The nearest equivalents were *superintendents* of asylums for the mentally ill and *neurologists* who specialized not only in organic diseases, like multiple sclerosis, but also in what are now designated as psychoneuroses. This essay focuses on the physicians' definitions of mental health. See also Barbara Sicherman, "The Quest for Mental Health in America, 1880–1917" (Ph.D. diss., Columbia University, 1967), pp. 78–152.

2. For the relationship between definitions of mental health and values, see Marie Jahoda, *Current Concepts of Positive Mental Health* (New York: Basic Books, 1958), pp. 3–4; M. Brewster Smith, " 'Mental Health' Reconsidered: A Special Case of the Problem of Values in Psychology," *American Psychologist* 16 (1961): 299–306.

3. D. A. Gorton, *An Essay on the Principles of Mental Hygiene* (Philadelphia: Lippincott, 1873), p. ix.

4. The career patterns and personalities of George M. Beard and Mary Putnam Jacobi differed in several important respects. He was a physician of modest scientific training, an individualist, and an eager controversialist more interested in philosophy than in meticulous research—tendencies viewed with alarm by some colleagues. She was an exceptionally well trained physician who wrote closely reasoned papers and worked actively in New York's medical schools and hospitals. Despite barriers against women, Jacobi's brilliance and no-nonsense approach gained her entry into the city's most prestigious scientific and medical institutions. But in their commitment to mental hygiene and in the emotional or religious motivations for their choice of vocation, the similarities between them significantly outweigh the differences. In the early 1880s both also participated in an organization that aimed to prevent mental illness as well as to reform mental hospitals. He was treasurer; she was vice-president.

5. These generalizations derive from an analysis of the works and biographies of fifty-eight mental hygienists, all physicians. George M. Beard and Mary Putnam Jacobi went further than most mental hygienists in rejecting religion, but

the others also had been affected by the religious training of their childhood. Among those exposed to Calvinism, a number suffered from religious terrors, nervousness, or both. Several chose medicine only after seriously considering a career in the ministry. Even S. Weir Mitchell, who was the son of a "liberal" Philadelphia physician and who ultimately became a broad church Episcopalian, was exposed to the rigors of Presbyterianism by his maternal grandfather. See also Margaret A. Cleaves, *The Autobiography of a Neurasthene as Told by One of Them* (Boston: Badger, 1910).

6. Charles E. Rosenberg and Carroll S. Rosenberg suggest the essential continuum between religion and health reform in two antebellum reformers. See Charles E. Rosenberg and Carroll S. Rosenberg, "Pietism and the Origins of the American Public Health Movement: A Note on John H. Griscom and Robert M. Hartley," *Journal of the History of Medicine and Allied Sciences* 23 (1968): 16–35. The choice of career is always a complex matter, related not only to childhood imperatives, but also to opportunities and exposure. The intricate relationship between individual values, evangelical religion, faith in progress, and the choice of a scientific career (for instance, agricultural chemistry in the 1850s) is sensitively discussed by Charles E. Rosenberg, "Science and Social Values in Nineteenth-Century America: A Case Study in the Growth of Scientific Institutions," in *Science and Values: Patterns of Tradition and Change*, ed. Arnold Thackray and Everett Mendelsohn (New York: Humanities Press, 1974), pp. 21–42.

7. H. Wardner, "Thoughts on Insanity and Its Preventable Causes," *St. Louis Medical and Surgical Journal* 40 (1881): 388–89. On the distinction between "minimal" and "extended" conceptions of health, see Smith, " 'Mental Health' Reconsidered," p. 305.

8. Women's Medical Association of New York City, ed., *Mary Putnam Jacobi: A Pathfinder in Medicine* (New York: Putnam, 1925), p. xxiii.

9. Henry Maudsley, *The Pathology of Mind* (New York: Appleton, 1880), p. 85; Samuel Osgood, "Health and the Higher Culture," American Public Health Association, *Public Health Papers and Reports* 2 (1874–75): 202.

10. George M. Beard, *American Nervousness: Its Causes and Consequences* (New York: Putnam, 1881). For an analysis of George M. Beard's work, see Charles E. Rosenberg, "The Place of George M. Beard in Nineteenth-Century Psychiatry," *Bulletin of the History of Medicine* 36 (1962): 245–59.

11. Henry Putnam Stearns, *Insanity: Its Causes and Prevention* (New York: Putnams, 1883), p. 47.

12. F. M. Turnbull, "Education as a Means for the Prevention of Insanity," *Journal of Nervous and Mental Diseases* 9 (1882): 296.

13. Wardner, "Thoughts on Insanity and Its Preventable Causes," pp. 389–90; Peter Bryce, "The Mind, and How to Preserve It," *Transactions of the Medical Association of the State of Alabama* (1880), p. 255; Charles K. Mills, *Toner Lectures, Lecture IX: Mental Over-work and Premature Disease among Public and Professional Men* (Washington: Smithsonian Institution, 1885), p. 21.

14. Charles W. Page, "How Can We Escape Insanity?" *Report of the State Board of Health of the State of Connecticut* 5 (1882): 187; Mary Putnam Jacobi, "Some Consid-

erations on the Moral and on the Non-Asylum Treatment of Insanity," *Journal of Social Science* 15, pt. 2 (1882): 86; Beard, *American Nervousness,* p. 119. The idea that all experiences of great intensity, even those generally considered pleasurable, can cause stress is currently being revived. See *New York Times,* 10 June 1973.

15. John P. Gray, "Thoughts on Hygiene," New York State Lunatic Asylum, Utica, *Annual Report* 32 (1874): 59; James F. Hibbard, "The Hygienic Value of Rational Irregularities in Habits of Living," American Public Health Association, *Public Health Papers and Reports* 16 (1890): 189. Even in the 1950s, neuroses were still attributed to such extremes as poverty and wealth, overwork and underwork. See Lawrence S. Kubie, "Social Forces and the Neurotic Process," in *Explorations in Social Psychiatry,* ed. Alexander H. Leighton, John A. Clausen, and Robert N. Wilson (New York: Basic Books, 1957), pp. 78–79.

16. For the pre–Civil War emphasis on environmental factors in mental illness, see Norman Dain, *Concepts of Insanity in the United States, 1789–1865* (New Brunswick, N.J.: Rutgers University Press, 1964), pp. 84–113; and David J. Rothman, *The Discovery of the Asylum: Social Order and Disorder in the New Republic* (Boston: Little, Brown, 1971), pp. 109–29. The views of mental hygienists on success resemble those of the "Genteel Reformers"; both groups came from similar social backgrounds.

17. See S. Weir Mitchell, *Wear and Tear, or Hints for the Overworked* (Philadelphia: Lippincott, 1887); Page, "How Can We Escape Insanity?" pp. 192–93; Stearns, *Insanity,* pp. 104–5; J. S. Jewell, "Influence of Our Present Civilization in the Production of Nervous and Mental Diseases," *Journal of Nervous and Mental Diseases* 8 (1881): 14–17; Eugene Grissom, *Mental Hygiene for Pupil and Teacher. A Lecture* (Raleigh, N.C., 1877), p. 34; Henry M. Hurd, "Predisposing Causes of Insanity," *American Journal of Insanity* 48 (1887): 357–60.

18. Page, "How Can We Escape Insanity?" p. 197; Robert T. Edes, "High-Pressure Education; Its Effects," *Boston Medical and Surgical Journal* 106 (1882): 220–21.

19. C. F. Folsom, "The Prevention of Insanity," American Public Health Association, *Public Health Papers and Reports* 7 (1881): 88.

20. Jacobi, "Some Considerations," pp. 77–96.

21. W. H. DeWitt, "Education, Its Relation to Insanity," *Cincinnati Lancet and Observer* 19 (1876): 998. See also Page, "How Can We Escape Insanity?" p. 194; Joseph F. Kett, "Adolescence and Youth in Nineteenth-Century America," *Journal of Interdisciplinary History* 2 (1971): 287.

22. John Favill, "Mental Hygiene," Wisconsin State Board of Health, *Annual Report* 1 (1876): 52–53; John P. Gray, "Insanity: Its Frequency: And Some of Its Preventable Causes," New York State Lunatic Asylum, Utica, *Annual Report* 43 (1885): 57–60.

23. Turnbull, "Education as a Means for the Prevention of Insanity," pp. 295–96; James McLachlan, *American Boarding Schools: A Historical Study* (New York: Scribner, 1970), p. 178. The view that masturbation had been overemphasized as a cause of insanity appeared in "Reports of Societies: New York Neurological Society," *Boston Medical and Surgical Journal* 116 (1887): 12–14; Folsom, "Prevention of Insanity," p. 89; and Nathan Allen to Dr. [Edward] Hitchcock, 20 January 1862, College Archives, Amherst College, Amherst, Mass.

24. Daniel Hack Tuke, *Insanity in Ancient and Modern Life, with Chapters on Its*

Prevention (London: Macmillan, 1878), p. 176; Stearns, *Insanity*, p. 195; R. T. Edes, "The New England Invalid," *Boston Medical and Surgical Journal* 133 (1895): 102. The relationship between ill health and the declining birthrate was a favorite medical subject in the late nineteenth century. See Carroll Smith-Rosenberg and Charles Rosenberg, "The Female Animal: Medical and Biological Views of Woman and Her Role in Nineteenth-Century America," *Journal of American History* 60 (1973): 332–56.

25. Mitchell, *Wear and Tear*, pp. 35–36, 32. For divergent interpretations of Mitchell's treatment of women, see Ann Douglas Wood, " 'The Fashionable Diseases': Women's Complaints and Their Treatment in Nineteenth-Century America," *Journal of Interdisciplinary History* 4 (1973): 25–52; Regina Markell Morantz, "The Lady and Her Physician," in *Clio's Consciousness Raised: New Perspectives on the History of Women*, ed. Mary S. Hartman and Lois W. Banner (New York: Octagon, 1974), pp. 38–53. See also Carroll Smith-Rosenberg, "The Hysterical Woman: Sex Roles and Role Conflict in 19th-Century America," *Social Research* 39 (1972): 652–78.

26. Mary Putnam Jacobi, "Modern Female Invalidism," *Boston Medical and Surgical Journal* 133 (1895): 174–75; Jacobi, "Some Considerations," pp. 77–96. See Mary Putnam Jacobi, *The Question of Rest for Women During Menstruation* (New York: Putnams, 1877).

27. A thoughtful interpretation of the medical literature on sexuality suggests the diverse social and personality needs this advice may have served. See Charles E. Rosenberg, "Sexuality, Class and Role in 19th-Century America," *American Quarterly* 25 (1973): 131–53; Rothman, *Discovery of the Asylum*, pp. 109–54, 206–36; Peter T. Cominos, "Late-Victorian Sexual Respectability and the Social System," *International Review of Social History* 8 (1963): 18–48, 216–50.

28. For a critique of the practice of defining health or normality on the basis of evidence drawn from patients, see Daniel Offer and Melvin Sabshin, *Normality: Theoretical and Clinical Concepts of Mental Health* (New York: Basic Books, 1966). The subjects of a 1958 study of "normal" young men virtually embodied the Gilded Age definition of mental health. They were little inclined to introspection or fantasy, had fairly strong impulse control, mild emotional responses, and had acquired a realistic self-image without an identity crisis. See Roy R. Grinker, Sr., Roy R. Grinker, Jr., and John Timberlake, " 'Mentally Healthy' Young Males (Homoclites): A Study," *Archives of General Psychiatry* 6 (1962): 405–53.

29. For suggestive data on mortality, see Frederick I. Hoffman, "American Mortality Progress during the Last Half Century," Mazÿck P. Ravenel, ed., *A Half Century of Public Health* (New York: American Public Health Association, 1921), pp. 94–117; and Edgar Sydenstricker, "The Vitality of the American People," *Recent Social Trends of the United States: Report of the President's Research Committee on Social Trends* (New York: McGraw-Hill, 1933), 1: 602–60. Obviously a high death rate was not unique to this generation, but its impact may have been increased by its conjunction with diminishing birthrates and the erosion of religious reassurances about death.

30. For the effects of loss, see John Bowlby, "Separation Anxiety," *International Journal of Psycho-Analysis* 41 (1960): 89–113. For Charles Darwin's efforts to "cut down on his emotional intake" (a need related to his turning away from

religion), see Donald Fleming, "Charles Darwin, The Anaesthetic Man," *Victorian Studies* 4 (1961): 219–36. The life of Mary Putnam Jacobi's husband provides a particularly telling example of the high incidence of infant and maternal death. It is ironic that Abraham Jacobi, considered by many the founder of American pediatrics, outlived two wives, and of the eight children he fathered, only one lived to adulthood.

31. Mary Putnam Jacobi, [Address Twelfth-St. School Reunion], 1902, Folder no. 35, p. 6, Mary Putnam Jacobi Papers, Schlesinger Library, Radcliffe College, Cambridge, Mass.

32. S. Weir Mitchell, *Dr. North and His Friends* (New York: Century, 1901), p. 389.

33. Erik H. Erikson has suggested that neurotic anxiety can be avoided sometimes by "concentration on limited goals with circumscribed laws." Erik H. Erikson, *Childhood and Society* (New York: Norton, 1963), pp. 308–9.

34. Rosenberg, "The Place of George M. Beard in Nineteenth-Century Psychiatry"; Charles L. Dana, "Dr. George M. Beard: A Sketch of His Life and Character," *Archives of Neurology and Psychiatry* 10 (1923): 427–35; "George Miller Beard, A.M., M.D.," *Encyclopaedia of Contemporary Biography of New York*, 6 vols. (New York: Atlantic, 1883), vol. 3; A. D. Rockwell, *Rambling Recollections. An Autobiography* (New York: Hoeber, 1920).

35. [Mary Ann Fellows Beard] to George M. Beard, 15 July 1862, George M. Beard Papers, Yale University Library, New Haven, Conn. See also W. H. Beard to George M. Beard, 16 February 1863, Yale University Library. For evidence of the family's separation, see "Rev. Edwin Spencer Beard" [Windham County], transcript, n.d., Archives of the Andover Newton Theological School, Newton Center, Mass.

36. George M. Beard, Private Journal, pp. 73–76, 82–83, 90, 103–4, 143, 172, 180, 181, 193, 200, 201, Beard Papers. See also Spencer Field Beard to George M. Beard, 14 March 1866, Beard Papers.

37. George M. Beard, Private Journal, pp. 75, 95, 90, 107, 112–13, 164–65, 182, Beard Papers.

38. Beard Papers, pp. 154, 88, 125, 139–40, 84. For the quotation on sinful pleasures, see Rockwell, *Rambling Recollections*, p. 185.

39. Spencer Field Beard to George M. Beard, 1 December 1856, Beard Papers.

40. George M. Beard, Private Journal, pp. 87, 88, 96, 98, 109–10, 185–86, 201–2, Beard Papers.

41. Beard Papers, pp. 183, 204, 203.

42. Rockwell to C. L. Dana, 3 November 1905, Beard Papers; letter inserted in A. D. Rockwell, *The Late Dr. George M. Beard. A Sketch* (New York: American Academy of Medicine, 1883). George M. Beard's journal ends in 1863, shortly after he joined the church. Unfortunately, there is no surviving evidence that indicates his reasons for leaving it again. Probably his medical studies and conversion to evolutionary theory played a part. Even before completing his medical studies, he had begun to direct his energies into popular lectures and articles on hygiene. Beard, Private Journal, pp. 80, 101, 145, 189, 194–95, Beard Papers.

43. C. L. Dana, "Dr. George M. Beard," pp. 429–30; George M. Beard, Private

Journal, p. 76, Beard Papers. For his views on treatment, see George M. Beard, *A Practical Treatise on Nervous Exhaustion (Neurasthenia), Its Symptoms, Nature, Sequences, Treatment* (New York: Treat, 1880). For his need for recognition, see George M. Beard, *Herbert Spencer on American Nervousness. A Scientific Coincidence* (New York: Putnams, 1883); "George Miller Beard," *Encyclopaedia of Contemporary Biography*.

44. George M. Beard, Private Journal, p. 157, Beard Papers. Beard, *American Nervousness*, pp. 313–14, 336–38; George M. Beard, "Medical Education and the Medical Profession in Europe and America," pp. 35, 23, Beard Papers.

45. George M. Beard, *Sexual Neurasthenia (Nervous Exhaustion). Its Hygiene, Causes, Symptoms, and Treatment*, ed. A. D. Rockwell (New York: Treat, 1884), pp. 102–3, 117–28; Beard, *American Nervousness*, pp. 313–14; Rockwell, *Rambling Recollections*, p. 186; E. C. Spitzka, Review of *A Practical Treatise on Nervous Exhaustion (Neurasthenia); Its Symptoms, Nature, Sequences, Treatment*, by George M. Beard, *St. Louis Clinical Record* 7 (1880): 93. For George M. Beard's views on food and drink, see George M. Beard, *Eating and Drinking, A Popular Manual of Food and Diet in Health and Disease* (New York: Putnams, 1871), pp. 84–96; George M. Beard, *Stimulants and Narcotics; Medically, Philosophically, and Morally Considered* (New York: Putnams, 1871); *Scientific Reform, a Letter to Rev. Theodore L. Cuyler, D.D. on the Attitude of Physicians and Scientists Toward the Temperance Cause* (New York: Putnams, 1872).

46. Walter E. Houghton, *The Victorian Frame of Mind, 1830–1870* (New Haven: Yale University Press, 1957), pp. 61–77.

47. For material on Mary Putnam Jacobi, see Ruth Putnam, ed., *Life and Letters of Mary Putnam Jacobi* (New York: Putnams, 1925); Roy Lubove, "Mary Corinna Putnam Jacobi," in *Notable American Women 1607–1950: A Biographical Dictionary*, ed. Edward T. James, Janet Wilson James, and Paul S. Boyer, 3 vols. (Cambridge, Mass.: Harvard University Press, 1971), 2:263–65; Eugene P. Link, "Abraham and Mary P. Jacobi, Humanitarian Physicians," *Journal of the History of Medicine and Allied Sciences* 4 (1949): 382–92; Victor Robinson, "Mary Putnam Jacobi," *Medical Life* 35 (1928): 334–54; Rhoda Truax, *The Doctors Jacobi* (Boston: Little, Brown, 1952).

48. Putnam, *Life and Letters of Mary Putnam Jacobi*, pp. 23–28, 32–33; Jacobi, Address [Twelfth-St. School Reunion], 1902, Folder 35, Mary Putnam Jacobi Papers.

49. Putnam, *Life and Letters of Mary Putnam Jacobi*, pp. 28–30, 35–42, 53–59. See also "Conversations with Dr. Anderson, June, 1862," Folder 12, "M. C. Putnam to George H. Putnam, 1857," Folder 9, Mary Putnam Jacobi Papers; George Haven Putnam, *Memories of My Youth: 1844–1865* (New York: Putnams, 1914), pp. 77–78.

50. Putnam, *Life and Letters of Mary Putnam Jacobi*, pp. 31, 29.

51. Women's Medical Association of New York City, *In Memory of Mary Putnam Jacobi, January 4, 1907* (New York: Academy of Medicine, 1907), p. 5; Putnam, *Life and Letters of Mary Putnam Jacobi*, pp. 16, 106. For Mary Putnam Jacobi's defense of Positivism, see Mary Putnam Jacobi, *The Value of Life: A Reply to Dr. Mallock's Essay "Is Life Worth Living?"* (New York, 1879).

52. Putnam, *Life and Letters of Mary Putnam Jacobi*, pp. 80–82, 322–23, 110–11. Victorine

Haven Putnam was eighteen when Mary Putnam was born; the next child arrived eighteen months later. Ibid., p. 15. Joyce Cushmore, "Abraham Jacobi: Father of American Pediatrics," *American-German Review* 25 (1959): 29–31, 37.

53. Jacobi, "Modern Female Invalidism," p. 174; Jacobi, "Some Considerations," p. 89; Putnam, *Life and Letters of Mary Putnam Jacobi*, pp. 203, 105–6.

54. Putnam, *Life and Letters of Mary Putnam Jacobi*, pp. 117, 141–42, 123, 203.

55. Mary Putnam Jacobi, "Effeminacy," Folder 3, "Fugitive Papers Before 1873," Mary Putnam Jacobi Papers. A reference to "dying ones" suggests that the piece may have been written in the early years of the Civil War.

56. Mary Putnam Jacobi, ed., *Women's Medical Association of New York City*, p. 504; Jacobi, *Value of Life*, pp. 229, 237.

57. Stearns, *Insanity*, p. 216.

58. S. Weir Mitchell, *Doctor and Patient* (Philadelphia: Lippincott, 1904), p. 6; S. Weir Mitchell, *Address on Opening of the Institute of Hygiene of the University of Pennsylvania* (Philadelphia: University of Pennsylvania Press, 1892), p. 4.

59. Tuke, *Insanity in Ancient and Modern Life*, p. 196. By the late nineteenth century, ministers, too, favored less restrictive child-rearing methods.

60. Page, "How Can We Escape Insanity?" p. 198; Beverley R. Tucker, *S. Weir Mitchell: A Brief Sketch of His Life with Personal Recollections* (Boston: Badger, 1914), p. 48; Folsom, "The Prevention of Insanity," p. 89; Wardner, "Thoughts on Insanity and Its Preventable Causes," pp. 385–86.

61. Nathan Allen, "Physical Culture," College Archives, Amherst College, Amherst, Mass.; Gray, "Insanity," pp. 54–55; Folsom, "The Prevention of Insanity," p. 90.

62. Like George M. Beard and Mary Putnam Jacobi, Mitchell also suffered from religious terrors, ill health in adolescence, and had at least two severe bouts of nervousness as an adult. His brother died of tuberculosis in Weir Mitchell's youth. See Anna Robeson Burr, *Weir Mitchell: His Life and Letters* (New York: Duffield, 1929); Ernest Earnest, *S. Weir Mitchell: Novelist and Physician* (Philadelphia: University of Pennsylvania Press, 1950); Margaret C.-L. Gildea and Edwin F. Gildea, "Personalities of American Psychotherapists: Mitchell, Salmon, Riggs," *American Journal of Psychiatry* 101 (1945): 464–66.

63. Mary Putnam Jacobi suggested that superior individuals, including scholars, poets, and statesmen, were ready to sacrifice their health for higher goals. Jacobi, *Value of Life*, p. 201.

64. Donald Meyer, *The Positive Thinkers: A Study of the American Quest for Health, Wealth and Personal Power from Mary Baker Eddy to Norman Vincent Peale* (Garden City, N.Y.: Doubleday, 1965).

65. William James, *The Energies of Men* (New York: Dodd, 1914); William James, *Talks for Teachers on Psychology and to Students on Some of Life's Ideals* (New York: Holt, 1962), pp. 99–112. On mental health in the Progressive era, see Sicherman, "The Quest for Mental Health," pp. 391–410.

BONNIE ELLEN BLUSTEIN

10 "A Hollow Square of Psychological Science": American Neurologists and Psychiatrists in Conflict

"The modern science of psychology," declared the American neurologist William Hammond in 1876, "is neither more nor less than *the science of mind considered as a physical function.*"[1] Because he and other physicians with a special interest in diseases of the nervous system believed this, they threw open their office doors to patients suffering from such "nervous" complaints as insomnia, dyspepsia, and general malaise. Because many lay persons in the bustling and often bewildering urban centers also believed it, clinical neurology prospered in America, and especially in New York City, in the decades after the Civil War.[2] The specialty began to acquire an organizational apparatus with the formation of the New York Neurological Society in March 1872, its rival New York Society for Neurology and Electrology in 1874, and the American Neurological Association (initially dominated by New Yorkers) in 1875. Three years later, New York neurologists—or at least some of their most outspoken leaders—were ready to make a bid for control of the institutions that could serve as a base for their teaching and research: the large and crowded asylums for the insane. They therefore launched a public attack on the professional organization that had virtually monopolized these institutions since 1844, the Association of Medical Superintendents of American Institutions for the Insane (AMSAII).[3] However, in bringing to the fore the issue of scientific reform in the study and practice of psychiatry, they also exposed their own work to more concentrated and critical scrutiny. It is an irony of the asylum reform movement of 1878–83 that the neurologists who helped to initiate and lead it were ultimately unable to meet the challenge that they had themselves invited.

No specialty within nineteenth-century American medicine corresponds precisely to the psychiatry of our own time, and the distinction then existing between neurologist and superintendent was no simple division of labor. Rather, responsibility for the care of the insane lay at the intersection of the crosscutting concerns of two distinct and very different sections of the profession. One psychiatric tradition, "developed out of a growing medical response to patients sufficiently ill or aged or 'difficult' to require hospitalization," was practiced almost exclusively by the superintendents who were represented in the Asylum Association.[4] The views of these men on asylum construction and management (their main shared concerns) owed much to British psychiatric practice and psychological thought, particularly the tradition of "moral treatment" of the insane.[5] In contrast, American neurology was based largely on Civil War experience with gunshot wounds of the nerves; the expertise of its practitioners originally centered on the diagnosis and treatment of organic disorders. But their postwar civilian practices quickly grew to include "the still functioning though symptom-bearing psychiatric patient outside of institutional settings."[6] The theory that underpinned this style of work was drawn largely from French and German sources: it was a conception of neurology as one discipline that studied a range of problems from normal psychology to insanity, to functional and finally to organic nervous disorders. Neurologists styled themselves as scientists above all, deliberately (but not cynically) employing the most up-to-date medical technology and the most vigorous denunciation of metaphysics. This was a role with obvious appeal in a metropolis whose citizens were busily striving to make it into a modern cultural and scientific as well as a commercial center.[7] New York neurologists, therefore, had many reasons to believe that they could successfully challenge the well-established superintendents who still dominated the field of psychological medicine in America.

Historians of American medicine who have discussed the contest between neurologists and superintendents have usually placed it in the context of the development of psychiatry rather than neurology.[8] By the middle of the 1870s, many asylum superintendents had come to see neurology as an increasingly serious threat. The AMSAII was by then already under attack by such leaders of medical psychology as John C. Bucknill of England for its failure not only to make good its extravagant claims of the curability of insanity in the asylum context, but also to apply consistently its own theoretical principles. In addition, its exclusion of all but superintendents of insane asylums left an increasing proportion of American alienists (including assistant superintendents and directors of institutions for the feebleminded) outside the fold, and fostered a limited and conservative outlook among the members of the association.[9] While the rise of neurology did not create these problems, it undoubtedly aggravated them. Neurologists have sometimes been seen as obstructionists whose narrowly physicalist conceptions inhibited the development of psychotherapy.[10] Alternatively, some neurologists—such as the iconoclastic George M. Beard and the influential James Jackson Putnam—have been recognized for their often prophetic psychiatric insights.[11] The neurologists' attack on abusive practices they claimed were prevalent in American asylums and their sharp criticism of the superintendents' presumed ignorance of the latest work in medical science have been seen as a stimulus —perhaps the key one—to psychiatric innovation. Barbara Sicherman, for instance, has written that "medical specialists in neurology provided . . . probably the decisive . . . impetus to asylum reform."[12] More recent work, however, has stressed emerging conflicts within psychiatry itself as the critical factors in its largely self-imposed reforms toward the end of the nineteenth century. While not denying that external challenges influenced the behavior of the superintendents, this view does reopen the question of the significance of their conflict with the neurologists.

It would be an oversimplification at best to view the neurologists' involvement in the asylum reform movement as a manipulative policy of a coterie selfishly wishing to extend its influence and income, a charge frequently articulated by contemporaries and echoed by a few historians.[13] It is probable, although undetermined empirically, that to some extent private-practice neurologists and asylum superintendents competed for the same "insane" patients. But there is also strong reason to believe that most asylum inhabitants would have been inappropriate and unwanted candidates for outpatient neurological attention: they were simply either too crazy or too poor.[14] We are thus led to consider other professional reasons neurologists offered or might reasonably have had for pursuing the asylum reform issue. Some, notably Edward Spitzka (recently returned from European study), decried the "waste of material" occasioned by the superintendents' neglect of scientific investigation; they suggested that their own researches would be greatly facilitated by access to asylum patients. Such access, they noted, would also allow more thorough clinical instruction for medical students and thus would benefit the profession as a whole.[15] Beyond this, the insane occupied a central band of the spectrum of neurological patients that I have just described. Reflective neurologists frequently asserted that any rigid distinction between "nervous" and "mental" diseases was theoretically impossible, although at times obvious and even necessary in practice.[16] To such men, the existence of large asylums for the insane, often publicly supported and usually beyond neurological influence, may well have appeared to be a visible contradiction of the main principles of their science.

In the present essay, I recount the story of the contest between neurologists and superintendents in some detail in order to illustrate the somewhat paradoxical situation of American neurology a century ago. The events of the years 1878–83 began to reveal many of the stresses and strains

that were emerging within the specialty as neurologists attempted to incorporate clinical experience and scientific preconceptions into a unified
body of knowledge. The story also suggests the extent to which the limits
of such a medical debate may be set by the interests and opinions of the
lay public. While the private-practice neurologist typically relied neither
on political patronage nor on the massive financial support which came to
be necessary for medical research in the twentieth century, he was inescapably dependent on how Americans "with means" decided whether or not
to entrust themselves and their relatives to his care. Thus the controversy
addressed here was not simply a jurisdictional dispute among professionals
that happened to spill over into the popular press, but an example of the
interrelations of lay and professional concerns in the establishment of a
working definition of insanity and a workable specialty of neurology.

In the end, neurologists of the 1880s were scarcely more successful
than their contemporaries in the Asylum Association in constructing a
usable and consistent science of abnormal psychology. Moreover, they had
to contend with mounting public skepticism (and perhaps with their own
private doubts) about their central claims, despite the partial success of the
asylum reform campaign. The distinguished otologist D. B. St. John
Roosa, for example, a former officer of several neurological societies, jocu-
larly told an alumni dinner of the University Medical College (New York)
in 1882 that

> our bosoms swell with pride when we come to our alienists. With our
> Kiernan, our Spitzka, our MacDonald and our Hammond, we present
> a hollow square of psychological science that can successfully resist
> any charge that the rough riders of the law may make upon us. There
> is no question of insanity that we cannot get on both sides of, and
> illustrate the resources of medical minds and the independence of
> thought inspired by the chairs of neurology and medical jurispru-
> dence.[17]

Resourcefulness and originality, however, were unsatisfactory substitutes
for the standards of precision and objectivity that were considered by all
concerned to be the hallmarks of scientific medicine.

Open conflict between neurologists and superintendents began early
in March 1878 with the presentation before the New York Neurological
Society of Spitzka's paper on "The Study of Insanity Considered as a
Branch of Neurology, and the Relations of the General Medical Body to
This Branch," published soon after by the twenty-five-year-old author
under the title "Reform in the Scientific Study of Psychiatry."[18] As a
program for the advancement of neurological science, Spitzka's remarks
resonated with many current ideas for the upgrading of medicine as a

profession. First, he stressed the need for scientific study (not just humane care) of the insane, and in explicating this he relied on a prevalent conception of science as both materialist and reductionist. " 'Mental disease' is merely a symptomatic term," he declared, "as 'mental' and 'moral' are adjectives founded on abstractions. With the abstract, medicine does not profess to deal, and accordingly the great masters of modern science have ever sought for a proper material basis for such symptomatic conceptions." Investigation had proved that "the topographical area within which the mental pathologist is to conduct his difficult and interesting researches, constitutes but a segment of that great system which comprises the legitimate domain of the general neurologist." Spitzka therefore concluded that "from a pathological and clinical point of view . . . the study of insanity should be considered a subdivision of neurology."[19]

Spitzka looked to the insane asylum for an appropriate context in which to pursue this research, probably with the example in mind of the European general and mental hospitals in which he had recently studied. He was disturbed, therefore, that "it is only under exceptional circumstances, if ever at all in America, that the teacher of nervous diseases can command the material essential to a thorough clinical and pathological demonstration of insanity." Asylum reform was thus necessary and proper, and neurologists would not be the only beneficiaries. "There is hardly a specialty in medicine," Spitzka asserted, "which will not profit by the opportunities thus given of extending the scope of its investigation." And the general practitioner, given the chance to study insane patients as part of his education, could "be taught insanity sufficiently thoroughly as not to be at a loss when mental alienation occurs in his practice as a complication of other diseases." In urging the appointment of visiting physicians to asylums, especially "neurologists, and by preference, of such neurologists as are engaged in instruction in our regular medical schools," Spitzka could thus anticipate support from outside the circle of his own specialty. His goal of the full use of hospitals for teaching purposes, in particular, was frequently articulated by the leaders of the profession. However, it was infrequently realized. "The material of our asylums is a rich material, but it will remain a dead material unless the general medical body examines the subject of asylum management from a medical and philanthropic point of view," he wrote. He recommended "uniting psychiatry with neurology, in our college courses, and . . . liberally providing the teachers of these subjects with the requisite material. This should be effected by the same mechanism which is employed in the utilization of the material collected in our general hospitals."[20]

Spitzka's analysis of the obstacles in the way of this program was not only advanced but controversial: it was a call to arms against what he considered to be an unscientific monopoly enjoyed by a small clique of asylum superintendents. He suggested that the problem was at root "that spirit, dominating the Asylum Association, which systematically shuns inquiry, excludes competition, avoids open discussion, and opposes supervision, because it has the best reasons for fearing such inquiry, competition, discussion and supervision." He admitted that he did not oppose monopoly in principle: "If capable, zealous and honest scientists establish a monopoly in scientific matters, even a monopoly may become endurable." But he insisted that the present crop of superintendents, many of them political appointees, had violated the public trust by failing to use the opportunities that were available to them to advance the science of psychiatry.[21]

The young neurologist eloquently expressed his outrage at the sins against science that were allegedly committed by asylum superintendents. They concerned themselves with obituaries of their fellows and reminiscences of their patients, with roofing and drainpipes and agricultural prizes, with inaccurate historical digressions and "impassioned glorifications of 'mechanical restraint.'" They were, "in short, experts at everything except the diagnosis, pathology and treatment of insanity." Their infrequent and perfunctory autopsies were conducted for the coroner, not for science. Their institutions lacked ophthalmoscopes, electrical apparatus, microscopes, and other essential instruments; their published clinical lectures lacked accuracy, and their occasional attempts at research lacked elementary honesty. Citing in particular the large sums of public money spent at an unnamed asylum in New York State (undoubtedly Utica), Spitzka concluded that "the work there done is not only without value, but absolutely misleading; that the claims advanced are founded on that happy combination of effrontery and ignorance, which currently passes under the designation of, and is certainly kin to, charlatanism; in short, that the State has paid $50,000 for what is little better than the private advertisements of one medical superintendent."[22]

Spitzka's animadversions on the superintendents' scientific attainments were elaborated by others in the discussion following the reading of his paper. Superintendent Wilbur of the Asylum for Idiots in Syracuse (who would later become a key leader of the asylum reform movement) had prepared an extended critique of the misuse of medical statistics in the Annual Report of the Utica Asylum, a report which had received favorable newspaper publicity.[23] Edward C. Seguin, president of the New York Neurological Society, "could strongly endorse the position taken by Dr. Spitzka. . . . He had several years previous been present at a meeting of the Asylum Association, and had noticed that no scientific papers or discussions there occurred, in fact there was absolutely no provision for scientific contributions made." He also noted, perhaps smugly, that "in the preamble of their Constitution, we look in vain for the word 'Science.' "[24]

The scientific outlook, then, was the critical distinction—from the neurologists' point of view—between themselves and the superintendents. Spitzka had added, almost as an afterthought, that unscientific asylum superintendence also led to many "features revolting to humanity," and suggested that (contrary to the repeated pronouncements of superintendents) home treatment was often more conducive to rapid recovery than were "the grated windows, crib-beds, bleak walls, gruff attendants, narcotics and insane surroundings of an asylum."[25] Although such humanitarian considerations were secondary, at best, in this initial report, they would become the main issues in the public debate which was to follow.

Spitzka's paper was referred by the Neurological Society to a three-man committee, which in April 1878 reported its recommendations for launching a crusade for "asylum reform." The neurologists were by no means unanimous as to the desirability of this project, but the group endorsed the conclusions that Spitzka had

> brought forward much that is worthy of the earnest attention of the Neurological Society and demanding its active interference to rectify if possible the evils complained of and which the committee believed to exist.
> The committee would especially urge . . . a determined effort toward the prohibition of mechanical restraint . . . believing as they do that such means are unworthy of the age, contrary to sound medical science and discountenanced by the experiences of many years in Great Britain, France and Germany.[26]

The group also adopted the recommendations that the society support and urge other physicians to support a resolution before the State Assembly along the same lines, and voted to submit the report for publication in the widely read *Medical Record*. Three members were delegated to solicit endorsements of the legislative petition from other physicians. And in the elections that were held later that evening, the society chose leading anti-asylum activists to serve as president, first and second vice-presidents, treasurer, and to fill three seats on its council.[27]

While Spitzka and a few associates (notably Hammond) were mobilizing the Neurological Society for this fight, they were attempting to do the same in the New York Medico-Legal Society. This body, composed of lawyers and doctors (including several prominent neurologists), had frequently interested itself in such legal issues as the testamentary capacity of allegedly insane persons, the "insanity defense" for persons accused of violent crimes, and procedures for commitment to the asylum. Spitzka's paper on "Real Asylum Abuses," which was read before the group in March 1878, was thus not out of place, and again the audience was sympathetic to his plea and to Hammond's call for action. "In accordance with

a unanimously carried motion, a committee was appointed, with powers
to memorialize the Legislature regarding the alleged abuses, and instructed to append a copy of Dr. Spitzka's paper to the memorial in question."[28]

It was not to be expected that the superintendents would remain silent
in the face of this onslaught. An editorial written by Hammond and
published anonymously in the *New York Herald* soon provided an occasion
for a much-publicized attack on the author, who was already known to the
public as a controversial figure.[29] Eugene Grissom's speech "True and
False Experts," which was read before a large audience at the annual
meeting of the Asylum Association in the nation's capital, was reported the
next day in the Washington *National Standard*. Grissom chose to ignore
Hammond's allegations of abuses at John P. Gray's model Utica Asylum
and his call for a state senatorial investigation, concentrating his fire on
Hammond's moral character and skirting the issue of scientific expertise.
He accused Hammond of lack of sympathy for the insane on the grounds
of the neurologist's narrow construction of the notion of "legal insanity"
and his insistence on the punishability of insane criminals in many cases.
The superintendent of the North Carolina State Asylum hinted that his
rival cared less for the consistency of his expert testimony than for the
large fees he might receive from either defense or prosecution in any legal
case. He was "a moral monster whose baleful eyes gleamed with a delusive
light," and atheistic to boot. Grissom reminded his Washington audience
that Hammond had left that city in disgrace fifteen years earlier, having
been found guilty by court martial of misconduct as Surgeon General of
the United States Army.[30] Thus Grissom conveyed the clear impression
that traditional morality, rather than a scientific orientation, was the main
desideratum for the caretaker of the insane.

"True and False Experts" was featured in the July issue of the *American Journal of Insanity,* prompting Hammond to press libel charges. He did
not sue Grissom (saying that it was not worth his while to travel to North
Carolina to do so), but the editor, John P. Gray of Utica, who was widely
suspected of having instigated Grissom's speech in addition to publishing
it. In his substantive response to Grissom, published in pamphlet form,
Hammond defended his practice of accepting large monetary rewards for
the valuable services that his scientific knowledge enabled him to render.
He did not deny the charge of infidelity; rather, he cited this allegation as
evidence that his opponent was not only ignorant but, more importantly,
unscientific.[31] Hammond had already castigated the asylum system as inhumane in principle, saying that it was wrong to degrade insane persons
by depriving them of their liberty and dignity when they were not dangerous. He thus argued both from the neurologists' point of view, which
placed scientific qualifications first, and from Grissom's, which empha-

sized humanitarian values. He suggested as well that Grissom himself might possibly be insane.

The vituperative tone of Grissom's fusillade, and Hammond's equally colorful rejoinder, attracted wide notoriety. But the general support received by each of these self-appointed champions from his professional organization indicated serious concern for the issues which lay beneath the abusive rhetoric of the sort that was described in the nineteenth century as "indulgence in personalities." The occasional dissenter—such as Superintendent Wallace of Texas, who criticized other members of the Asylum Association for their enthusiastic endorsement of Grissom—only highlighted the lines that had been drawn.[32]

The superintendents had other means of defense at their disposal, as a second incident will illustrate. Dr. A. E. MacDonald, a member of both the New York Neurological Society and the Asylum Association, had listened quietly to Spitzka's denunciation of his asylum colleagues as "shallow pretenders and ignorant indifferentists," and had declined to comment even when invited directly to do so. But then he fired his young assistant at the Ward's Island Asylum, Dr. James Kiernan, who had told the Neurological Society only that "with regard to most of the points in the paper he was not at liberty to deliver an opinion" but that "he could confirm many of the writer's statements, especially as he had himself had the honor of conducting Superintendents through the asylum at which he served, who did not know what progressive paresis was."[33] The superintendents, under attack for their monopolistic domination of the asylums, could still use that power to defend themselves.

Spitzka summed up the summer's controversy in a paper read before the New York Neurological Society in October 1878, "Merits, Motives and Progress of the Reform in Asylum Abuses." The rules of the society were suspended to permit reporters to hear Spitzka's remarks and the comments —doubtless supportive—of Hammond, Kiernan, and Seguin. The next day's *New York Times* contained a not unfavorable summary of this medical press conference.[34] The neurologist pointed out that the superintendents had had ample opportunity to defend themselves, yet they had provided no satisfactory rebuttal to the charges that they were apt to "neglect or distort the pathological study of insanity," that they were "*not* appointed to their positions on grounds of special proficiency or ability," and that they "treat[ed] their patients with a neglectful and cruel routine, and cause[d] damage by employing unphysiological methods of restraint." Instead, they had endorsed Grissom's invocation of "religious and sectarian prejudices" and resorted to "an appeal to indifferentism" on the question of autopsies. "We need not ask the question of any enlightened body of colleagues," Spitzka declared, "whether such a procedure could be employed by any Association which has the shadow of a right to call itself a scientific one."[35] It was clear then, at least to the neurologist, that the medical profession—and especially those members who had made a special study of the nervous system—had not only a right but a duty to investigate the asylums.

The experience of the past months had convinced Spitzka that the existence of abuse was no longer a matter of doubt. Moreover, no protection was to be expected from the State Lunacy Commissioner, who appeared to consider his job to be the protection of "the interests of the asylum circle." What was now needed would be an official inquiry and examination to move the controversy beyond bitterness and charges of personal hostility. Then the present asylum critics would be called upon "not only to elevate science, to raise the tone of an important branch of the medical profession, to benefit both the practitioner, student and clinical teacher, and to ameliorate the condition of the insane, but even to improve on the asylums of the Old World, and to render ours models." Spitzka expressed his hope—as well as his allegiance to the political values of patriotism and the free enterprise system—that American physicians, freed from the interference of "a close [sic] corporation and an unfortunate fusion of political with medical interests," would make rapid progress in psychiatry to the credit of both the profession and the nation.[36]

Spitzka concluded by outlining a twenty-point program that was directed toward "working out the problem of a scientific and liberal management of our asylums." Most points called for reform in supervision, management, and financial accountability; only a few dealt with scientific research. One detailed suggestion would have mandated compulsory, accurate, and minute autopsies on all patients who died in an asylum. Several others concerned the collection of reliable medical statistics of insanity. Above all, the earnest young researcher was sure that in months and years to come, doctors (especially neurologists) would rectify all present shortcomings by approaching the problem of asylum care of the insane with "accuracy as to reported facts, correct logic in forming conclusions, and a liberal scientific spirit."[37]

This offensive soon struck a responsive chord in many general practitioners. Hammond appeared by invitation before the New York State Medical Society at its annual meeting in February 1879 to read a paper on "The Non-Asylum Treatment of the Insane." Here he stressed his opinion that "the medical profession is, as a body, fully as capable of treating cases of insanity as of any other disease." He assured his audience that

> there is nothing surprisingly difficult, obscure, or mysterious about diseases of the brain which can only be learned within the walls of the asylum. . . . A general practitioner of good common sense, well-grounded in the principles of medicine, with such a knowledge of the

human mind and of cerebral physiology and pathology as can be obtained by study, and familiar with all the clinical factors in his patient's history, is more capable of treating successfully a case of insanity than the average asylum physician.[38]

It was, he said, mainly the medical officers of asylums who had "very diligently inculcated the idea that they alone . . . are qualified to take the medical superintendence" of insane patients.[39]

There is reason to believe that Hammond's remarks were not mere cynical attempts to win the support of general practitioners to the cause of asylum reform. His view as to the desirability of the nonasylum treatment of the insane was the natural and logical consequence of a firm belief in the somatic pathology (as well as etiology) of the disease and an equally firm belief in its almost epidemic proportions. As early as 1871—when John P. Gray could still praise the appointment of Hammond to a chair of medical psychology—the neurologist had suggested placing insane patients in the homes of private physicians for treatment, although he still considered asylums necessary and even compared American institutions favorably to European ones.[40] In 1876 he stated that "it is not a matter of doubt that many insane persons are sent to lunatic asylums who could with regard to every consideration affecting their comfort and health be better attended to in their own homes under the care of the family physician."[41]

This opinion did not rest on charges of asylum abuse or mismanagement but on the assumption that the patients were suffering from an ordinary physical disease of the brain. And Hammond apparently never rejected the idea that asylums would always be necessary for the less prosperous patients whose families and friends could not afford private care.[42]

However, while appealing—as Spitzka had done—to the professional pride of the New York general practitioners who may have distrusted the specialism of the superintendents, Hammond was careful to point out the many "eminent alienists," including Seguin, Spitzka, Beard, S. Weir Mitchell, and J. S. Jewell, who practiced the "science and art of psychiatry" without asylum affiliation.[43] He thus left ample room for the claims of neurological expertise: If the average physician could treat diseases of the brain like any others, it was logical to suppose that the expert on diseases of the nervous system could do so still better. The family doctor who encountered a case of insanity would be well advised to arrange for a neurologist's consultation, rather than surrender the patient to an asylum in despair. At least one medical reviewer interpreted Hammond's speech in just this way. It was "a carefully and well-written article," he said. "Dr. Hammond says that a good practitioner is as well able to treat the insane as the superintendent of an asylum. . . . His eminent position as an authority in nervous diseases entitles this paper to a very special consideration, and any physician having such a patient on his hands will do well to consult this paper before taking decided measures relating to an asylum."[44]

Connecticut physicians, too, were actively concerned with the issue of asylums for the insane. With state legislation on asylum construction pending in 1879, Dr. C. M. Carleton, the president of the Connecticut Medical Society, wished his members to "receive proper information relating to the question." The New York Neurological Society was therefore invited to send a representative to address the Connecticut society's annual meeting in Hartford. Again Hammond spoke for the neurologists. Formerly, he said, asylums had been built as prisons and the insane had been treated as criminals; current practice was unfortunately little better. In future years, he predicted, physicians "may even come to the conclusion that asylums are but sorry substitutes for the skill and care which should be exercised towards lunatics in their own homes." Meanwhile, there was much that could be done. Since insanity was a disease like any other, "the absolute and irresponsible power of the superintendents must be taken away, and hospitals for the insane must be organized exactly as are all other hospitals." The repetitive and tedious discussions of asylum construction that characterized meetings of the Asylum Association were unscientific and irrelevant, since neither hospitals nor asylums were in themselves curative. The highest priority for legislation should not be new construction, but reorganization: "It is just here that reformation must begin."[45]

The reform crusade—at least in Hammond's opinion—had achieved considerable success in the few months since the meeting of the New York State Medical Society. The "hundreds of letters I have received from eminent physicians in all parts of the country," he declared, "convince me that the seed then planted has taken root." He urged the Connecticut group to initiate a petition calling for an investigation of the asylums of their state, as the New Yorkers had done. The remainder of his talk underlined this appeal with tales of mechanical restraint, forced feeding, and other alleged abuses. The Neurological Society, hearing that Hammond had been "kindly received" in Hartford, elected Carleton as an honorary member. But several influential Connecticut alienists had taken affront at the New Yorker's remarks, and the paper was not published in the *Transactions* of the Connecticut society as originally intended. Dr. Rufus Barker and Dr. D. D. Cleaveland, whose views on the "cottage system" the neurologist had especially endorsed, joined with six of their Connecticut colleagues to urge Hammond to publish the paper himself, and it appeared in his short-lived journal, *Neurological Contributions.*[46]

Neurological science, however, was not progressing as rapidly as the agitation for asylum reform. Perhaps most conspicuous to the public were the continual wrangles of neurological experts on the witness stand, for such behavior displayed to a large audience their disturbing lack of consensus. In 1879, for example, when the convicted murderer John Reynolds tried to plead mental incompetence, Hammond appeared for the prosecution while his friend and fellow neurologist M. González Echeverría testified for the defense. An editorial in the *Medical Gazette* called the attention of the profession to this disagreement "to indicate the inevitable conclusion that psychological medicine is as yet wanting in the first elements necessary for any branch of scientific investigation, viz., exact methods of observation. Of two observers whose positions should entitle their opinions to equal weight, either one has been deceived by assumed symptoms which the other was shrewd enough to detect, or else both combine to show the uncertainty of the very groundwork on which these opinions rest."[47] Neither interpretation, surely, could be considered a compliment to neurology.

Moreover, the New York asylum reform crusade was by this time—about a year after its inception—in some trouble. In June 1878 the Neurological Society had formed a committee that was to compose "a statement of facts and presumptions regarding insane asylums." This body was to include ten members "with power to add to its number medical men not members of the society." The summer had been occupied with these tasks, and at the October meeting, which Spitzka addressed, the society had accepted the report of its committee and had voted to have copies printed for distribution. The petition prepared and circulated by the Committee on Insane Asylum Abuses of the Neurological Society was submitted to the state Senate in March 1879, and referred to a committee of that body. The two members of the committee (one of whom represented the district including Utica) then brought back a "piece of special pleading, miscalled a report," as the neurological committee described it, "so unfair, so one-sided, and so grossly misrepresenting the real facts of the case, that we feel called upon to solemnly protest against its being received by the profession and public as even remotely embodying the results of a *bona fide* examination."[48]

The senators had acquitted the New York superintendents of all charges of misconduct; their report was seen by many as an implicit indictment of the neurologists. Moreover, some signers of the petition had withdrawn their endorsements. This gave rise to further allegations that the neurologists had used names without permission or had misrepresented their case. In rebuttal, the Neurological Society claimed that "a few of the signers became alarmed when they received a *quasi* threatening summons from the Senate committee . . . and that still a few others withdrew theirs at the personal solicitation of the superintendents."[49] Whatever the merits of these charges and countercharges, the neurologists were clearly on the defensive.

By the fall, the neurologists saw even a greater need of vindication. Hammond indignantly reported to his colleagues in October that "a board of consulting physicians had been appointed to the insane asylums under the charge of the Commissioners of Charity and Corrections [of New York City] not one member of which was noted in any way as a psychologist; while all of them were either as medical officers of other institutions under the control of the commissioners or as Deans of Colleges bound to the Commission by ties which would hamper any attempt on their part to independent action."[50] The appointment of such a board, of course, had been one of the neurologists' original demands; its composition was for this reason all the more offensive. Hammond offered the resolution "that in the opinion of the Neurological Society the Board of Consulting Physicians . . . is not so constituted as to represent the science of psychological medicine being composed as it is of physicians and surgeons who however distinguished in other directions have had little or no experience with insanity and who have not made special study of the subject."[51]

The mood of the meeting, with Spitzka in the chair, is suggested by the fact that the motion was seconded by L. C. Gray and carried before Dr. McBride thought to ask for the names of the appointees in question. Hammond's reply was doubtless satisfactory: while the new board included such outstanding clinicians as Edward G. Janeway, A. L. Loomis, and Austin Flint, Jr., the only member with any claim to psychological expertise was the young Allan McLane Hamilton, an asylum employee whom Hammond was suing for plagiarism. But still Hammond saw fit to modify his rhetoric. He "did not by any means intend to cast a reflection on the appointees," he said diplomatically, although it is difficult to understand how else his remarks about their lack of independence could be construed. "There were distinguished surgeons, pathologists and physiologists among them. But it stood to reason that, just as it would be absurd to appoint a consulting board entirely composed of psychologists to a Women's Hospital, so it was absurd to appoint to lunatic asylums a board containing not a single psychologist." He then remarked with unmistakable personal animus that the board "could not have been more favorable to the superintendents than if the latter had themselves as was very likely selected the names of the appointees."[52]

The society was apparently convinced that their specialty had been slighted by the Commissioner. The Committee on Asylum Abuses was continued, despite its difficulties in the spring, and a motion that Hammond's resolution be published was referred to the council for action. Not only that, but the chair moved that a minute of the meeting of 9 January

1877, which reported a vote of thanks to Dr. MacDonald (still superintendent of the city asylum on Ward's Island but no longer a member of the society), be stricken from the record as incorrect. No one present seemed to recollect the passage of such a motion, nor the reading of such a minute. MacDonald's former associates resolved unanimously that the note was "an improper record."[53]

In the following weeks, however, several members of the society came to believe that approval of Hammond's resolution had been precipitous. Dr. Seguin stated at the November meeting that "he himself, and he believed also other members of the Society, had labored ... under a wrong impression . . . that as he now understood the question from private conversations the Board . . . [was] not expected to pass judgment upon cases of insanity, but that, on the contrary, each member was to restrict himself to opinions upon the special branch of medicine of which he was considered a specialist." He therefore moved reconsideration. After some discussion it was decided to ask the Commissioner of Charities and Corrections for more information.[54]

By December no satisfactory answer to this request had been received. Moreover, the *New York Times* had confirmed Hammond's worst apprehensions. Not only did it declare flatly that the board did "represent all the important specialties," as Spitzka took pains to point out to the other neurologists, but it attacked the very idea that insanity was a disease of the brain. New Yorkers were informed that

> a belief has been strongly growing up among the best medical practitioners . . . that insanity, although registered as a disease of the brain and nervous system, arises, in the majority of instances, from causes not primarily nervous in their origin. . . . It may be regarded as a demonstrated fact, said a member of the board yesterday, that, as a rule, there is no primary lesion of the brain in insanity. . . . Direct medicament of the brain and nervous system is malpractice in [many] cases; and yet the system has been to dose with bromides and narcotics.[55]

Such a direct challenge to their specialty could scarcely have been ignored by the Neurological Society, whether or not asylum reform was an issue. Eight months earlier the *Times* had expressed skepticism about the materialistic claims of neurology. "No accurate definition of insanity is now, or is ever likely to be, possible," the editor commented. "Although usually co-related with brain disease, it by no means follows that a man is to be pronounced insane because brain disease exists in his case. . . . The thing to be established is a mental phenomenon (an intangible thing). . . . Experts are always liable to err by confounding the cerebral disease with the mental disturbance."[56] And as the investigation of the city asylums got

under way in November, the *Times* presented a still more damaging indictment of neurology:

> The members of the Board [it stated] pretty unanimously express the
> conviction that the cant of psychological medicine and the eloquent
> talk about the wonderful properties of nerve-cells and their laws of
> action have held the attention of medical men altogether too long, and
> that the time has come to dismiss this high-sounding rigmarole from
> the literature of science, and to place insanity where it belongs—as a
> symptom of disease which may or may not have its primary seat in
> the nervous system. . . . [T]he institution of the board represents a
> turning-point in the doctrines, literature, and treatment of insanity.[57]

It was contrary to the canons of scientific inquiry, as well as medical
ethics, to debate medical matters in the popular press. However, a correspondent signing himself "D" wrote to the *Times* to rebut this pernicious
view, which he said was "as old as the hills." D. carefully explained that
"while no specific lesion of the brain has always been found in insanity
. . . it is generally supposed that the morbid changes are too subtle, our
instruments and tests, etc., too gross to determine the fact positively one
way or the other." In such cases, besides, lesions were rarely found elsewhere in the body to account for the insanity. In "replacing" insanity
among the noncerebral diseases, D. concluded, "the committee will be
doing nothing new or original, for that is where insanity is already placed
for the last 40 or 50 years, and with almost as little success as when it was
placed in the misty regions of metaphysics."[58]

This was an unusual debate for the public newspapers, and one which
suggests the importance attached to lay opinion by the neurologists, despite their commitment to the elite scientific culture.

The *Times* editor chose to respond to D. on a less theoretical plane.
"One of the difficulties to be encountered" by the asylum investigators, he
said, "lay in the fact that a crusade, led by one of our so-called experts, had
already been commenced, and was being prosecuted with more vigor than
regard for precision of statement or the public good," by "a clique of
physicians who are radically opposed to everything in existing asylum
management because they are not themselves the managers at liberal salaries." However, he reported cheerfully, "a combination, evidently formed
for the purpose of obtaining possession of these institutions in the interest
of a small society of so-called experts, holding monthly meetings of mutual
compliment, has been signally defeated," despite the efforts of "a single
filibustering expert and his hungry followers."[59] The uncomplimentary
reference to Hammond and the New York Neurological Society, whether
or not deserved, must have been unmistakable.

Landon Carter Gray, of the Neurological Society, rebutted these allegations in a letter he wrote to the *Medical Record*. This organ of the profession, he said, and not the daily press, was the proper place in which to discuss the asylum issue. He claimed, moreover, that the intellectual qualifications of the Neurological Society justified its leadership of the reform crusade.[60] In fact, Beard and Seguin had already assumed prominent roles in a broad-based reform movement—in which neurologists united with lay charity workers—growing out of a mass meeting held at Cooper Union in December 1879. This National Association for the Protection of the Insane and the Prevention of Insanity (NAPIPI) was formally organized in July of the following year, its leaders having already promoted a bill in Albany for the creation of a State Lunacy Commission. The editors of the *Record* probably spoke for many New York physicians in agreeing with the goals of the Neurological Society without condoning its "newspaper notoriety" and "unhappy mode of getting signers" to its petitions. They regretted that "any influential member of the profession" would endorse a petition *against* lunacy reform.[61] But they clearly did not accept the leadership of the Neurological Society, nor the tone of its crusade.

Seguin, along with some other members of the Neurological Society, hesitated initially to take part in what promised to be a sordid fray. Further official action, beyond the inquiry to the commissioner, was therefore deferred to the meeting of January 1880. As if to disprove the *Times*'s disparaging remarks, the members of the society opened that meeting with a lively discussion of Newton Shaffer's paper on "The Hysterical Element in Orthopedic Surgery." They then turned to the consideration of a draft response to the report of the Senate committee. This document, prepared by Hammond, Spitzka, and Morton and read after prefatory remarks were made by McBride in which he outlined the history of the controversy, apparently convinced the group to act. Seguin said that "at first he had hesitated about the use of such strong language but that analysis of the Senate Committee's report had convinced him that strong language had to be used." L. C. Gray made similar comments. Finally, it was decided to approve the report of the Asylum Abuse Committee and to authorize the publication of three thousand copies for distribution.[62]

Meanwhile, neurologists and superintendents continued to clash as expert witnesses in the courtroom, for example, in the much-publicized case of the elderly Abraham Gosling, who was brought to trial in the spring of 1880 for smashing the windows of a hotel at which he had been kept waiting by a clerk. To Hammond, a clearer case of paralytic insanity could not have been found, and he so testified both at the trial and in a paper read before the New York Medico-Legal Society at its April meeting. "If Mr. Abraham Gosling does not die of General Paresis within three years," the neurologist proclaimed, "I will burn my diploma and retire from the medical profession." Gosling had been an inmate of a series of

asylums in Great Britain, New York, and Pennsylvania, and had been
discharged "cured" from each in succession. Several superintendents testified for the prosecution that Gosling was sane enough to be held responsible for his destructive acts.[63] They could scarcely have admitted his lunacy,
for to do so would have undercut the claims of curability on which the
superintendents insisted and which were already facing serious challenges
both within and without the profession. (It would also, of course, have
impugned the prognostic competence of those who had discharged Gosling.) Thus Dr. Hannah declared that if Gosling were insane it must be
"emotional insanity or a transitory mania"—in his opinion, not really
insanity at all.[64] But to the neurologists, these conditions were (and had to
be) considered genuine clinical entities.

Spitzka cited this disagreement as evidence that the true representative of psychological medicine was the physician who, like Hammond,
could read subtle neurological signs, and not the superintendent who
confined his attention to gross behavior. Obviously sensitive to the skepticism with which expert neurological witnesses were often met, Spitzka
told the Medico-Legal Society that "there is no reason why the disrepute
into which expert testimony has fallen owing to such exhibitions as the
present one, should be a *permanent incubus on the medical profession*, if all of
you . . . will unite in condemning patently defective testimony whenever
occasion offers."[65] Rebuffing a lawyer's perhaps naïve attempt to smooth
things over, Spitzka insisted that cases such as that of Gosling could not
be regarded as matters of honest difference. Psychological medicine was,
he firmly believed, an exact science. "If the evidence [for the prosecution]
was given with a full knowledge on the part of the witnesses of the teach-
ings of science then it was not honest, but if it was honest it was not
scientific but given in ignorance."[66] Yet, by his own admission, not all lay
persons or physicians were convinced that neurology had a corner, or even
a hold, on scientific psychology.

This incident illustrated that the neurologists' critique of asylum
management remained a stronger weapon than their positive knowledge
claims in their fight against the superintendents, and the asylum reform
issue correspondingly remained a subject for discussion (alongside clinical
reports and other scientific papers) at regular meetings of the Neurological
Society. In May, for example, W. R. Birdsall read a paper containing his
"Observations on the Insane Asylums of California and Nevada," with
Spitzka as commentator.[67] Closer to home, an alleged homicide at New
York City's Blackwell's Island Asylum—the Maria Ottmer case—had
added impetus to the society's work. Spitzka was delegated to represent the
group at the inquest, after permission was obtained from the coroner.[68]
But before he could report that the incident "illustrated the defects in the
medical management of our County Asylums," a new Senate investigating

committee had been appointed. The question of how the Neurological Society would conduct itself with respect to the forthcoming inquiries was placed on the agenda of its meeting of 5 October 1880.

Hammond suggested that the society prepare to prove its allegations in testimony before this new committee, and he came to the meeting armed with pamphlets which could be distributed to the members in order to equip them for this ordeal. But Gray and Seguin were again inclined to be cautious. Should the Senate committee summon him to testify, Seguin remarked, he would refuse to appear and would resign from the Committee on Asylum Abuses. Spitzka, who was at least as eager as Hammond to see the fight through but who was also more alert to the sensibilities of his colleagues, attempted to smooth things over. He said that "it was unfortunate that Dr. Hammond had not given a more accurate idea of the manner in which the Committee proposed to act. There had not been the slightest intimation that the members of the Society would be placed in the witness box, on the contrary they were to act as counsel and make suggestions; he would add that the Senate committee was a body of unusual intelligence and superior to anything he had expected to see come from Albany."⁶⁹

The society unanimously agreed to refer the matter to the Committee on Asylum Abuses, expressing the sense that there was no need to alter the composition of that committee.

When the Senate committee hearings began on Thursday, December 2, the neurologists were ready. Drs. McBride, Spitzka, Beard, Seguin, Kiernan, Morton, Hammond, and L. C. Gray appeared on the witness stand, after all, during the week. Hammond, who took the stage on the afternoon of the first day's hearings, led the way with remarks on a wide range of topics. Conceding that most patients' complaints were not based in fact, he nonetheless discoursed at length on the evils of forced feeding, forcible restraint ("except in the most extreme cases"), and the withholding of patients' mail. He admitted that some superintendents were fit to hold their posts, mentioning in particular Dr. Shaw, who had obtained his appointment at the Kings County Hospital through the recommendation of the Neurological Society. But he considered these cases exceptional, "more by accident than otherwise." The experienced and confident witness drew appreciative laughter with his remark that "he thought, with Dr. Spitzka, that the office of Medical Superintendent should be abolished and a lay Superintendent appointed to raise turnips, lobby in the Legislature, and entertain the friends of visitors."⁷⁰

The omissions in Hammond's testimony are also interesting. He apparently did not elaborate on his views of the pathology and prevalence of insanity, except to criticize a new law by which persons with a single harmless delusion could be committed. Nor did he expound on the theme of the noninstitutional treatment of the insane. Perhaps this was because the asylums under investigation housed indigent patients, who would not be able to afford private care at home. Perhaps he had been convinced that to espouse such radical positions would damage his credibility. In any case, he contented himself with the declaration that "he was in favor of the employment of the insane in some suitable labor, and thought that such a course tended greatly to modify the violence of their malady."[71]

Hammond did not stress the lack of scientific attainments which, the neurologists agreed, characterized most superintendents. From his remarks the senators and their large audience would have concluded that his charges of incompetence referred primarily to the management of their institutions, not to their contributions to the science of psychological medicine. Spitzka, in contrast, made a point of the expenditure of $30,000 of the taxpayers' money for scientific investigations at Utica. He repeated his earlier claim that these funds had been wasted by John P. Gray, who had thus provided an additional basis for foreign criticism of American medical psychology. George Beard devoted much of his testimony to a description of European asylums, which he thought could serve as admirable models for American reformers, and the remarks of William J. Morton on the asylums at Geel and Fitz-James emphasized the same point. Hammond, too, later responded to these points after his former assistant, Allan McLane Hamilton (a great grandson of Alexander Hamilton), announced that unfavorable comparisons of American with European institutions were unpatriotic, and after MacDonald had impugned Hammond's and Spitzka's motives and expertise. Hammond's answer was a loyal declaration that Dr. Spitzka knew more about the anatomy, physiology, and pathology of the insane than any other man in the country.[72]

When the dust settled, the Senators and the public seem to have been less impressed with the neurologists' testimony, after all, than with that of Reverend William G. French, whose work for the Protestant Episcopal City Mission had taken him to the city asylums for many years. French had kept a diary since 1874 in which he described the abuses and neglect he had observed. Although he had received a subpoena, his superiors attempted to prevent him from testifying before the committee. The Senators' rebuke of the mission for this intimidation was the high point of the hearing.[73] Further details, obtainable from newspaper accounts, are amusing and horrifying, in turn, but not especially helpful. The investigation suggested that the major abuses charged by the Neurological Society did not generally exist, but many thought that the hearings themselves had prompted recent reforms. The defenders of the asylum incumbents weakened their credibility with conflicting testimony: for example, some claimed that mechanical restraint was not used, while others (including Hamilton) had to be prevented by the chair from using the witness stand to deliver extended speeches on the necessity of the restraint system. The neurologists, however, failed to establish themselves as the sole authorities on the treatment of the insane, and even appeared to be somewhat irresponsible and sensationalist.

Hammond and Spitzka expressed their general satisfaction with the proceedings, nonetheless, and toward the end of the week of hearings the Neurological Society committee could report to the members that "the movement for the amelioration of the condition of the insane has been furthered by the organization of the National Association for the Protection of the Insane and the Prevention of Insanity," itself a result of "the initiative which the committee of the Neurological Society began in 1878." The sense of the meeting seems to have been that it would be both proper and desirable to leave further activity in this sphere to the new national association. And nothing more was said of "reform in the scientific study of psychology."[74]

The regular November 1880 meeting of the Neurological Society had been postponed from Tuesday, November 2 (election day) to the following Friday, as the nation chose James A. Garfield to be its next president. Anticipating a favorable outcome of the upcoming senatorial hearings, the neurologists had turned their attention to improvements of their own work which would enable them to move confidently into the positions of authority—intellectual even more than managerial—from which they hoped the superintendents were soon to be dislodged. A committee was already revising the constitution and bylaws of the society, with the goal of legal incorporation. More significant was the presentation of Spitzka's "Remarks on the Nomenclature of Certain Chronic Insanities," discussed by Drs. Kiernan, L. C. Gray, W. R. Birdsall, and Mary Putnam Jacobi, for this represented a step toward a full-scale theoretical treatment of insanity from a neurological point of view. Gray had even proposed the formation of a committee that would make a classification of the varieties of insanity. However, his motion was tabled: perhaps the neurologists were simply too busy preparing for the next month's investigation, or perhaps they sensed that their science was still unequal to such an ambitious task.[75]

Eight months later, President Garfield was shot, and the trial of his assassin, Charles J. Guiteau, in 1882 provided a new public forum for outspoken alienists in both camps.[76] Prominent superintendents denounced the defendant and the "insanity dodge" by which he might have avoided punishment; to them, as to the general public that was anxious for revenge, the apparent insanity of Guiteau's act could be seen instead as the result of habitual viciousness. But those neurologists who chose to comment on the case—including Spitzka, Hammond, and George Beard, all active in asylum reform work—took the opposite view. Exhibiting greater concern for theoretical consistency (and hence scientific respectability) than for popular approval, they insisted that Guiteau presented an unmis-

takable case of "reasoning mania." Although their diagnosis was probably
not far from the truth, this position did little to enhance their credibility
with the public or their standing within the medical profession. The
medical editor E. S. Gaillard, for example, thought that George Beard's
statement in the case had helped to convince lay persons that their views
on insanity were as valid as those of the experts, and that "alienists,
neurologists, [and] psychologists" did more harm than good by raising a
public clamor.[77] Hammond's compromise position, which held Guiteau to
be medically insane but also legally responsible for his acts, might have
done more to popularize neurology than did a narrower insistence that the
medical specialist was to be the supreme authority in the courtroom.[78] But
this view was unacceptable to most alienists, and in any case would have
undermined the sweeping claims which seemed to follow logically from
the assumption that neurologists possessed the scientific key to psychology. Despite the wide publicity afforded by the Guiteau trial, therefore,
the neurologists could scarcely have considered the affair an unqualified
success.

In New York, meanwhile, the Senate investigating committee had
continued its deliberations throughout 1882; its report was finally released
in 1883 and legislation which created a State Lunacy Commission was
enacted. Although vindicating the neurologists' claims that reform had
been needed, these results simultaneously defused the issue. The National
Association for the Protection of the Insane was by then faltering: it lost
three key members (Wilbur, Seguin, and Beard) in personal tragedies
during the year, and could not resolve internal differences between the
remaining physicians and lay members who were generally hostile to
medical experts. Besides, the Asylum Association, whose strong and organized opposition had impeded the work of NAPIPI all along, was believed
by Kiernan and others to be on the verge of self-reform. More and more,
therefore, "neurologists and psychiatrists could agree that professional
experts alone should care for the insane."[79] Unity against lay interference
in their work brought the two groups closer together, more firmly committed than ever to a "medical model" of insanity but still far from the goal
of explicating such a model in a scientifically rigorous way.

Neurologists' best efforts at this time to place their science of psychology on a firm basis proved to be unhappily inadequate. Spitzka admitted
in his textbook on insanity, which was published in 1883, that "in the
present state of our knowledge, it is impossible to frame a definition of
insanity which, while it meets the practical everyday requirements, is
constructed on *scientific* principles." His provisional, carefully worded
attempt was a full paragraph long, yet he acknowledged that it was actually
"merely a paraphrase of the dictum that insanity is a deficiency or perversion of the mental faculties, not provoked by any external cause, but

arising and developing within the *ego.* "[80] Neither the author nor his critics were particularly satisfied with this, and one reviewer suggested that Spitzka might have done better to follow the lead of the German alienists whom he so admired, omitting any definition of his subject matter whatsoever.[81]

Hammond's attempts at a definition were scarcely more successful. "I regard insanity," he wrote in 1870, "as a manifestation of disease of the brain characterized by a general or partial derangement of one or more faculties of the mind, and in which, while consciousness is not abolished, mental freedom is perverted, weakened, or destroyed."[82] In his own *Treatise on Insanity* (published in the same year as Spitzka's), he restated this, adding, however, the alternate definition that insanity was "a psychic manifestation of brain disease unattended by loss of consciousness."[83] Even these definitions did little more than invoke the assumption that the behavioral disorders which he classified in terms of mental functions had a physical basis in the brain.

Neither Hammond nor Spitzka could provide an adequate classification scheme for insane patients, a deficiency perhaps the more conspicuous since asylum superintendents, faced with the practical problem of assigning their patients to wards, routinely dealt with this issue.[84] Hammond recognized that his somaticism logically called for a classification of the forms of insanity based on their morbid anatomy and physiology, analogous to the plan employed in his discussion of other diseases of the nervous system. This he was patently unable to supply. "It is to be regretted," he wrote apologetically, "that the present state of cerebral anatomy and physiology is such as to prevent our making any precise localizations of the several forces and faculties which go to make up the mind."[85]

Spitzka also devoted considerable attention to this insoluble and rather embarrassing dilemma. In physical conditions of the brain, he asserted, "must we seek for the groundwork of a scientific nomenclature and classification of the morbid states underlying mental derangement. Unfortunately, sufficient positive observations on which to base a thorough pathology of these diseased states are, as yet, desiderata." He listed the sophisticated instruments which the skilled neurologist had at his disposal, but noted that

> these appliances and the most elaborate methods of the laboratory have more frequently failed than succeeded in revealing the organic conditions responsible for mental disturbance.
>
> It is for this reason that while the ideal aim of the progressive alienist will continue to be the solution of the great problem of the physical foundation of insanity, he is commonly limited . . . to a recognition of disease manifestations, and not of disease . . . to a

classification of symptom groups; and . . . to the treatment of symptomatic states.[86]

In short, Spitzka admitted, "the conceptions and processes of mental science are . . . traditional and empirical to a great extent."[87] And many reviewers of both his and Hammond's books agreed with this estimate, probably reflecting the sentiments of most of the profession. While convinced that the neurologists were eminent scientists and distinguished physicians, they came to reject the idea that neurology was the proper science with which to understand insanity. One critic commented, for example, that Spitzka "underrates the importance of the psychological treatment of his subject throughout. Such a treatment is assuredly more truly scientific, and can be made as completely practical as one more distinctively clinical or pathological."[88] Another, a lay person writing in the *New York Times,* was less hopeful. "To attempt to review critically any works treating of insanity would be an unprofitable task in the absence of aught resembling an accepted standard of judgment," he complained. "The doctors cannot please the lawyers, the lawyers cannot suit the doctors, and neither of them can satisfy the public at large."[89]

To some neurologists, the discomfiture of Spitzka and Hammond in their systematic attempts to treat the subject of insanity suggested the wisdom of a policy of avoiding this branch of medicine, at least for the time being. "Science has not yet made up its mind," declared the *Journal of Nervous and Mental Diseases,* "as to what is, and what is not, insanity."[90] The specific disagreements between Hammond and Spitzka on such questions as the relation between medical and legal definitions of insanity and the form and nature of the criticism to be leveled against the asylums provided further reason for cautious agnosticism. Thus it is not surprising to find that even a superficial examination of the neurological work of the late 1880s and of the 1890s shows a marked trend toward the separation of psychiatric concerns from the study of demonstrably organic nervous disorders. For example, the *Journal of Nervous and Mental Diseases* changed its policy when Bernard Sachs took charge in 1886, thereafter excluding polemical articles and stressing more detailed and specific studies and, according to a recent analysis, showing "a marked decline in the publication of purely psychiatric contributions." When the policy changed again, thirty years later (under the editorship of Smith Ely Jellife), and the *Journal* came to serve briefly as an organ for the psychoanalytic movement, several senior neurologists—including Charles L. Dana, C. K. Mills, and M. Allan Starr—resigned in protest from the editorial board.[91] This was not simply conservatism on the part of the older men, but a logical response given their experience with the crisis of the 1880s. Dana's *Textbook of Nervous Diseases,* published in 1892, had contained no chapter, section, nor even index reference to *insanity*, and the same was true of Mills's more extensive *Nervous System and Its Diseases* which had appeared six years later.[92] While no less impressed than Hammond and Spitzka had been with the prospects for modern science, men like Dana and Mills came to see the best possibilities for research in the application of the newer pathological doctrines (especially bacteriology) and surgical techniques (notably asepsis) to the study of nervous diseases, rather than in an apparently vain attempt to find a physiological or anatomical basis for mental functions and their disorders.[93]

The "crisis of psychiatric legitimacy" faced both by neurologists and by superintendents around 1880 has yet, a century later, to be resolved.[94] At the time, superintendents dealt with the disparity between their abundance of cases and their deficiency of theoretical knowledge by searching aggressively for new and usable scientific theories, by reorganizing their professional association in 1895 on a broader basis as the American Medico-Psychological Association (later the American Psychiatric Association), and by cooperating in the administration of legislatively mandated reforms in the management of their institutions.[95] Some neurologists joined them in this work, particularly in the first aspect, and they were often influential. Other neurologists considered an alternative resolution of the parallel crisis that emerged in their own situation during those years: they redefined their specialty to emphasize those areas in which existing theories were most promising, and they abandoned those in which the theoretical defects were most obvious. In doing so, however, they merely circumvented the dilemmas which have been seen by many observers as inherent in any "medical model" of insanity.[96] Thus this chapter in the history of American neurology lends some support to the argument that such a model may never suffice to clarify such problems as the sensitivity of psychiatry to social values and needs, the relationship of psychiatry as a specialty to medicine as a whole, and the internal structure of the psychiatric community.[97] In the words of David Morgan, "In the field of psychological medicine we must face the disconcerting fact that after a century or more of clinical experience, the medical model of mental disorder remains little more than a speculative, if paradigmatic hypothesis that is still the subject of contentious debate."[98] Despite an abundance of "true experts," psychological medicine is, in the opinion of many, still an unfilled square.

Notes

I would like to thank Charles E. Rosenberg, Andrew Scull, Philip Hesser, and especially John T. Cumbler for their helpful comments on earlier drafts of this essay.

1. Unsigned review of John P. Gray, *The Dependence of Insanity on Physical Disease* (Utica, N.Y.: Utica Asylum Press, 1871), in *Journal of Psychological Medicine* 5 (1871): 576, italics in the original.
2. For a fuller discussion of this theme, see Barbara Sicherman, "The Uses of a Diagnosis: Doctors, Patients and Neurasthenia," *Journal of the History of Medicine and Allied Sciences* 32 (1977): 33–54; and Bonnie Ellen Blustein, "New York Neurologists and the Specialization of American Medicine," *Bulletin of the History of Medicine* 53 (1979): 170–83.
3. On the formation of the AMSAII, see John Albert Pitts, "The Association of Medical Superintendents of American Institutions for the Insane, 1844–1892: A Case Study of Specialism in American Medicine" (Ph.D. diss., University of Pennsylvania, 1979); and Constance M. McGovern, " 'Mad Doctors': American Psychiatrists 1800–1860" (Ph.D. diss., University of Massachusetts, 1976).
4. Charles E. Rosenberg, "The Crisis in Psychiatric Legitimacy: Reflections on Psychiatry, Medicine and Public Policy," in *American Psychiatry: Past, Present, and Future*, ed. George Kriegman et al. (Charlottesville: University Press of Virginia, 1975), pp. 135–48.
5. See Norman Dain, *Concepts of Insanity in the United States, 1789–1865* (New Brunswick, N.J.: Rutgers University Press, 1964); and Nancy J. Tomes, "The Persuasive Institution: Thomas Story Kirkbride and the Art of Asylum Keeping" (Ph.D. diss., University of Pennsylvania, 1978).
6. Rosenberg, "Crisis in Psychiatric Legitimacy," p. 141.
7. On post–Civil War American neurology, see Sicherman, "Uses of a Diagnosis"; Blustein, "New York Neurologists"; and Bonnie Ellen Blustein, "A New York Medical Man: William Alexander Hammond, M.D. (1828–1900), Neurologist" (Ph.D. diss., University of Pennsylvania, 1979), esp. pp. 121–57. On scientific activity in New York during this period, see Douglas Sloan, "Science in New York City, 1867–1907," *Isis* 71 (1980): 35–76.
8. See, for example, Nathan G. Hale, Jr., *Freud and the Americans: The Beginning of Psychoanalysis in the United States, 1876–1917* (New York: Oxford University Press, 1971); Barbara Sicherman, "The Quest for Mental Health in America" (Ph.D. diss., Columbia University, 1967), pp. 35–45, 162–75; and Pitts, "Association."
9. Pitts, "Association." English alienists had already, by 1870, confronted such a crisis of confidence: see Peter McCandless, " 'Build! Build!': The Controversy

Over the Care of the Chronically Insane in England, 1855–1870," *Bulletin of the History of Medicine* 53 (1979): 553–74.

10. For example, see D. S. Werman, "True and False Experts: A Second Look," *American Journal of Psychiatry* 130 (1973): 1351–54.
11. For example, Sicherman, "Quest for Mental Health," and Charles E. Rosenberg, "The Place of George M. Beard in Nineteenth-Century Psychiatry," *Bulletin of the History of Medicine* 36 (1962): 245–59.
12. Sicherman, "Quest for Mental Health," p. 35.
13. For example, Werman, "True and False Experts"; cf. editorial, "Asylum Abuses," *New York Medical Journal* 31 (1880): 160–62.
14. See Rosenberg, "Crisis in Psychiatric Legitimacy."
15. This argument was thoroughly consistent with the movement within the profession for reform of medical education generally. See Robert P. Hudson, "Abraham Flexner in Perspective: American Medical Education 1865–1910," *Bulletin of the History of Medicine* 46 (1972): 545–61.
16. Blustein, "New York Neurologists," esp. pp. 173–76.
17. Quoted in Thomas L. Stedman, "Our New York Letter," *New England Medical Monthly* 1 (1882): 228.
18. E. C. Spitzka, "Reform in the Scientific Study of Psychiatry," *Journal of Nervous and Mental Diseases* 5 (1878): 200–229. The manuscript minute books of the New York Neurological Society (hereafter cited as NYNS Minutes) and of its council, as well as those of the American Neurological Association, are on deposit in the Rare Book Room, New York Academy of Medicine. I am grateful to Dr. Fletcher H. McDowell and Dr. Peritz Scheinberg for permission to use these materials, and to Mrs. Alice Weaver for her assistance in locating them. On Spitzka's paper, see also NYNS Minutes, 4 March 1878.
19. Spitzka "Reform," pp. 202–4.
20. Ibid., pp. 204, 216–19.
21. Ibid., pp. 214, 205.
22. Ibid., pp. 206–10.
23. "The Utica Insane Asylum. Annual Report of Dr. Gray," *New York Times*, 18 March 1878, p. 5, col. 5.
24. "Neurological Correspondence," *Journal of Nervous and Mental Diseases* 5 (1878): 331–37.
25. Spitzka, "Reform," p. 224.
26. NYNS Minutes, 4 March and 1 April 1878.
27. NYNS Minutes, 1 April 1878. However, only eleven members voted in this election.
28. "Medico-Legal Society," *Journal of Nervous and Mental Diseases* 5 (1878): 337.
29. On Hammond, see Blustein, "New York Medical Man," esp. pp. 11–12, 17.
30. Eugene Grissom, "True and False Experts," *American Journal of Insanity* 35 (1878–79): 1–36.
31. William A. Hammond, *An Open Letter to Eugene Grissom*, 2d ed. (New York: Trow, 1878); William A. Hammond, *To the Medical Profession* (New York: n.p. 1879).
32. See review and analysis of the controversy in *St. Louis Clinical Record* 5 (1878): 158–65; and editorial note, *American Journal of Insanity* 35 (1878–79): 480–83. The influential medical editor E. S. Gaillard remarked that while "the animus of

[Grissom's] paper is objectionable . . . it is useful and entertaining" (Rev. of Grissom, "True and False Experts," in *American Medical Bi-Weekly* 9 [1878]: 56). See also Werman, "True and False Experts."

33. "Neurological Correspondence," p. 331; Spitzka, "Reform," p. 214.

34. "A Plea for Asylum Reform," *New York Times*, 8 October 1878, p. 2, col. 5; E. C. Spitzka, "Merits, Motives and Progress of the Reform in Asylum Abuses," *Journal of Nervous and Mental Diseases* 5 (1878): 694–714; NYNS Minutes, 7 October 1878.

35. Spitzka, "Merits," p. 701.

36. Ibid., p. 709.

37. Ibid., p. 714.

38. William A. Hammond, "The Non-Asylum Treatment of the Insane," *Transactions of the Medical Society of New York* (1879), pp. 280–97 (esp. pp. 292–93); also published in *Neurological Contributions* 1, no. 1 (1879): 1–22.

39. Ibid., p. 281.

40. William A. Hammond, *A Treatise on the Diseases of the Nervous System* (New York: Appleton, 1871), pp. 383–84.

41. William A. Hammond, *A Treatise on the Diseases of the Nervous System*, 6th ed. (New York: Appleton, 1876), p. 376.

42. William A. Hammond, *A Treatise on Insanity in Its Medical Relations* (New York: Appleton, 1883), pp. 720–21.

43. Hammond, "Non-Asylum Treatment," pp. 281–82.

44. Unsigned review, *American Medical Bi-Weekly* 10 (1879): 181–82.

45. NYNS Minutes, 5 May 1879; "Special Report for the Medical Record," *Medical Record* 15 (1879): 566–70; William A. Hammond, "The Construction, Organization and Equipment of Hospitals for the Insane," *Neurological Contributions* 1, no. 2 (1880): 4–6, 13.

46. Hammond, "Construction," pp. 1, 13–14; NYNS Minutes, 2 June 1879.

47. *Medical Gazette* 4 (1870): 222–23; cf. review of M. G. Echeverría, *The Trial of John Reynolds, Medicolegally Considered*, in *Medical Gazette* 5 (1870): 69–71.

48. See "To the Legislature of New York," *Neurological Contributions* 1, no. 1 (1879): 92–96; "Provisional Report to the Committee of the New York Neurological Society, Relative to the Subject of Insane Asylum Abuses," "Insane Asylum Investigation," and "Suggestions for Improvements in the Management of the Insane and of Hospitals for the Insane in the State of New York," *Neurological Contributions* 1, no. 2 (1880): 26–28, 59–60, 61–67.

49. Ibid.

50. NYNS Minutes, 6 October 1879.

51. Ibid.

52. Ibid. The members of the board were Austin Flint, Jr., whose psychiatric interests dated from the appointment; Charles Inslee Pardee, who lectured on diseases of the eye and ear; Alfred L. Loomis, a specialist in physical diagnosis and diseases of the chest; Edward G. Janeway, a pathologist who would later specialize in neurology; Montrose A. Pallen, a gynecologist; J. R. Wood, a surgeon; J. P. P. White, W. D. White, and Allan McLane Hamilton.

53. NYNS Minutes, 6 October 1879.

54. NYNS Minutes, 3 November 1879.
55. "Treatment of the Insane," *New York Times*, 14 November 1879, p. 3, col. 1; NYNS Minutes, 2 December 1879.
56. Editorial, commenting on a talk given by George Beard before the Medico-Legal Society, *New York Times*, 9 March 1879, p. 4, cols. 6–7.
57. "Treatment of the Insane."
58. "The City Lunatic Asylum," letter to the editor, *New York Times*, 17 November 1879, p. 3, col. 4.
59. Editorial, *New York Times*, 18 November 1879, p. 4, col. 6.
60. L. C. Gray, "Lunacy Reform," *Medical Record* 17 (1880): 132–33.
61. Editorial, "Discussing Lunacy Reform," *Medical Record* 17 (1880): 124; "A Petition Against Lunacy Reform," *Medical Record* 17 (1880): 192; and W. C. Church et al., "Lunacy Reform," *Medical Record* 17 (1880): 246. On the subsequent development of the NAPIPI, see Sicherman, "Quest for Mental Health," pp. 45–72.
62. NYNS Minutes, 2 December 1879 and 6 January 1880.
63. William A. Hammond, "General Paralysis of the Insane, with Special Reference to the Case of Abraham Gosling," in "Proceedings of Societies," *Gaillard's Medical Journal* 29 (1880): 652–55, with report of discussion in the Medico-Legal Society, pp. 655–63. Cf. William A. Hammond, "Remarks on Paralytic Insanity or General Paralysis of the Insane with Special Reference to Abraham Gosling," *Medical Gazette* 7 (1880): 289–91; also, "The Case of Abraham Gosling," *Medical Record* 17 (1880): 444; and "Medical News," *American Medical Bi-weekly* 13 (1881): 286. Hammond's prognosis proved correct: Gosling did die not long after the affair.
64. "Proceedings of Societies," pp. 655–56.
65. Ibid., pp. 662–63.
66. Ibid.
67. NYNS Minutes, 4 May 1880.
68. See E. C. Spitzka, "The Maria Ottmer Homicide as Illustrating the Defects in the Medical Management of the Asylums under the Administration of the Commissioners of Charities and Corrections," in "Proceedings of Societies," *Gaillard's Medical Journal* 30 (1880): 506–19; NYNS Minutes, 3 February 1880.
69. NYNS Minutes, October 5, 1880.
70. "Insane Asylum Methods, Alleged Abuses Laid Before the Senate Committee," *New York Times*, 2 December 1880, p. 8, col. 1.
71. Ibid.
72. "Insane Asylum Methods"; "Ward's Island Asylum. Answers to Charges," *New York Times*, 5 December 1880, p. 2, cols. 4–5; "Investigating Asylums," *New York Times*, 7 December 1880, p. 12, cols. 1–2; "The Care of the Insane," *New York Times*, 8 December 1880, p. 2, cols. 2–3.
73. "Investigating Asylums" and "The Care of the Insane"; "The Rev. Mr. French Heard," *New York Times*, 10 December 1880, p. 3, cols. 1–2.
74. NYNS Minutes, 7 December 1880.
75. NYNS Minutes, 5 November 1880; Minutes of Council, 12 December 1880.
76. For a full discussion of the medicolegal issues in the case, see Charles E.

Rosenberg, *The Trial of the Assassin Guiteau: Psychiatry and Law in the Gilded Age* (Chicago: University of Chicago Press, 1968), esp. pp. 226–28.

77. [E. S. Gaillard], "Guiteau and the Neurologists," *American Medical Weekly* 14 (1882): 625–27.

78. See Blustein, "New York Medical Man," pp. 288–93.

79. Sicherman, "Quest for Mental Health," esp. p. 71.

80. Edward C. Spitzka, *Insanity: It's* [*sic*] *Classification, Diagnosis and Treatment* (New York: Bermingham, 1883), pp. 18, 21.

81. Unsigned review of Spitzka, *Insanity,* in *Boston Medical and Surgical Journal* 109 (1883): 543–44.

82. William A. Hammond, *Insanity in Its Medico-Legal Relations: Opinion Relative to the Testamentary Capacity of the Late James C. Johnston, of Chowan County, N. C.* (New York: Bake, Voorhis, 1866), p. 5.

83. Hammond, *Treatise,* p. 266.

84. Neurologists, of course, objected that superintendents arranged their patients unscientifically.

85. Hammond, *Treatise,* pp. 33, 285–86.

86. Spitzka, *Insanity,* p. 18.

87. Ibid.

88. Review of Spitzka, *Insanity,* in *Medical Record* 24 (1883): 442.

89. "Dr. Hammond on Insanity," *New York Times,* 24 June 1883, p. 10, col. 3.

90. Review of Spitzka, *Insanity,* in *Journal of Nervous and Mental Diseases* 10 (1883): 551.

91. See Eugene Brody, "The Journal of Nervous and Mental Diseases: The First 100 Years," *Journal of Nervous and Mental Diseases* 158 (1974): 6–17; idem, 159:1–11; L. S. Kubie, "The Journal of Nervous and Mental Diseases: The First 100 Years," *Journal of Nervous and Mental Diseases* 159 (1974): 77–80; and J. B. Mackie, "The Journal of Nervous and Mental Diseases: The First 100 Years," *Journal of Nervous and Mental Diseases* 159 (1974): 305–18.

92. Charles L. Dana, *Textbook of Nervous Diseases* (New York: Wood, 1892), esp. p. [iii]; C. K. Mills, *The Nervous System and Its Diseases* (Philadelphia; Lippincott, 1898). Mills did, however, suggest that insanity might find a place in a projected second volume.

93. See Charles L. Dana, "Therapeutics and Neurological Therapeutics," *Quarterly Bulletin of the Clinical Society of the New York Post-Graduate Medical School and Hospital* 1 (1886): 244. I expect to discuss this further in a subsequent paper.

94. See Rosenberg, "Crisis."

95. See Sicherman, "Quest for Mental Health."

96. For a discussion of these dilemmas, see David Morgan, "Explaining Mental Illness," *Archives Européennes de Sociologie* 16 (1975): 262–80. For defenses of medical model-making in the analysis and treatment of insanity, see Miriam Siegler and Humphry Osmond, *Models of Madness, Models of Medicine* (New York and London: Macmillan, 1974); and J. K. Wing, *Reasoning About Madness* (New York: Oxford University Press, 1978).

97. Rosenberg, "Crisis."

98. Morgan, "Explaining Mental Illness," p. 267.

Michael J. Clark

11 The Rejection of Psychological Approaches to Mental Disorder in Late Nineteenth-Century British Psychiatry

It is not our business, it is not in our power, to explain *psychologically* the origin and nature of any of [the] depraved instincts [manifested in typical cases of insanity] . . . it is sufficient to establish their existence as facts of observation, and to set forth the pathological conditions under which they are produced; they are facts of pathology, which should be observed and classified like other phenomena of disease. . . . The explanation, when it comes, will come not from the mental, but from the physical side—from the study of the *neurosis*, not from the analysis of the *psychosis*. [1]

In thus forcibly stating one of the most widely held and seemingly incontrovertible propositions in later Victorian medical psychology, Henry Maudsley was for once not self-consciously distancing himself from the slipshod and mediocre views of his fellow psychologists, but rather affirming what had become almost a basic article of faith for British psychiatrists in the latter decades of the nineteenth century. Historically speaking, the last four decades of the century were characterized by a growing preponderance of somatic-pathological approaches to almost every aspect of "psychological medicine," and by a corresponding tendency to disparage any kind of "psychological" approach to the problems of mental disorder, at least within the context of legitimate medical practice; to the extent that already, by the time Maudsley was writing in the early 1870s, most practitioners of psychiatry had grown accustomed to taking the superior efficacy and scientificity of somatic approaches almost entirely for granted. [2] Leading psychiatrists such as David Skae, George Savage, George Blandford, J. Batty Tuke, and Thomas Clouston called repeatedly for a reclassification of mental disorders on systematic and "scientific" (that is, etiological and somatic-pathological) principles, [3] while leading clinical-psychiatric textbooks of the period, such as Bucknill's and

Tuke's *Manual of Psychological Medicine*, urged that the clinical psychological categories of psychiatric nosologies should be reformulated in order to conform better to the findings of recent experimental researches in cerebral localization.[4] Except for purely diagnostic purposes, the psychological interpretation of the "mental" and behavioral symptoms of insanity was emphatically rejected, and the medical treatment of insanity generally regarded as consisting almost entirely in the treatment of concurrent bodily disease by ordinary medicinal and regimenal means—in what Maudsley called "attack[ing] the mental through the bodily humours."[5] Yet, as a long tradition of somewhat naïve historiography of "moral treatment" and its pioneers, and more recently the very differently conceived work of Bynum, Scull, and McCandless, remind us, this had not always been the case.[6] In the first three decades of the century, orthodox medicine's claim to exercise exclusive control over the domain of insanity had appeared briefly to be in jeopardy;[7] and even in the second half of the century, its dominant position did not go entirely unchallenged, even from within the established system of psychiatric social administration.[8] And (as contemporary psychiatrists themselves sometimes admitted), somatic-pathological approaches to insanity had yielded remarkably little in the way of tangible gains for psychological medicine. They could hardly be said to have increased scientific understanding of the causes and pathology of insanity; nor could it plausibly be claimed that they had been any more effective in curing insanity than "moral treatment" or other, more purely empirical and "unscientific" methods that were practiced by laymen.[9] Viewed in this light, the question: Why did Victorian psychiatrists so deliberately and consistently eschew psychological approaches to the interpretation and treatment of mental disorder?[10] may appear rather less of an "unhistorical" anachronism than might first have been imagined. Indeed, I believe that this question can be the starting point for an interesting and fruitful historical inquiry into some of the most important aspects of later Victorian medical psychology, and that this essay will serve to give some credence to this view.

Before commencing this inquiry, however, it is necessary to explain more fully the terms of reference and the mode in which it is to be conducted. This essay does not attempt to give a *complete* answer to the question posed, that is, it does not attempt to give an exhaustive account of *all* the medical-theoretical, sociocultural, socioinstitutional, and other factors which conspired to prevent later Victorian psychiatrists from experimenting with more psychologically oriented approaches to the problems of interpreting and treating mental disorder. Rather, it attempts to understand how this was legitimated by the medical-psychological theory of the time—that is, it focuses primarily on the implicit and explicit reasons given in later Victorian psychiatric theory to explain and justify the orthodox medical approach to these problems. This is not intended to imply any disregard or disrespect for sociological explanations in the history of psychiatry, or any neglect of recent work on the social-institutional reasons for the failure of Victorian psychiatry to fulfill its early promises of effective "individual treatment."[11] On the contrary, it stems from the belief that the peculiar constitutive fusion between moral judgments and positive knowledge-claims so characteristic of Victorian psychiatric theory in general (and of medical attitudes toward psychological approaches to mental disorder in particular) itself comprises one of the most interesting and important aspects of the social history of psychiatry in this period, and that this fusion enables us to draw important social-historical conclusions from analysis of the content of the theory itself. It also reflects partly the more specifically historical consideration that the social-institutional factors invoked by (for example) Scull and McCandless to explain institutional psychiatry's failure to realize the early Victorian ideal of an individuated system of "moral treatment" in pauper asylums cannot satisfactorily account for the failure to employ an individualized system in private consultancy practice either, where no such constraints were operative.

Investigators of the "origins," "antecedents," and "anticipations" of modern psychoanalytical and "dynamic-psychiatric" theories have long since familiarized us, at a relatively superficial level, with the development of concepts of unconscious mentation, and with the significance attributed to sexuality, dreams, early childhood experiences, and so forth, in the works of leading Victorian physiological and medical psychologists.[12] But in their overriding determination to present these conceptions as precursors of modern theoretical views, these investigators have almost entirely failed to ask what role these "insights" actually played in the medical psychology of their own time. However, I shall not consider this body of evidence directly in this essay, but rather, by approaching the problem from a quite different angle, seek to suggest that the mere existence of such insights, in an isolated and largely unrelated form, is largely irrelevant to the question of why they failed to herald any more general reorientation of psychiatry toward more psychologically informed approaches. I shall argue that their relationship to the central organizing concepts of Victorian medical psychology was so marginal and so intrinsically negative in its practical implications that they could hardly have constituted a viable basis for any systematic body of interpretative knowledge, much less for any system of "psychotherapeutics." The reasons for the remarkably deliberate and consistent rejection of such approaches to mental disorder in later nineteenth-century British psychiatry are, I believe, to be found more in an analysis of its basic conception of what caused and constituted mental disorder, and of the implications for the nature and proper scope of medical intervention in such cases that were believed to stem from this view. Accordingly, the next section of this essay will endeavor to define briefly the principal elements of this view. This attempt to generalize about Victorian medical views concerning the nature and causation of mental disorder may seem somewhat unhistorical, in its apparent neglect of individual differences, and of changes through time. But the considerations that tended to predispose later Victorian psychiatrists against any kind of psychological approach to the interpretation or treatment of mental disorders made constant reference to a common heritage of received medical ideas about the nature and causation of mental disorder, and the responsibilities and duties of physicians in such cases, which persisted almost unchanged from the first emergence of "psychological medicine" as a recognized medical specialty down to the end of the nineteenth century and beyond. Some initial attempt to formulate this common heritage of received ideas in general terms seems, therefore, desirable, if not essential, for understanding these considerations more fully.[13]

The Basic Victorian View of Mental Disorder

The essence of the Victorian medical view of mental disorder may be described as the interpretation of dualism not so much in the sense of a particular statement or hypothesis about mind-body relations, but more as a kind of rough yardstick or readily applicable criterion of physical and mental health. From at least the first quarter of the nineteenth century— that is, from the period in which (as Bynum and Scull have shown) medical men had succeeded in winning widespread acceptance and authoritative status among the most influential strata of society for their professionally interested view of insanity as basically a bodily disease—it had been customary for physiological and medical psychologists to regard insanity and other supposedly analogous states, such as dreams, mesmeric and "electrobiological" trances, and hysteria, as morbid intervals of a kind of psychophysical interaction. These abnormal mental states were seen as lapses from a dualistic (or later, "parallelist") norm of healthy bodily and mental functioning into diseased states affecting the whole physical and psychological person, in which the Ego or psychical person lost its power of self-determination and regressed to "lower," more automatic levels of psychological functioning, the mind becoming increasingly absorbed either by delusive constructions based on internal, "subjective" sensations (as in hysteria and hypochondriasis) or by externally suggested dominant ideas (as in hypnosis).[14] Put crudely, it was believed that in conditions of mental health, states of consciousness were the outcome of *normal psychological processes*, subject to the control of the rational Will and its power determinately to focus the Attention on particular sensations, ideas, motivations, and so forth (more precisely, on external impressions, moral ideas, and altruistic motivations). The salient qualities of such healthy states of mind were the capacities to perceive external reality correctly, form correspondingly exact and intelligent judgments, and adjust one's conduct accordingly; and the criterion of mental health was the degree to which the "powers" that served to sustain this objective mental orientation (that is, the control of the Will over the Imagination and instincts, and the power of the reason to make accurate perceptions, just comparisons and correct judgments) were retained.[15] Similarly, in states of physical well-being, "vital" phenomena were the outcome of *normal physiological processes*, characterized by the absence of any painful internal sensations attending either bodily or mental functioning, and by the smooth, frictionless performance of "automatic" and reflex actions without the intervention or arousal of consciousness.[16] In the completely healthy individual, these two conditions, mental and physical, coexisted and maintained a certain relational equilibrium between themselves, but did not normally interact with or otherwise influence each other *directly*. (There were, however, certain very important kinds of *indirect interactions*, such as those involved in the execution of voluntary movements or the expression of the emotions, which, nevertheless, did not invalidate the general proposition.) "Normal" mentation and voluntary behavior were thus self-determined, although subject to the uniform and universal "laws of mind" given by the association psychology, while normal "vital" processes and phenomena were more or less fully determined, in a quite separate and distinct sphere, by the physical "laws of organization" given by the biological and physiological sciences.[17]

In states of mental ill health, however, this normal or "natural" autonomy of psychical life was severely reduced, or even lost altogether. Thought and feeling were progressively removed from the sphere of volitional control, deprived of their self-determined character, and eventually reduced to the level of mere epiphenomena of underlying morbid states (whether structural or "functional") of the brain and nervous system or other implicated viscera, or even abolished altogether; while conduct underwent a corresponding degeneration and became more impulsive, "automatic," and irresponsible in character. With this regression to lower, more automatic modes of mental action, the mind increasingly lost its accustomed objective orientation, and became increasingly preoccupied with erroneous subjective constructions of incorrectly perceived external objects or suggestions, and with morbid subjective feelings, which arose more or less indirectly from the diseased impressions that were made upon it; while the individual's behavior became progressively less well adapted to objective circumstances, and more and more the unmediated expression of instincts, external suggestions, and dominant ideas.[18] Diseased physical processes, as it were, spilled over from their ordinary sphere of action in the physical organism into the normally separate and closed domain of mind, impairing or suspending the action of the normal psychological processes that were ordinarily responsible for mental phenomena. And further, in the course of this morbid transformation, the mental phenomena lost their customary law-governed character, and thus became inaccessible to rational inquiry and interpretation, since the normal psychological processes of causation had become disordered and even superseded by the irruption into their proper sphere of action of extraordinary causal powers of an altogether different order, whose effects could not confidently be predicted from any knowledge of the laws governing their normal action in states of health.[19] Mental disorder and other related abnormal mental states thus represented not merely the antithesis of mental health, but also the negation of the possibility of scientific understanding which, however hypothetically, seemed to exist for healthy states of mind. And dualism stood not only for a particular view of mind-body relations, but also for a practical view of what constituted mental health and ill health, as well as comprising the only acceptable epistemological basis for rational scientific inquiry in physiology and psychology.[20]

The history of this view of psychopathology is also the history of medicine's appropriation and cultivation of mental disorder as part of its rightful and "natural" sphere of professional involvement. Almost all of its constitutive elements are to be found more or less fully developed not only in specialist medical works on insanity, but also in more "popular" expositions, and in phrenologically inspired commentaries on insanity in the 1820s and 1830s—the period in which (as we have already noted) the orthodox medical view of insanity was gaining widespread acceptance among elite opinion.[21] With the almost universal acceptance of the view that insanity was a disorder of mind resulting from a structural or functional lesion of the "organ of mind," the brain, these somewhat crude underlying notions were given much less prominence in medical writings on insanity, and tended to appear in more sophisticated and less explicit forms. But much the same *implicit* view of abnormal mental states and their physical concomitants may be traced in the treatment of certain major themes in physiological and medical psychology throughout the remainder of the century. In particular, the numerous works published in the second and third quarters of the century on "mental physiology" (itself a suggestive title) were all, to a greater or lesser degree, implicitly founded on such a view of the differential relations between body and mind in sickness and health. This may be inferred even from a cursory persual of their contents—discussions of mesmeric, hypnotic and "electrobiological" trances, dreaming, toxic and narcotic hallucinations, sleepwalking, and, in general, of all those abnormal mental and bodily states that occupied the borderland between the wholly "physical" and the wholly "psychical," in which dualistic (or parallelist) norms of physiological and psychological functioning no longer held, and both "mental" and "vital" phenomena testified more or less plainly to some kind of extraordinary psychophysical interaction.[22] Similar views were more or less apparent in the recurrent controversy over the civil and criminal responsibility, or degree of responsibility, of the mentally disordered, in which the whole burden of the alienists' view consisted simply in the proposition that certain forms or phases of mental disorder could impair or destroy the normal freedom of the will, and thereby at least diminish temporarily or annul their victims' normal responsibility for their own thoughts and conduct.[23] And they may equally be inferred from Victorian mental-hygienic prescriptions, which may be interpreted as attempts to prescribe the optimal physiological conditions for the full assumption and exercise of individual moral responsibility in conduct, in order to make the body into a more perfect instrument of the rational will.[24]

Implications of the Victorian Medical View of Mental Disorder

This differential view of mind-body relations in normal and abnormal mental states had numerous implications for the whole theory and practice of psychiatry in Britain throughout the Victorian period. But three of these stand out as of particular significance for the present inquiry: (1) the need for established scientific (and, more especially, physiological) rationales to legitimate any medical use of "psychological" methods in treatment; (2) the restriction of legitimate medical psychology to the sphere of diagnosis; and (3) the definition of the necessary conditions for individual accessibility to psychological methods of treatment themselves comprised a form of mental disorder.

1. Scientific Rationales and the Legitimation of "Psychological" Methods of Treatment

Throughout the period during which psychological medicine was striving to gain recognition as an accredited specialty of "scientific medicine," the increasing reluctance of Victorian science and medicine to accept any form of explanation which did not closely conform to received ideas of what constituted scientific naturalism manifested itself in a growing insistence upon the necessity for adequate *physiological* explanations in psychology.[25] This increasing epistemological rigidity was to have profound implications for the acceptability of psychological methods of interpretation and treatment in psychiatry. Since mental disorder was defined as a morbid state of the whole organism, in which the operation of normal psychological processes was impaired or suspended by the action of pathological physical processes, it seemed to follow that any therapeutic attempt to restore the "dualistic" (or parallelist) norm of healthy physical and mental functioning must also operate, at least in the first instance, through *physical* processes of causation. The brain and nervous system comprised the "organ" or "material instrument" of Mind, conditioning all its manifestations in sickness as in health. Therefore, it was argued, since according to the medical view of insanity there could be no "disease of Mind" itself (and therefore no medical therapy either), but only of its organ or material instrument, the medical treatment of insanity properly resolved itself into the restoration of the normal functioning of these same organs or instruments, that is, essentially into a question of the art of *physic* (which was, after all, the professionally congenial conclusion toward which the whole medical view of insanity was tending).[26] Attempts to operate directly upon the patient's mind could not, therefore, win medical acceptance until they had conclusively demonstrated some convincing *physiological* as well as psychological rationale for whatever degree of efficacy they appeared to possess. Unless they did so, whatever their empirical effectiveness might appear to be, they were likely to be dismissed as quackery, unscientific impostures, or worse—as were mesmerism, "phreno-mesmerism," homeopathy, faith healing, and (at least, until the very end of the century) hypnotism—and their practitioners ostracized, if not outlawed, from the profession of legitimate medicine. This was not necessarily to say that such methods might not actually "cure" illnesses—only that they could not be accepted as parts of the legitimate therapeutic armory of a truly "scientific" psychological medicine, and could not, therefore, be practiced without loss of professional integrity by any qualified practitioner.

The enduring force of this attitude may be illustrated by a brief review of the fortunes of mesmerism and hypnotism as therapeutic techniques that were available to orthodox psychological medicine during the Victorian period. At the beginning of the nineteenth century, Dugald Stewart (who, like Braid, held a naturalistic view of mesmeric phenomena) had urged that mesmeric manipulation be admitted to the therapeutic armory of legitimate medicine, at least on a trial basis: "why not make use of [the mesmerist's] facts, and lay aside his theory?—Why not excite the frame for the purposes of health . . . by an appeal to the imagination, and the principle of imitation, which . . . are the real magnetic instruments?"[27] But the atmosphere of deliberate mystification, quackery, and dubious

morality that surrounded both the practitioners and the subjects of mesmeric experiments, the growing association of mesmerism with
phrenology, and the bitter internecine quarrels in University College,
London, and in the Royal College of Physicians, which culminated in the
professional ostracism and martyrdom of Elliotson and his associates, were
to engender an inflexible and enduring hostility in the ranks of the medical
establishment not just toward anything that seemed to smack of mesmerism, but (as we shall have repeated occasion to observe) toward "psychological" methods of treatment generally. This hostility, which strongly
permeated the mental climate of orthodox medical education as well as of
medical literature throughout the period, was to persist almost undimin-
ished to the end of the century and even beyond. Thus even as early as 1838,
Robert Ferguson had addressed himself explicitly to Dugald Stewart's call
for the therapeutic use of mesmerism only in order to be able to reject it
decisively: "As a therapeutic agent, the magnetic manipulations are either
dangerous or uncertain, or inferior to remedies in common use in medicine."[28] More important than these practical considerations, however,
were the demoralization and loss of professional integrity that would
result from its use, so long as no plausible medicoscientific explanation
could be given for its effects:

> Its use would create on the one hand a despotism so entire, and on the
> other, a mental degradation so absolute, as has never yet been wit-
> nessed. . . . The physician demands the confidence [of his patients]
> . . . but he asks it for days and nights devoted to a conscientious pursuit
> of his profession, for multiplied experience, for probity, for all those
> qualities which . . . call forth the esteem of mankind—and not for acts
> which mystify and admit of no investigation, establishing power on
> the most dangerous of all foundations, that of a debasing superstition,
> a miserable amalgam of faith and fear.[29]

Ferguson's proscription on the use of mesmerism extended not merely to
cases of mental disorder, but also to ordinary cases of physical illness, and
even to its use as an anesthetic in surgical operations.[30]

In the next few years, medical opposition to mesmerism or "animal
magnetism" hardened still further, following the publicity given to the
Elliotson affair and to the extravagant claims made on behalf of phreno-
mesmerism by Elliotson and his associates, so that when James Braid came
to publish the results of his experiments with "hypnosis," he was almost
painfully conscious of the need to emphasize his wholly naturalistic view
of mesmeric phenomena, and to underline the consequent acceptability of
his methods to even the most cautious and skeptical of practitioners.

> I have now [Braid hastened to assure his medical readers] entirely
> separated Hypnotism from Animal Magnetism. I consider it to be
> merely a simple, speedy, and certain mode of throwing the nervous

system into a new condition, which may be rendered eminently available in the cure of certain disorders. I trust [he went on rather ingenuously] that it may be investigated quite independently of any bias either for or against the subject, as connected with mesmerism; and only by the facts which can be adduced.[31]

But in attempting to establish the arousal of "expectant attention" as a scientifically plausible explanation for all mesmeric phenomena,[32] Braid appeared to be basing his therapeutic use of hypnotism, in the class of diseased conditions most interesting to psychological medicine, on perhaps the most controversial and least reputable of possible foundations—that of "phreno-hypnotism."[33] Admittedly, he rejected the mesmerists' "explanation" for phreno-mesmeric phenomena.[34] But his own preferred explanation can scarcely have been any more acceptable to many of his professional colleagues than that of the mesmerists—since his admission that "during hypnotism, we [hypnotists] acquire the power, through the nerves of common sensation, of rousing any sentiment, feeling, passion, or emotion, and any mental manifestation, according to our ['phreno-hypnotic'] mode of manipulating the patient," once again raised the specter of the operator exercising a "mental despotism" over the hypnotized subject.[35]

But whether because of these adverse implications of his psychophysiological theories, whether because of his comparative youth and obscurity, or simply because of the sheer weight of authoritative prejudice massed against him, Braid's reasoned advocacy of hypnotism was conspicuously unsuccessful in both the short and the medium terms. In October 1843, Thomas Wakley had declared in the *Lancet* that "mesmerism is too gross a humbug to admit of any further serious notice. We regard its abettors [among whom he was to include advocates of hypnotism] as quacks and impostors. They ought to be hunted out of professional society. . . ."[36] And from the publication of *Neurypnology* in 1843 until Braid's death in 1860, Wakley was steadfastly to ignore the appearance of all of Braid's subsequent works.[37] Commenting on the revival of medical interest in hypnotism at the end of the 1870s, almost forty years after the British Medical Association had met in Manchester in 1842 and had refused to hear a paper by Braid on hypnotism, his admirer Daniel Hack Tuke observed that "Mr. Braid appears likely to have justice done to him at last";[38] but *Neurypnology* itself did not reach a second edition until 1899, and even then largely as the result of a revival of interest in Braid's work in Europe and North America, rather than in Britain. Although he left a name to posterity, both during his own lifetime and for much of the remainder of the century Braid enjoyed the unenviable distinction of being alternately ignored and vilified by both orthodox medicine and orthodox mesmerism.

Given such a hostile climate of opinion, it was scarcely surprising that when Hack Tuke came to review all the available evidence concerning psychosomatic phenomena with a view to deriving a systematic "psycho-therapeutics" some thirty years later, he was forced to stress the purely pragmatic argument in favor of giving hypnotism a trial. "Better cure a disease under a name [mesmerism or hypnotism] which is associated with an unproven theory than refuse on that account to employ it," he urged.[39] Starting out from what he regarded as the empirically incontrovertible, if inexplicable, fact that "certain purely psychical agencies produce certain physical results,"[40] Hack Tuke proceeded to argue that the use of hypnotism was sufficiently justified by its undoubted instrumental efficacy in harnessing the obscure but undeniably powerful influence of the mind on the body. Stressing that in the long term hypnosis was much less harmful as a sedative or anesthetic than chloral or bromide of potassium, and much more economical than other, more conventional "moral" methods of treating disease,[41] he urged that metaphysical scruples over the precise modus operandi involved in hypnotic therapeutics should not be allowed to stand in the way of a due recognition of their empirical efficacy: "We may employ [hypnotism], if found to be beneficial; and until convinced to the contrary, attribute its success to the operation of any mental state [such as, for example, expectant attention] which we . . . believe, from the effects produced in those cases in which extraneous agencies are excluded, to be sufficient to explain the result."[42]

Hack Tuke was concerned with far more than the mere judicious advocacy of hypnotism, however. His intention was to establish an acceptable scientific basis for a systematic "psychotherapy," and thus to encourage his fellow physicians "to employ Psychotherapeutics in a more methodical way than heretofore, and thus copy nature in those interesting instances, occasionally occurring, of sudden recovery from the spontaneous action of some powerful moral cause, by employing the same force designedly, instead of leaving it to mere chance."[43] In this way, he hoped to rescue admittedly efficacious psychological modes of treatment from the toils of quackery, and to make them more acceptable to orthodox medicine: "I want medical men who are in active practice to utilize this force [that is, the influence of the 'Mind' upon the 'Body'] . . . and rescuing it from the eccentric orbits of quackery, force it to tread, with measured step, the orderly paths of legitimate medicine."[44] But this attempt to succeed where men such as Braid had failed seems to have shared much the same fate as its predecessors. In his article "Hypnotism," which appeared in Hack Tuke's *Dictionary of Psychological Medicine* (1892), A. T. Myers observed that in spite of the advocacy of Braid and Hack Tuke, and the naturalistic explanations of hypnotic phenomena given by these physicians and by such eminent physiologists as William Carpenter, there had been a virtual prohibition placed on the medicoscientific investigation of hypnosis until after the establishment of the impeccably orthodox Society for Psychical Research in 1882.[45] With the exception of Milne Bramwell's experiments at Bethlem, and some in private practice in London, hypnotism had been almost entirely neglected by orthodox medicine in Britain since the mid-century demonstrations of Braid and Esdaile.[46] Ten years later, in spite of the publicity given to the use of hypnotism in the treatment of hysteria and neurasthenia in Europe and North America, and to the work of the "Nancy School" in establishing an acceptable psychophysiological rationale for hypnosis and discrediting the invariable association of hysteria and hypnosis as related morbid conditions,[47] and in spite of the British Medical Association's own cautious reconsideration of the merits of hypnotism in 1892–93,[48] John Milne Bramwell still felt it necessary to repeat Braid's assurances of 1843 in almost the same words. In his "Hypnotism; and the Treatment of Insanity and Allied Disorders by Suggestion," he took great pains to insist that the therapeutic efficacy of hypnotism depended wholly upon the operation of natural causes, and not on the operator's possession of any esoteric knowledge or occult powers of psychological dominance.[49] Once again, however, equally authoritative voices were to be heard in the contrary sense. Thus Joseph Ormerod, in his "Hysteria," elsewhere in the same volume of the *System of Medicine*, reaffirmed the traditional orthodox-medical opposition to both the psychological interpretation and treatment of the "psychoneuroses" in general, and of hysteria in particular; and insisted upon the necessary primacy of somatic-pathological modes of explanation in medicine: "granting that it may be necessary, in consequence of our present state of ignorance of the workings of the highest cerebral centres, to speak of these in transcendental terms, yet psychology alone cannot supply an explanation of disease, which, to satisfy the physician, must be physical."[50] And given such psychophysiological conclusions as did seem reliably to be established concerning the relationship between hypnotic and hysterical states, the verdict on hypnotism, he argued, could only be adverse, whatever its apparent instrumental efficacy as a method of treatment.[51]

This debate over the medico-psychological use of hypnotism was never conclusively resolved during this period. Perhaps only the dramatic decline in the incidence of classic cases of hysteria coming to the attention of medical practitioners has rendered it so largely an historical affair. For few conceptual associations in Victorian medical psychology were as strong, as tenaciously resistant to change, and as effective in narrowing down the perceived range of choice open to orthodox practitioners, as that between the use of "psychological" techniques, such as hypnotism, without acceptable natural-scientific rationales, and quackery, immoral practices and the loss of professional integrity and self-esteem. Perhaps the only closely comparable case is that of the association between susceptibility to external suggestion (particularly as manifested in hysteria and hypnosis) and essential mental and moral morbidity—an association which I shall discuss in more detail at a later stage.[52]

2. *The Restriction of Medical Psychology to the Sphere of Diagnosis*

This view of the nature and causation of insanity seemed to suggest further that while psychological approaches to mental disorders might be acceptable and even useful as aids to clinical diagnosis, they could make no significant contribution either to the interpretation or the treatment of such disorders. This point may perhaps best be explained in a specific context—that of late nineteenth-century neuropsychiatry. The conclusion that psychological approaches were admissible for diagnosis but not for interpretation or treatment had always been strongly implicit in the underlying Victorian medical view of insanity, but in the last three decades of the century it assumed a much more definite, even dogmatic form in the light of the growing acceptance of Jacksonian evolutionary-neurological ideas in medical psychology. For all his insistence on the real autonomy of psychological processes,[53] on the existential reality or "objectivity" to their subjects of abnormal perceptions and cognitions in nervous and mental disorders,[54] and on the significance of dreams and of other forms of abnormal mentation,[55] Hughlings Jackson seems never really to have regarded abnormal psychological phenomena as worthwhile or even legitimate objects of medicoscientific inquiry *for their own sakes.* Indeed, his "doctrine of concomitance" or hypothesis of strict psychophysical parallelism, understood as an epistemological and methodological rule to demarcate the exclusive spheres of competence of neurology, psychology, and philosophy, was propounded with the express intention of enabling physicians to set aside philosophical and psychological questions in order to conduct wholly "materialistic" inquiries into the physiology and pathology of the nervous system.[56] While frequently stressing the importance, and even the necessity, of psychological inquiry as an aid to medicine in a general way,[57] Jackson was even more emphatic in consistently dissuading his colleagues and pupils from undertaking such inquiries in their characters of physiologists and physicians. He repeatedly emphasized that his own concern with abnormal mental phenomena, like that of any other physician, was purely diagnostic, not interpretative. "Psychical symptoms," he wrote, "are to medical men only signs of what is wrong in a material system."[58] In his view, all such "mental symptoms" in nervous and "mental" diseases were the result either of *deficiency,* of local or general "dissolution" of the highest cortical centers (producing "negative" mental symptoms such as loss of volitional control, loss of speech, and loss of general or special sensibility), or of *defective inhibitory control* of "lower" by "higher" functional "levels" of the central nervous system (producing "positive" mental symptoms, such as hallucinations, delusions, or conspicuous behavioral automatism).[59] But whether "positive" or "negative," all mental symptoms ultimately partook of the same fundamental quality—that of deficiency or defect. As Jackson's colleague, disciple, and close friend Charles Mercier stated, "In every case of insanity the essential feature is defect. In no case does disease make a real, a fruitful addition to function. The affection of function is always in the direction of loss, of deficit, of diminution . . . in all cases of insanity, the real and important aberration is not necessarily the most conspicuous feature—the over-action— . . . but the degradation of activity to a lower plane. . . ."[60]

In this view, mental symptoms were indicative of a general diseased condition affecting the entire physical organism, of a regression to lower evolutionary levels, manifesting itself principally in a failure of inhibitory control of the lower by the higher functional levels of the central nervous system. Even though Jackson himself had insisted that the very extravagance of insane thought and conduct was merely indicative of the continued healthy functioning of lower centers whose powers of "expressive" functional action had remained unimpaired by the dissolution of the next highest, controlling centers,[61] his medicopsychological interpreters chose rather to regard all such phenomena as mere semblances of healthy part-functioning, scarcely concealing the underlying diseased state of the organism. As Mercier stated, "In most cases [of insanity] there is some other element which is more conspicuous than the mere defect, and in accordance with this more conspicuous element the form is named. . . . But . . . defect is in every case . . . the underlying disorder upon which the other [symptoms] are superimposed, and around which they are clustered. . . ."[62] Maudsley similarly observed of cases exhibiting exotic systematized delusions, that "it is surprising what mindlessness may be revealed at the back of what looks like very partial mental disorder."[63] But this view further implied that no attempt directly to come to terms with positive mental symptoms could possibly add anything of significance to the physician's understanding of the diseased states that they testified to. Not only did they all share in this negative quality of defect or deficiency, but, arising as they did from what Mercier described as "an inability to appreciate the true circumstances in which the individual is, and his true relation to these circumstances,"[64] they could scarcely be expected to become any more intelligible in the light of the patient's life experiences either. Such positive symptoms were, in Jackson's phrase, only "indirectly caused, or rather permitted,"[65] and could not, therefore, immediately be interpreted within any causal system of explanation. They were mere *epiphenomena,* which bore no direct or immediately intelligible functional relations to the underlying somatic-pathological realities to which, indirectly and unsystematically, they testified. They could be noted, enumerated, and classified as aids to diagnosis, but as "subjective data" they could form no part of the "objective" sciences of physiology and medicine, and could not constitute, therefore, the direct objects of any legitimate medicoscientific inquiry, let alone comprise a viable basis for any system of positive knowledge in medical psychology.[66] Mental symptoms were, indeed, of no particular interest or importance to the alienist physician, except insofar as they served to indicate the underlying diseased states of the nervous system that were always his ultimate concern. As Jackson stated, "Availing ourselves of abnormal affections of consciousness as signs of states of the central nervous system, we next, so to speak, put them on one side in order to study the [pathological] process [in mental or nervous disorders] in a purely materialistic manner."[67]

Thus, denied the status of eligible objects of rational inquiry, and artificially set aside on grounds of clinical expediency by the methodological rule of strict psychophysical parallelism, mental symptoms were effectively consigned to a kind of extrascientific limbo where they could have no significant influence on either the theory or the practice of psychological medicine.[68] Excluded almost by definition both from the domain of "objective" science and from the sphere of legitimate medical concern, they could not constitute a serious problematic for so self-consciously naturalistic and positivistic a branch of "scientific medicine" as later Victorian psychological medicine.

Given these assumptions about the essential nature of mental and behavioral symptoms in mental disorders, there seemed to be only two appropriate ways of dealing with such phenomena. They could either be understood teleologically, as indicative of the probable future course of development and final outcome of the disorder, or as more immediately indicative of certain definite concomitant physical-pathological states and processes of the organism. In neither case, however, did the implications of the approach extend beyond diagnosis to either interpretation or treatment—indeed, these possibilities were more or less expressly excluded. In the first case, whatever possibilities of interpretative insight or therapeutic guidance the teleological mode of interpretation might have had to offer were largely unrealized in practice, due to medical psychology's strongly held conviction that all cases of mental disorder, if not rapidly arrested, would sooner or later evolve inexorably into cases of chronic dementia. Much emphasis was given in later Victorian clinical-psychiatric texts to the characteristic mental and behavioral symptoms believed to presage the imminent onset of general conditions of progressive dissolution—to the telltale improprieties of the early stages of general paralysis, the "morbid introspection," "solitary habits," and emotionally self-indulgent religiosity of the "insanity of adolescence," and to the re-crudescence of sexual desire in incipient senile dementia.[69] But none of these characteristic patterns of symptomatic behavior was regarded as possessing any particular interest or significance, since they all partook of the same fundamental character of defect, and all pointed unmistakably toward the "common goal" of dementia, "the common form of all insanity," as Mercier described it.[70] Sir Thomas Clouston went as far as to define mental disease as "a tendency to dementia,"[71] and Mercier, too, argued that "every form of insanity is dementia with superadded symptoms," explaining that "usually . . . the onset of the insanity is attended by active symptoms . . . only after it is laid bare by their subsidence does the dementia come into clear view. . . ."[72] In this view, dementia was, so to speak, the "explanation" of the symptoms, which thus only acquired significance when interpreted retrospectively, in the light of the subsequent development of the diseased state toward dementia. But dementia was, by definition, a state in which the very possibility of meaning, let alone of particular meanings, had been lost—in which the mental manifestations signified only the chaotic disintegration or even extinction of mind itself. Therefore, with its onset the phenomena of mind and behavior passed once and for all beyond the reach of rational interpretation, regardless of whatever intelligible meanings they might once have possessed in previous life-historical contexts.[73] Dementia was an extreme case, but one which dominated the attitudes of medical psychologists toward the interpretation of much less severe forms of mental disorder by reason of its teleological importance. What was true of dementia was, however, to a greater or lesser extent true also of all its various incipient manifestations—namely, that (as Mercier said) "we cannot dive into the illogical mental processes of the insane."[74]

In the second case, the interpretation of mental symptoms as the psychological correlates of diseased states and processes of the physical organism was largely deprived of its potential psychological interest by the absence of any real commitment on the part of medical psychologists to the serious investigation of abnormal mental phenomena as worthwhile objects of study in themselves, even within the framework of the "correlative method." Later Victorian medical psychology proceeded largely upon the basis that, as Maudsley put it, mental disorders were "neither more nor less than nervous diseases in which mental symptoms predominate"—that they differed only in degree, not in kind, from ordinary nervous diseases such as epilepsy and chorea, and should therefore be studied in conjunction with them on comparative principles.[75] In this way, the complex and poorly differentiated mental symptoms encountered in the "psychoses" could be reduced to the same terms as their simpler and more readily intelligible counterparts in the "neuroses."[76] Viewed in this light, the problems of diagnosis and interpretation of mental disorder seemed to resolve themselves into questions of *correlation*—of tracing out systematically the correspondences between particular recurrent groups of symptoms and particular underlying diseased states of the organism, and of classifying these correspondences according to some consistent nosological criteria. This was the "correlative method" of medico-psychological inquiry so well described by Maudsley:

> Accepting the exact parallelism which there is the best reason to believe to exist between physiological . . . and mental processes, [the "mental pathologist"] will make it his scientific aim to trace out patiently the exact correspondences between the two, and so . . . arrive at such a precise and full knowledge of both as to be able to say with certitude; This physiological state . . . being manifest to observation, of necessity this psychological experience will be sensible to consciousness; and to say that of every mental function of the brain and of every affection of consciousness.[77]

But even when undertaken on the basis of adherence to the Jacksonian hypothesis of strict psychophysical parallelism, this did not in practice imply any very serious attempt to come to terms with abnormal-psychological phenomena as such, since (as we have already seen) mental and behavioral symptoms could not themselves constitute an acceptable scientific basis for interpretative knowledge-claims in medical psychology. They could be enumerated diagnostically, as indirect indications of underlying morbid states of the central nervous system, but not interpreted psychologically as immediate manifestations of abnormal states of mind. As Jackson said, "On the basis of mere concomitance, mental symptoms (synonymously abnormal states of consciousness) are, strictly speaking, only signs to physicians of what is not going on or of what is going on wrongly in part of a patient's material organisation . . . the physical process in these and all other kinds of [nervous and 'mental' disorder] is our proper concern as medical men."[78] Nor (since they all partook uniformly of the quality of defect or deficiency) could their investigation make any significant contribution toward determining the *normal* psychological "functions of the brain" and nervous system: "Negative and positive mental symptoms are for us only signs of what is not going on, or of what is going on wrong, in the highest sensori-motor centres."[79] They could not be interpreted in their own terms, or for their own sakes, but only appreciated insofar as they helped physicians to infer "the [diseased] physical conditions [of the central nervous system] implied by the psychical states," which were "in all cases the things we [physicians] have ultimately to deal with."[80] Once more, then, the phenomena of mental pathology were set aside in a kind of extra-scientific domain of their own, and prevented from making any effective contribution to either medical or normal psychology; and a "method" which seemed to admit the possibility of more generous recognition and more serious investigation of the psychological aspects of mental disorder instead served merely to confirm and strengthen their habitual neglect by orthodox psychological medicine.

3. The Definition of the Necessary Conditions for Individual Accessibility to Psychological Methods of Treatment as Themselves Comprising a Form of Mental Disorder

Since loss of the subjective sense of effective personal agency, morbid vulnerability to suggestions (whether internal or external in origin), and tendencies toward mental and behavioral automatism were normally regarded par excellence as symptoms of mental and moral decay, it seemed to follow that any state of the organism evincing these characteristics, arising from whatever apparent cause and in whatever context, must necessarily constitute a form of mental disorder. Viewed in a slightly different perspective, however, these same "symptoms" or tendencies were precisely those characteristics of the mental constitution that seemed most conducive to the success of "psychological" modes of therapeutic manipulation, such as hypnosis. Both the advocates of psychological methods of treatment and the more cautious physicians to whom they addressed their appeals were thus brought face to face with the possibility that the very conditions on which the success of such methods of treatment seemed to depend might themselves constitute a *morbus in se*, so similar in its essential characteristics to the original morbid state that the apparently "successful" application of these methods might actually worsen rather than relieve the disorder. Indeed, the very arguments used by medical psychologists attempting to give naturalistic explanations for the efficacy of such techniques as hypnosis often seemed to lend fresh support to this conclusion. Thus James Braid, even while assuring his medical readers that mere susceptibility to hypnosis was quite distinct from actual neurosis, nevertheless took great pains to distinguish hypnotic states from "common sleep" in such a way as to suggest strongly that while the latter was healthy and "natural," the former was morbid and unnatural, and not far removed from states of mental disorder characterized by dominant or obsessive ideas.[81] Noting that "bodily disease, and even insanity, frequently arises from allowing the mind to be occupied inordinately by one particular object or pursuit,"[82] Braid went on to admit that, in hypnosis, "I *rivet* the [subject's] *attention* to *one idea,* and the eyes to *one point,* as the *primary* and *imperative conditions.* . . . I endeavour to rid the mind *at once* of all ideas *but one,* and to fix *that* one in the mind *even after passing into the hypnotic state.* "[83] Nor were the implications for the patient's mental and moral autonomy any better—rather the reverse, for as Braid himself admitted, subjects could systematically be conditioned by means of "phreno-hypnotic" manipulation.[84] Braid presented this discovery as an incalculably beneficial acquisition for education, as well as for medicine;[85] but his readers, attuned as they were to the prevailing early Victorian moral climate of voluntarism and sturdy individualism, can scarcely have regarded Braid's vision of man as an aggregate of perfectly plastic stimulus-response arcs without grave misgivings. Much the same might be said of Daniel Hack Tuke's consistent pleas for the revaluation of hypnosis by orthodox medicine during the latter decades of the century. While reaffirming Braid's naturalistic view of hypnosis, Hack Tuke also stressed "the remarkable parallelism" to be discerned between the symptoms of certain forms of mental disorder (especially "some cases of quiet delusional insanity") and the "symptoms" of hypnosis, whether artificially or spontaneously induced;[86] and regarded hypnosis as the principal type of that large class of abnormal mental states described by Laycock, Carpenter, and Hughlings Jackson in which "the will and consciousness are suspended, and the brain is placed in the condition of the true spinal or reflex system."[87] Indeed, he seems to have regarded mental automatism as the most essential psychological characteristic of hypnosis,[88] and repeatedly drew attention to the complete subjection or "mental slavery" of the "hypnote" to the will of the operator,[89] to an extent which seriously alarmed even the most sympathetic of his professional colleagues.[90] That Hack Tuke himself was aware of the adverse conclusions that could be drawn from his analysis may perhaps be inferred from his growing tendency to advocate the use of hypnotism as a scientific aid to physiological and medical psychological inquiry, rather than as an efficacious mode of treatment for some forms of mental disorder.[91]

If works so apparently favorable as these to the use of techniques such as hypnotism could, nevertheless, be interpreted in a contrary sense, it is scarcely surprising to find that medical authors who were opposed to the use of such techniques should have based their opposition on the more or less explicit and detailed affirmation of an essential pathological kinship between mental disorder and susceptibility to "psychotherapeutics" of whatever kind. Thus Sir Henry Holland argued that persons of "nervous" or hysterical temperament were peculiarly susceptible to hypnosis, and that hypnotic and hysterical trances, if not actually identical, were nevertheless closely related states of mental and moral degeneracy: "The nervous or hysterical temperament is that most prone to be thus acted upon [mesmerically or hypnotically]. . . . In the extreme cases of such susceptibility this idiosyncrasy touches closely upon epilepsy, catalepsy, or other forms of cerebral disorder."[92] Speaking of the young, unmarried, impressionable and mostly female subjects of Reichenbach's miraculous "Odyle" cures, he claimed that "all of them [were] admitted to have some peculiarity of nervous condition or habit, such as catalepsy, paralysis, somnambulism, or spasmodic affections. . . ." This circumstance, in his view, readily explained their apparent susceptibility to this mode of treatment.[93] Hypnosis, Holland conceded, might be induced wholly by the normal psychological process of "expectant [that is, externally captured and focused] attention," as Braid and Carpenter had argued.[94] But he insisted that its induction required a degree and duration of this influence that could only be termed *pathogenic.*[95] This adverse view continued to be affirmed by most authorities on "mental physiology" and medical psychology throughout the remainder of the nineteenth and even into the twentieth century. Thus Hack Tuke's *Dictionary of Psychological Medicine* (1892) included two articles on hypnotism by Charcot and his collaborators Marie and La Tourette, both of which stressed the close pathological kinship between hysteria and hypnosis, and warned that the use of hypnotism as a method of treatment for neuralgia or neurasthenia might actually precipitate an attack of hysteria instead.[96] Tuke's *Dictionary* also included an article, "Hysteria," by Horatio Donkin which emphatically affirmed the "pathological kinship" hypothesis: "Not only is there a morbid similarity between many of the spontaneous phenomena of hysteria and the induced or suggested ones of hypnotism, but also it is among hysterical sufferers that many instances of natural somnambulism and most of the subjects of induced hypnotism are found. . . . It is certain from general experience that human beings are hypnotizable in direct proportion to their nervous instability."[97]

Just how strong and how widespread this orthodox medical view remained even in the early twentieth century may be inferred from Milne Bramwell's article on hypnotic therapeutics in Allbutt's and Rolleston's *System of Medicine.* In this article, Bramwell implicitly acknowledged the force and relevance of orthodox misgivings by attempting to prove that hypnotic treatment set out to counteract and suppress the very morbid characteristics whose presence in the subject was generally held to be necessary for its successful application. It was widely believed that hypnotic "cures" presupposed, and operated by virtue of, a morbid degree of suggestibility on the part of their subjects, and that such cures actually tended to aggravate this weakness in their subjects' mental and moral constitutions; but Milne Bramwell insisted that the opposite was in fact the case. Noting that: "Most of the diseases treated by suggestion—insanity, obsession, bad habits, involuntary muscular movements . . .—are due to want of control in one form or another,"[98] he affirmed that "the object of treatment by suggestion . . . should . . . be the development of the patient's control of his organism and of his own will-power."[99] Far from establishing any mental or moral despotism over the patient, the curative process was, he claimed, wholly voluntary and essentially cooperative.[100] Not only did hypnotic subjects "never accept suggestions which are contrary to their moral sense";[101] the whole object of hypnotic treatment was precisely to counteract any such suggestibility which the patient might evince: "The whole object of suggestion treatment ought to be the development of the patient's will-power and his control of his own organism. That idea, and that idea alone, should be instilled into his brain, and no experiment, however trivial, should be made which could possibly tend to make him believe that the operator was trying to dominate him."[102] As such, it went beyond the mere alleviation of symptoms to the true goal of "scientific" therapeutics—to a radical prophylaxis of the "disease" itself: "To this freedom [of the will], when gained, we owe not only the cure of disease, but also . . . freedom from relapse."[103]

Yet once again, the weight of authoritative opinion elsewhere in the same work seems to have favored the opposite view. Both Sir Clifford Allbutt and Joseph Ormerod pronounced themselves deeply distrustful of all modes of treatment that relied upon "confessional" or suggestive techniques, on moral as much as on medical grounds. Allbutt identified "psychotherapy" with suggestibility, and regarded both as primary symptoms of an hysterical constitution;[104] while according to Ormerod, there was no real difference between the "disease" hysteria, and the hypnotic "cure": "There are so many similarities between the hypnotic and hysterical states, that in hypnotizing for the cure of hysteria we may be said to favour the very condition we want to eradicate . . . a dreamy semi-conscious state, in which the subject's mental activities are removed from his own control; not a good training for an hysterical patient."[105]

This widely held view of the conditions that were necessary for effective psychological manipulation in cases of mental disorder, and especially for efficacious hypnotic suggestion treatment in cases of hysteria, seemed effectively to preclude the possibility of such techniques ever becoming acceptable to orthodox medicine. If mental impressionability, weakened or suspended volitional control, and tendencies to automatic obedience to the promptings of external suggestions or dominant ideas were primary symptoms of mental disorder, then any system of hypnotic treatment or "psychotherapy" that seemed to rely on the exploitation, indeed the positive cultivation, of these very same "morbid" characteristics, must be a veritable contradiction in terms. Hysterical or other "neurotic" patients might

be hypnotized, and their local symptoms transferred, transformed by suggestion, or even suppressed altogether, as they were in Charcot's Salpêtrière.[106] But this was not intended to show how easily such patients could
be cured, once the psychological dynamics of their conditions had been
understood, but rather, to show just how *ill* they really were, and how
inveterate their conditions had become.

The Moral-Pastoral Responsibility of the Physician for the Mentally Disordered Patient

The most important general conclusion which most physicians drew from
these implications of the orthodox-medical view of insanity was that since
the mentally disordered had been deprived of their normal moral and legal
responsibility by virtue of their unsoundness of mind, it was the duty of
the physician (in conjunction with other benevolent persons in authority)
to *assume* this responsibility on their behalf, and to exercise moral-pastoral
supervision over them until such time as the remission or cure of their
insanity permitted them to reassume the management of their own lives.
And the more morally abandoned and irresponsible the mentally disordered proved themselves to be, the more moral-pastorally responsible for
them the physician was. Moral-pastoral functions, of course, figured
largely in the duties of every Victorian physician. This was an age as yet
largely unprovided with effective treatments for the majority of the
diseased conditions, physical as well as mental, with which it was confronted; and there existed (as indeed, to some extent, there still does) a close
relationship between the maintenance of the physician's professional authority and the due performance of his pastoral functions. To an extent
unusual even for his own time, however, the Victorian "psychological
physician" bore a special burden of moral-pastoral responsibility, for not
only were his charges the most morally depraved of patients (according to
the prevailing contemporary view), but also he was even more bereft than
were his other medical colleagues of effective treatments for the conditions
he was supposed to deal with. Indeed, it may be argued that in the majority
of cases, and for most of the time, it was his exercise of moral-pastoral
functions, rather than any practice of medicine as such, which entitled him
to claim professional status and authority.[107] This view of the physician's
moral-pastoral responsibilities in cases of insanity seemed to suggest, however, that if (as was normally assumed to be the case) immoral behavior was
one of the most characteristic symptoms, as well as one of the principal
remote causes, of insanity, and if the cure of insanity consisted primarily
in the social and moral reconstruction and rehabilitation of the patient,
then discipline, chastisement, even punishment could be expected to play
important roles in the "therapeutic" process. Further, any action by the

patient that implicitly or explicitly tended to reduce or undermine the physician's credibility and moral authority should be severely reprobated. And therefore, the first principle of the physician's professional conduct should be to avoid undertaking any course of action, whether by himself, his patient, or both in conjunction, which would in any way tend to detract from the patient's moral integrity or from the physician's own moral and professional authority. The moral and professional authority of the physician, and his unswerving commitment to the practice of orthodox somatic medicine, were seen as bound together in a chain of common connection and mutual dependence; and anything which tended to weaken or undermine either of these interdependent elements would, it was firmly believed, eventually tend to weaken or undermine the other as well.

The Moral-Pastoral Responsibilities of the Psychological Physician and the Medical Treatment of the Psychoneuroses

In this section, I hope to bring out the full significance of these considerations for the psychological treatment of mental disorders by examining in more detail one particular aspect of the practice of psychological medicine, namely, medical attitudes toward the treatment of the so-called psychoneuroses, and of hysteria in particular.

Throughout the last century, and well into the twentieth century, the essential moral depravity, willfulness, and egoism of hysterics was one of the most widely accepted commonplaces of medical psychology. In one of the more temperate passages in his work, *On the Pathology and Treatment of Hysteria* (1852), Robert Brudenell Carter described the characteristic moral state of chronic hysterics as "a[n] union of selfishness and depravity,"[108] while according to Daniel Noble, writing at almost the same time, "the upright and intelligent physician . . . sees in the vagaries of hysterical women neither morbid viscera nor mental derangement . . . but he observes that he has to do with *spoiled children* 'of a larger growth,' whose diseased sensibility solicits the anxious care and consideration of the friends who are about them."[109] Nor were medical appreciations in later decades any kinder, in spite of the progressive "scientificization" of the medical study of hysteria during this period. According to Sir George Savage, "The characteristic of all hysterical cases is the tendency to laziness, want of will, getting into bad habits [etc.],"[110] a conclusion which was to be echoed by many other Victorian medical writers.[111] Even those physicians who were otherwise most sympathetic to the plight of the hysterical woman, and most anxious to have hysteria officially recognized as a genuine illness, were emphatic in reprehending the moral depravity, want of willpower, and morbid egoism that featured so conspicuously among the "symptoms" of the "disease." Thus Donkin, in his article "Hysteria," affirmed that "the cardinal fact in the psychopathy of hysteria is an exaggerated self-consciousness dependent on undue prominence of feelings uncontrolled by intellect . . . the hysteric is pre-eminently an individualist, an unsocial unit, and fails in adaptation to organic surroundings."[112] "Want of will-power," the "mental correlate to hysterical paralysis," was the clearest indicator of the hysterical condition; while "indolence" was "the foster-nurse of the hysterical temperament," since it "gives every opportunity to beget the worst results of self-consciousness."[113] Hysteria, Donkin insisted, was not malingering, but a genuine diseased condition; yet—

> the steps from the lowest [that is, most voluntary] to the highest [that is, most involuntary] grade of hysteria are imperceptible. . . . The most obvious cases of hysteria . . . where certain disorders of sensation and motion are demonstrably outside voluntary control, may also be marked by conduct which is the outcome of the subtlest craft; and the most typical of the physical affections of hysteria may be seen as well in those who are powerless to help themselves and rightly excite our pity, as in those whose actions occasion our contempt and aversion.[114]

There was, he argued, an essential difference between deserving and undeserving cases of hysteria; but how this distinction was to be made in practice remained unclear. Ormerod had the same difficulty in mind a few years later, when he took exception to the use of the word *hysteria* because, he said, "not only . . . has [it] become etymologically meaningless, but also . . . to many minds it has the disagreeable connotation of a certain moral feebleness in the patient, and of unreality in the symptoms."[115] In spite of this, he found himself describing the hysterical fit in terms which emphasized the essential cowardice, deceit, and histrionic character of hysterical behavior just as unmistakably as those of Carter or Donkin:

> In the [hysterical] fit the patient falls, apparently unconscious, but her fall is not so heedless or sudden as to result in serious injury; . . . the hysterical fit consists not so much of muscular spasm as of *coordinated purposive actions*. . . . Frequently a scene of violence is *enacted*. . . . Recovery from an hysteroid fit is more prompt and complete than in epilepsy; there is not the prolonged stupor, nor even the dazed and confused mental state. . . . During the fit itself . . . consciousness is less deeply affected . . . . The hysterical patient rarely suffers injury, can be brought around by appropriate measures, and can sometimes recall the circumstances of the fit. . . .[116]

But it was in relation to the treatment, rather than to the differential diagnosis or interpretation of hysteria, that the implications of the physician's moral-pastoral responsibility for the patient became most apparent.

Physicians regarded the treatment of hysteria almost as they might have done a game of chess—as a complex sequence of offensive and defensive maneuvers requiring elaborate strategic planning, in a situation where even the most trivial action, or inaction, could be productive of the gravest consequences. And the medical ideal of a full and radical cure took the form of a kind of moral checkmate—the complete submission of the patient to the physician's authority, with a full confession of moral wretchedness and of the various tricks and artifices involved in the presentation of the "symptoms." Later Victorian physicians and medical psychologists lavished a degree of attention on hysterical disorders wholly out of proportion to the actual seriousness of such conditions, endemic though they were in Britain as in other "advanced" European and North American societies during this period. This almost obsessive concern testified not so much to the seriousness or even the prevalence of hysteria, but rather to the peculiarly fundamental challenge which it seemed to present to orthodox medicine's basic conception of disease, and thus to the epistemological foundations on which the physician's claim to authority and prestige ultimately depended.[117] And it is with this anxious professional awareness of the seriousness of the issues and interests at stake in the doctor-patient encounter prominently in view that medicopsychological attitudes toward the treatment of hysteria should be interpreted.

Brudenell Carter's recommended course of "treatment" for hysterical disorders has acquired a certain notoriety for the extremity of its judgments and the ruthlessness of its prescriptions, but although no other medical authority on hysteria expressed himself in quite such uncompromising terms, the underlying principles of Carter's therapeutic approach do not differ essentially from those of many later authorities. The essence of his therapeutic regimen consisted not in any specifically medical mode of treatment, but rather in unmasking the basic mental state of deceit, imposture, and moral depravity which, as it were, constituted the underlying "pathological condition" in "voluntary" or "tertiary" hysteria, and then in using the psychological and moral ascendancy thereby acquired methodically to eradicate the patient's "symptoms," not by any conventional medical means or by persuasion, but by means of deliberate intimidation and even emotional blackmail.[118] The "treatment" was calculated to act "by wearing out the moral endurance of the patient, and . . . by taking from her all motives for deception," that is, by making the psychological costs of continued "illness" too great for the patient to persevere in such conduct.[119] Its object was to remove the patient's underlying motive for remaining in a state of chronic, self-induced hysteria (namely, her morbid craving for sympathy and attention), not by attacking the inherent strength of the motive, but rather by frustrating every means which might be adopted for its gratification, or by making such gratification available only at inordinate personal cost to the patient.[120] Apart from the administration of placebos and the (deliberately perfunctory) relief of any genuine intercurrent physical disorders (which were carefully to be distinguished from purely hysterical complaints),[121] there was little scope in Carter's system of treatment for any more specifically medical interventions by the physician. On the contrary, Carter took special care to warn physicians against being duped into prescribing complex medications for imaginary ailments, insisting that "the professional man who has once sanctioned imposture by sending medicines for the cure of self-produced illness, becomes at once an ally [of the hysterical patient], whose aid is the more important for being unconsciously rendered."[122]

Instead, the physician's principal weapon was to be studied indifference toward his patient's vagaries and extravagances, leaving her quite alone during her paroxysms, ignoring her attempts to introduce the subject of her illness into general conversation, and generally disappointing all her expectations of sympathetic attention.[123] This was certainly "psychological treatment" of a kind, but one calculated to operate by playing on the emotions of fear and shame to enable the physician to impose a general system of discipline and correction upon the patient, rather than through any serious attempt to come to terms with the patient's individual problems as such. Its preoccupation with the moral and psychological preparation of the physician for the ordeal of unmasking the patient to herself, and with the struggle for psychological dominance in the doctor-patient relation, effectively precluded any more sympathetic attitude toward the patient's own experiences.

Similar preoccupations with strategy, and with the paramount necessity of safeguarding the physician's moral and professional integrity, may be found in many later Victorian approaches to the treatment of hysteria. Thus both Donkin and Ormerod followed Carter in emphasizing the importance of correct differential diagnosis, and the larger considerations of medical credibility and authority which depended upon it. As Ormerod stated, "To overlook organic disease may do grave injury to the patient, and bring discredit on the physician; [while] to treat hysteria as organic disease may prolong and intensify the hysteria."[124] Both men stressed the virtues of what Donkin called "observant neglect" in treatment,[125] and both fully acknowledged the essential parts to be played by the physician's ability to project an authoritative image, and to call upon the resources of bluff and counterbluff, in the effective treatment of hysterical disorders. According to Donkin,

> Hysterical patients of many kinds may lose their symptoms, at least for a while, under almost any treatment which happens to be in fashion or to "impress their minds. . . ." The habit of many hysterical symptoms . . . of shifting their position . . . spontaneously or from

external suggestion or appliances, as . . . shown by the transference-phenomena in hemi-anaesthesia, indicates many modes of treatment to the reflecting physician. . . .[126]

Ormerod stressed that:

The relation of the physician to his patient is important . . . . She must believe in his superior knowledge and skill, that he possesses the clue to the puzzle of her symptoms. We know the advantage of this faith in the treatment of many diseases; but in hysteria it is essential that there should be no wavering assertions, no vacillating directions. . . . Doubts must be expressed to the friends only, or kept to ourselves.[127]

Once again, the emphasis was on the dramaturgic enactment of a necessary relationship between the physician's insight and authority and the patient's submission and compliance, rather than on any real attempt to come to terms with the patient's individual psychological problems as such. But while Carter's conception of strategy had favored the frontal assault, Ormerod commended a rather more oblique, pragmatic approach:

However sure we may be that symptoms are hysterical . . . we must not treat them as mere nonsense or matter for ridicule. This would merely put us out of touch with the patient; *we must enter into her point of view in order to convert her to ours* . . . it is safest not to attempt too sudden a conversion; for . . . a failure only makes future treatment more difficult. Time and steady pressure are more certain agents . . . there are patients who must be . . . urged and scolded, teased, bribed, and decoyed along the road to health.[128]

The strength and persistence of this overriding emphasis on the need to maintain the physician's moral and professional authority helps to explain how so many later nineteenth-century medical writers on hysteria could on the one hand insist that it *was* a genuine diseased condition (that is, belonging to a class of conditions normally conferring blame-free patient status), and could frequently show themselves to be sensitive and even sympathetic toward the psychosocial and sexual predicaments of their mainly young and female patients, yet on the other maintain so unbending an attitude of moral censure toward the hysterical patient.[129] To have adopted a more sympathetic or engaged approach would have constituted a neglect or evasion of the physician's moral-pastoral responsibility for his patient, and would almost certainly endanger the credibility of the system of medical knowledge and the reputation for strict probity upon which his professional authority in large measure depended. And the strength and persistence of these attitudes also help to explain why orthodox medicine should have been so unwilling to adopt any kind of individual psychological approach to the treatment of mental disorder in general,

and of the psychoneuroses in particular. For if moral depravity constituted
the underlying pathological state in conditions such as chronic hysteria,
then any kind of psychological approach involving operations such as
minute investigation of the patient's private affairs or hypnotic suggestion,
which were themselves regarded as essentially immoral, would merely
compound the patient's demoralization, thus betraying the trust vested in
the psychological physician, and undermining the entire basis of moral
rectitude and strict probity on which his authority depended.

Much of the same emphasis on the absolute priority of the physician's
moral-pastoral responsibilities can be found in the initial reactions of
British practitioners of psychological medicine to the nascent psychoanalytic and psychotherapeutic movements in Europe at the very end
of the century and in the early years of the present century. Inevitably,
psychoanalysis attracted unfavorable moralistic comment on account of its
apparent obsession with sexuality. Thus Mercier, even while admitting
that such practices were by no means uncommon, was nevertheless at
pains to observe (in his *Text-Book of Insanity*) that sadism, homosexuality,
and other sexual variations were "subjects which have of recent years been
treated with a lingering solicitude and a minuteness of detail out of all
proportion to their importance."[130] And in the bibliographical note to his
"Vice, Crime and Insanity," he was to commend the works of Krafft-Ebing
and his "imitators" to "the connoisseurs of pornography."[131] But although
there seems to have been a strong feeling that much of the new psychoanalytical literature was in decidedly bad taste,[132] mere prudishness
does not seem to have been the main reason for medicopsychological
disapproval of psychoanalysis and psychotherapy. Victorian medical writers had not, after all, normally avoided plain speaking about sexuality, and
even sexual abnormalities, when discussing, for example, the phenomena
of hysteria. A far more serious ground of objection seems to have been the
perceived incompatibility of the new methods of psychological analysis
and treatment with traditional professional conceptions of the physician's
moral-pastoral responsibilities. This argument was strongly urged in the
authoritative *System of Medicine* both by Ormerod and by Sir Clifford
Allbutt himself. In his "Hysteria," Ormerod gave a fairly detailed, generally correct, and not unsympathetic, account of Freud's and Breuer's views
on the psychogenesis of hysteria.[133] But he simultaneously evinced a grave
distrust of all suggestion treatments, and of psychotherapy in particular,
as tending to encourage the physician to play God, and the sinful patient
to exaggerate his or her moral depravity, in order to indulge a morbid
craving for masochistic gratification and subsequent medical absolution.

> This [method—that is, psychotherapy] curiously revives the old con-
> ception of the efficacy of the confessional . . . but in this novel confes-
> sional the doctor is the priest, listening to subjects of extreme privacy,

> while the penitent does not even know what he is about to confess, and his confession . . . may be purely the result of imagination or of suggestion received from without . . . we suspect that the treatment by inquisition and confession might sometimes do more harm than good.[134]

Allbutt, in his "Neurasthenia," lent strong support to this cautious and skeptical attitude toward the new psychological methods of interpreting and treating the psychoneuroses. In his view, "These secret introspective dramas, inflamed by reminiscent curiosity, are more than half factitious; and thirst for experience is confused with frailty of morals."[135] "In all we do, whether with adults or children," he warned, "we must beware of putting notions into the patient's head; . . . we must avoid giving the child, or the childish adult, the 'formula of his defects,' lest he act up to the character."[136] For Allbutt, psychoanalysis and psychotherapy as presently practiced were not just aesthetically and morally, but also methodologically and psychologically, unsound.

> To me [he wrote] . . . the recent introspective and confessional methods are odious. . . . It is true that our fundamental appetites, whether of sex, of eating and drinking, and so forth, do through all the gradual transformation into higher powers penetrate them; yet in health and sanity they are not carried up in the gross, but minister sub-consciously to higher ends . . . to endeavour to express the whole in terms of the foundations is a false debasement.[137]

He objected to them on precisely the same grounds on which orthodox Victorian psychological medicine had always objected to psychological approaches to mental disorder—namely, that they encouraged morbid introspection and egoism, heightened suggestibility, and aggravated existing deficiency of willpower. "In sexual neurosis," he argued, "this [exhibitionistic] merging of decency in egotism [in the presentation of symptoms to the physician], which differs from the argumentative or blatant obscenity which usually signifies insanity, is a part of the very loss of self-control which we seek to repair."[138] In Allbutt's view, the first priority of any "psychotherapy" ought to be the "*moral education* or re-education" of the patient, under the benevolent and responsible direction of the physician.[139] But judged by this standard the actual practice of psychotherapy stood condemned precisely because it seemed to ignore or deny any such responsibility, thereby compromising not only the patient's moral integrity, but also that of the physician and of medicine as a whole.

> Medicine [he insisted] . . . is not science only, but . . . the application of science to life . . . in the calling of medicine especially, moral values have always held their pre-eminence. If medical influences are to be kept sweet and wholesome, we must consider the wiles of the human heart, conscious and half-conscious, with a decent reserve and in gen-

eral terms, and in general terms brace the patient to rise superior to them; but this is not to be done by dabbling in them.[140]

This was also Sir James Crichton Browne's considered view. He objected strongly to the method of catharsis, on the grounds that "unburdening the mind of traumatic memories" might actually intensify rather than relieve the patient's sense of guilt and shame.[141] Instead, he argued that "in a vast majority of cases it should be the aim of a rational psycho-therapy to withdraw the patient's mind from the contemplation of an objectionable and painful past and from ferreting out verminous reminiscences, and to occupy it with prospective duties and wholesome pursuits, and sure and certain hopes."[142]

Once again, the apparent inseparability of the physician's discharge of his moral-pastoral responsibilities from the maintenance of the integrity and authority of medicine, and of the causes and essential nature of mental disorder from the ascription of moral depravity and diminished responsibility to its victims, seemed to constitute insuperable objections to the use of psychological methods for interpreting and treating cases of mental disorder. Until both of these interrelated and interdependent sets of conceptual associations had been dissolved or radically reformulated, there was no serious prospect of these objections being met and overcome. Orthodox medicine has always been notably reluctant to give due recognition to the importance of psychological factors in the causation and cure of ordinary "physical" illness; and not until medical psychologists felt assured that the use of psychological approaches would not jeopardize their precarious professional credibility and authority would they venture to employ any technique whose adoption implied a far greater security of professional identity than they had hitherto been able to enjoy.

Conclusion

The general conclusions to be drawn from this analysis of the underlying Victorian medicopsychological view of the nature and causation of mental disorder, and of its implications for the nature and scope of medical intervention appropriate in such cases, may briefly be summarized. Since mental disorder was conceived psycho-physiologically as a lapse from a dualistic or parallelist norm of physical and mental health, and psychologically as a state of dangerous moral irresponsibility, not only were psychopathological phenomena regarded as by definition inaccessible to rational scientific explanation, but also treatment was envisaged exclusively in terms of the restoration of this norm of health, and with it the patient's capacity for exercising individual responsibility. The medical treatment of mental disorder was to consist almost solely in the relief of intercurrent physical disorders, and the "moral" treatment in the repression of selfish instincts and emotions and the cultivation of more "altruistic" or "social" sentiments—that is, in the enhancement of the voluntary power of responsible self-determination; the discouragement of introversion and self-absorption; and the encouragement of a less subjective, more extraverted attitude toward external reality. And therefore, any mode of treatment which not only seemed (as did hypnotic suggestion and psychotherapy) to take for granted the morbid subjectivity and moral depravity of the mentally disordered, but actually to exploit and intensify them, while simultaneously undermining the whole basis of the physician's moral authority, could only be regarded as entirely contrary to the most fundamental principles of psychological medicine, and wholly unacceptable as an instrument of legitimate medicine. Finally, we can begin to understand why the considerable body of Victorian medicopsychological "insights" into unconscious or abnormal mentation and behavior could not constitute any serviceable body of interpretative or therapeutic knowledge for later Victorian psychiatry. These insights possessed the character not so much of possible objects of knowledge as of moral exemplars, or rather, of scientific exemplifications of well-established, *universal* moral truths which themselves contained all that was needful for the effective "moral treatment" of mental disorders, without need for further analysis or individuation. Their incorporation into medical psychology, and the profoundly negative significance ascribed to them within that body of knowledge, testified to the essentially moral-homiletic and didactic inspiration of much Victorian psychology.[143] In large measure, they owed their very existence as intelligible objects of discourse (at least, in the forms in which they were habitually recognized and discussed) to a system of ideas and moral values that necessarily cast them in an antithetical relation to the central organizing concepts of psychological medicine; and, in the very nature of things, it was scarcely probable that they could do other than confirm and strengthen, rather than question or undermine, the same ideas and values which had given them meaningful existence.

Notes

I should especially like to thank William Parry-Jones, of Linacre College, Oxford; Andrew Scull; Charles Webster, of the Wellcome Unit for the History of Medicine in Oxford; Ludmilla Jordanova, of the University of Essex; Karl Figlio, of Charing Cross Hospital Medical School, London; and Greta Ilott, for help, encouragement, and critical comments at various stages in the gestation and preparation of this work. The responsibility for all remaining errors of fact and judgment is entirely my own.

1. Henry Maudsley, *Responsibility in Mental Disease*, 2d ed. (London: Kegan Paul, 1874), p. 154 (italics in the original). For Maudsley's life and work, see G. H. Brown, comp., *Lives of the Fellows of the Royal College of Physicians of London 1826–1925* (London: Royal College of Physicians, 1955), pp. 172–73. (Continuation of William Munk, *The Roll of the Royal College of Physicians of London; Comprising Biographical Sketches of All the Eminent Physicians, Whose Names Are Recorded in the Annals, from the Foundation of the College in 1518 to Its Removal in 1825, . . .* 2d ed. rev. and enl. [London: Royal College of Physicians, 1878]; hereafter cited as *Munk's Roll*). See also Aubrey Lewis, "Henry Maudsley: His Work and Influence," 25th Maudsley Lecture, *Journal of Mental Science* 97 (1951): 259–77, reprinted in Sir Aubrey Lewis, *The State of Psychiatry: Essays and Addresses* (London: Routledge and Kegan Paul, 1967), chap. 4.

2. See, for example, James Crichton Browne, "The History and Progress of Psychological Medicine. An Inaugural Address," *Journal of Mental Science* 7, no. 37 (1861): 25–26, 29; Henry Maudsley, *Body and Mind: An Inquiry into Their Connection and Mutual Influence, Specially in Reference to Mental Disorders*, Gulstonian Lectures for 1870 (London: Macmillan, 1870), pp. 2–3; idem, *Responsibility in Mental Disease*, pp. 6–19; and Daniel Hack Tuke, "Progress of Psychological Medicine During the Last Forty Years," Presidential Address to the Medico-Psychological Association of Great Britain delivered at University College, London, on 2 August 1881, *Journal of Mental Science* 27 (1881–82): 321–26, 330–31. For Crichton Browne's life and work, see s.v. "Browne, Sir James Crichton," in the *Dictionary of National Biography 1931–1940*, pp. 106–7. For Hack Tuke, see s.v. "Tuke, Daniel Hack," in the *Dictionary of National Biography*, 19:1223–24, and in *Munk's Roll*, 4:237.

3. See David Skae, "A Rational and Practical Classification of Insanity," Presidential Address to the Association of Medical Officers of Asylums and Hospitals for the Insane (later the Medico-Psychological Association of Great Britain) delivered at the Royal College of Physicians of London on 9 July 1863, *Journal of Mental Science* 9 (1863): 310–11, 313–19; George H. Savage, *Insanity and Allied Neuroses: Practical and Clinical* (London: Cassells, 1884), chap. 2; George Fielding Blandford, *Insanity and Its Treatment: Lectures on the Treatment, Medical*

and Legal, of Insane Patients, 4th ed. (Edinburgh: Oliver and Boyd, 1892), pp.
91–103, 139–40; John Batty Tuke and German Sims Woodhead, "Pathology [of
Insanity]," in *A Dictionary of Psychological Medicine, Giving the Definition, Etymology and Synonyms of the Terms Used in Medical Psychology; With the Symptoms,
Treatment and Pathology of Insanity and the Law of Lunacy in Great Britain and
Ireland*, ed. D. H. Tuke (London: Churchill, 1892), pp. 892–99; and Thomas
Smith Clouston, *Clinical Lectures on Mental Diseases*, 5th ed. rev. (London:
Churchill, 1898), pp. 7–13. See also Hack Tuke, "Progress of Psychological
Medicine," pp. 328–31; and the discussions of different principles and systems
of classification in Maudsley, *Responsibility in Mental Disease*, pp. 78–86, and in
John Charles Bucknill and Daniel Hack Tuke, *A Manual of Psychological Medicine; Containing the History, Nosology, Description, Statistics, Diagnosis, Pathology
and Treatment of Insanity*, 4th ed. rev. (London: Churchills, 1879), pp. 27–53. For
Skae and his system of classification, see F. J. Fish, "David Skae, M.D.,
F.R.C.S., Founder of the Edinburgh School of Psychiatry," *Medical History* 9
(1965): 36–53; for Savage, see s.v. "Savage, Sir George Henry," in *Munk's Roll*,
4:306–7; for Blandford, see s.v. "Blandford, George Fielding," in the *Dictionary
of National Biography*, 2d supp., 1:176–77, and in *Munk's Roll*, 4:168–69; for Batty
Tuke, see "Obituary of Sir John Batty Tuke," *Edinburgh Medical Journal* n.s.
11 (1913); 431–37; and for Clouston, see s.v. "Clouston, Sir Thomas Smith," in
Who Was Who 1897–1916, pp. 143–44. It should be emphasized that, with the
possible exception of Skae, none of these alienist physicians advocated the
exclusive adoption of systems of classification based on etiological, pathological,
or developmental principles. Indeed, they all expressed more or less grave
misgivings about their immediate practicability, given the paucity of existing
scientific knowledge about the exact causation and pathology of mental disorders. Rather, they advocated their progressive adoption as guides to scientific
research to serve alongside more traditional, symptomatological classifications, in the hope that future research would gradually permit the existing
clinical systems to be brought into closer correspondence with more "scientific" arrangements of mental disorders.

4. Bucknill and Tuke, *Manual of Psychological Medicine*, pp. 34–35, 47–48, For
Bucknill, see s.v. "Bucknill, Sir John Charles," in the *Dictionary of National
Biography*, 1st supp., 1:331–32, and in *Munk's Roll*, 4:102–3.

5. Henry Maudsley, *The Pathology of Mind: A Study of Its Distempers, Deformities and
Disorders* (London: Macmillan, 1895), p. 363.

6. William F. Bynum, "Rationales for Therapy in British Psychiatry, 1780–1835,"
chap. 2 of this book; Andrew T. Scull, "From Madness to Mental Illness:
Medical Men as Moral Entrepreneurs," *European Journal of Sociology* 16 (1975):
225–34; idem, *Museums of Madness: The Social Organization of Insanity in Nineteenth-
Century England* (London: Allen Lane, 1979), pp. 129–41; Peter McCandless,
"Insanity and Society: A Study of the English Lunacy Reform Movement"
(Ph.D. diss., University of Wisconsin, 1974), pp. 106–7. See also Michael Fears,
"The 'Moral Treatment' of Insanity: A Study in the Social Construction of
Human Nature" (Ph.D. diss., University of Edinburgh, 1978), chap. 2.

7. See Bynum, "Rationales for Therapy," chap. 2 of this book; Scull, "From
Madness to Mental Illness," pp. 225–34, 236–37, 240–41; idem, *Museums of Madness*,
pp. 130–41.

8. See, for example, Sir James Coxe, *On the Causes of Insanity and the Means of Checking Its Growth* (Edinburgh: Neill, 1872), pp. 5, 7–11, 17–18. For Coxe, see his obituary in *Edinburgh Medical Journal* 23 (1878): 1139–41. See also Andrew T. Scull, *Decarceration: Community Treatment and the Deviant—A Radical View* (Englewood Cliffs, N.J.: Prentice-Hall, 1977), pp. 104–9, 110–12, 124–29.

9. See, for example, Hack Tuke, "Progress of Psychological Medicine," pp. 328–31, 333; Maudsley, *Pathology of Mind*, pp. 515, 545; and Theophilus B. Hyslop, *Mental Physiology, Especially in Its Relation to Mental Disorders* (London: Churchill, 1895), pp. 6–7. For Hyslop, see his obituary, *Journal of Mental Science* 79 (1933): 424–26. See also Scull, *Museums of Madness*, pp. 167–71, 173, 178.

10. Throughout this essay, I use the terms *mental disorder* and *insanity* interchangeably and in a very broad sense, to include the whole range of "mental" and "nervous" diseases, both "organic" and "functional," which came within the purview of alienist physicians either in asylum or in consultancy practice, or (in a few cases) in clinical neurological practice. However, in the latter sections I shall be concerned primarily with the treatment of those conditions which by the end of the nineteenth century had come to be designated the "psychoneuroses," especially hysteria, neurasthenia, and all those conditions characterized, in the eyes of contemporary practitioners of "psychological medicine," by more or less pronounced affective disorders, moral depravity, and a morbid degree of suggestibility. While this may appear willfully to ignore certain important clinical distinctions that are usually regarded as essential for any meaningful discussion of psychiatric treatments, it is one of the principal contentions of this essay that, even where such distinctions were ostensibly made in the literature of later Victorian "psychological medicine" itself, much the same framework of interpretative ideas was in fact employed, with much the same implications for treatment, in dealing with less severe "nervous" or "functional" complaints as with more severe, chronic "psychoses."

11. See McCandless, "Insanity and Society," chaps. 7, 8; Scull, *Museums of Madness*, pp. 186–204, 208–20.

12. See, for example, E. L. Margetts, "The Unconscious in the History of Medical Psychology," *Psychiatric Quarterly* 27 (1953): 115–38; Henri Ellenberger, "The Ancestry of Dynamic Psychotherapy," *Bulletin of the Menninger Clinic* 20 (1956): 288–99; idem, "The Unconscious Before Freud," *Bulletin of the Menninger Clinic* 21 (1957): 3–16; idem, *The Discovery of the Unconscious: The History and Evolution of Dynamic Psychiatry* (New York: Basic Books, 1970); Lancelot Law Whyte, *The Unconscious Before Freud* (New York: Basic Books, 1960); and Mark David Altschule and Evelyn Russ Hegedus (collab.), *The Roots of Modern Psychiatry: Essays in the History of Psychiatry*, 2d ed., rev. and enl. (New York: Grune, 1962), chaps. 4, 6.

13. The interpretation of Victorian medical conceptions of insanity that is given in the following section is somewhat similar to that recently developed by Roger Smith in his work on insanity pleas and forensic psychiatry in the mid-nineteenth century. See his article "Mental Disorder, Criminal Responsibility and the Social History of Theories of Volition," *Psychological Medicine* 9 (1979): 13–19, which was, however, unavailable at the time of writing.

14. See, for example, Maudsley, *Body and Mind*, pp. 72–75, 81–83, 93–97, 100–102, 108–9; idem, *Responsibility in Mental Disease*, pp. 133–34, 137–38, 149–54, 165–66, 172–73, 187–88, 193–95, 196–200, 236–39, 249–53; William Benjamin Carpenter, *Principles of Mental Physiology*, 6th ed. (London: Kegan Paul, 1881), pp. 391–93, 553, 657–60, 663–70; idem, *Nature and Man*, ed. J. Estlin Carpenter (London: Kegan Paul, Trench, 1888), pp. 171–72, 294–96; William Bevan Lewis, *A Textbook of Mental Diseases, with Special Reference to the Pathological Aspects of Insanity*, 2d ed. rev. (London: Griffin, 1899), pp. 143–49, 151–53, 172–76, 180–85, 190–95, 332–38, 346–57. For Carpenter, see J. Estlin Carpenter, "William Benjamin Carpenter—A Memorial Sketch," in Carpenter, *Nature and Man*, and s.v. "Carpenter, William Benjamin," in the *Dictionary of National Biography*, 9:166–68, and in the *Dictionary of Scientific Biography*, 3:87–89. For Bevan Lewis, see his obituary, *Journal of Mental Science* 76 (1930): 383–88.

15. One of the clearest and most comprehensive expositions of this classic Victorian psychiatric position, and of its implications for the interpretation of abnormal mental states, was given as early as 1830 by John Conolly in his *Indications of Insanity*. See John Conolly, *An Enquiry Concerning the Indications of Insanity, with Suggestions for the Better Protection and Care of the Insane* (1830; facs. reprint ed., with an *Introduction* by Richard Hunter and Ida MacAlpine, Psychiatric Monograph Series No. 4, London: Dawsons, 1964), pp. 40–60, 71–77, 84–85, 95–96, 113–14, 115–24, 127–29, 133, 135–36, 150, 154–56, 166–69, 222–32, 257–59, 299–305, 310–11, 323–26, 338–40. For Conolly's life and work, see Henry Maudsley, "A Memoir of the Late John Conolly," *Journal of Mental Science* 12 (1866): 151–74; Sir James Clark, *A Memoir of John Conolly, M.D., D.C.L., Comprising a Sketch of the Treatment of the Insane in Europe and America* (London: John Murray, 1869); s.v. "Conolly, John," in the *Dictionary of National Biography*, 4:951–54, and in *Munk's Roll*, 4:33–34; Denis Leigh, *The Historical Development of British Psychiatry* (Oxford: Pergamon Press, 1961), 1:210–70; and Richard Hunter and Ida MacAlpine, *Introductions* to Conolly, *Indications of Insanity*, pp. 1–35; idem, *The Construction and Government of Lunatic Asylums and Hospitals for the Insane* (1847; facs. reprint ed., Psychiatric Monograph Series No. 6, London: Dawsons, 1968), pp. 7–38; and idem, *The Treatment of the Insane Without Mechanical Restraints* (1856; facs. reprint ed., Psychiatric Monograph Series No. 5, London: Dawsons, 1973), pp. vii–xlvi.

16. See, for example, Maudsley, *Pathology of Mind*, pp. 6–9, 93–94; Bevan Lewis, *Mental Diseases*, pp. 148, 159–61, 172–73.

17. See, in particular, Sir Henry Holland, *Chapters on Mental Physiology*, 2d ed., rev. and enl. (London: Longmans, 1858), pp. 94–96, 133–38, 221–22; Daniel Noble, *The Human Mind in Its Relation with the Brain and Nervous System* (London: Churchill, 1858), pp. 150–51; Robert Dunn, *An Essay on Physiological Psychology* (London: Churchill, 1858), pp. 43–47; and Carpenter, *Mental Physiology*, pp. ix, 5–7, 22–26, 657. For Holland, see s.v. "Holland, Sir Henry," in the *Dictionary of National Biography*, 9:1038–39, and in *Munk's Roll*, 3:144–49; for Noble, see s.v. "Noble, Daniel," in *Munk's Roll*, 4:114; and for Dunn, see s.v. "Dunn, Robert," in the *Dictionary of National Biography*, 6:210.

18. See, for example, Holland, *Mental Physiology*, pp. 40, 42–43, 44, 46, 55–56, 95–96; Henry Maudsley, *Body and Will* (London: Kegan Paul and Trench, 1883), pp.

308–9; idem, *Pathology of Mind*, pp. 16–17, 145–50, 311–13; Bevan Lewis, *Mental Diseases*, pp. 142–53, 170–76, 332–35, 346–59.

19. See pp. 284–88 of this chap. and notes 73–74.

20. See pp. 274–76 of this chap. and notes 14–19; see also pp. 283–85 and notes 56, 66–68; Scull, *Museums of Madness*, pp. 159–61.

21. See pp. 272, 274 of this chap. and notes 6–7.

22. See, for example, John Abercrombie, *Inquiries Concerning the Intellectual Powers and the Investigation of Truth*, 5th ed. (Edinburgh: Waugh and Innes, 1835); Holland, *Mental Physiology*; Sir Benjamin Collins Brodie, *Psychological Inquiries*, 4th ed., 2 vols. (London: Longmans, 1862); Daniel Hack Tuke, *Illustrations of the Influence of the Mind Upon the Body in Health and Disease, Designed to Elucidate the Action of the Imagination* (London: Churchill, 1872); and Carpenter, *Mental Physiology*. For Abercrombie, see s.v. "Abercrombie, John," in the *Dictionary of National Biography* 1:37–38; for Brodie, see s.v. "Brodie, Sir Benjamin Collins, Bart.," in the *Dictionary of National Biography* 2:1288, and in *Plarr's Lives of the Fellows of the Royal College of Surgeons of England*, vol. 1, revised by Sir D'Arcy Power, assisted by W. G. Spencer and Prof. G. E. Gash, 2d ed. rev. (Bristol: John Wright, 1930); vol. 2 edited by Sir D'Arcy Power, continued by W. R. Le Fanu (London: Royal College of Surgeons, 1955), 1:144–48 (hereafter cited as *Plarr's Lives*).

23. See Maudsley, *Responsibility in Mental Disease*; Nigel Walker, *Crime and Insanity in England*, 2 vols. (Edinburgh: Edinburgh University Press, 1968–1973), vol. 1, chaps. 5–9; and Smith, "Criminal Responsibility."

24. See, for example, Robert Brudenell Carter, *On the Influence of Education and Training in Preventing Diseases of the Nervous System* (London: Churchill, 1855); Coxe, *On the Causes of Insanity*, pp. 13–28; Daniel Hack Tuke, *Insanity in Ancient and Modern Life, with Chapters on Its Prevention* (London: Macmillan, 1878), chaps. 1, 5, 6, 8, 9; James Crichton Browne, "Education and the Nervous System," in *The Book of Health*, ed. Malcolm Morris (London: Cassell, 1883), pp. 269–380; and Thomas Smith Clouston, *The Hygiene of Mind* (London: Methuen, 1906). For Carter, see pp. 293, 295–96 of this chap. and n. 108.

25. See, for example, Dunn, *Physiological Psychology*, "Prefatory Note," pp. 5, 91–92; idem, *Medical Psychology* (London: Churchill, 1863), pp. 3–4; Thomas Laycock, *Mind and Brain; or, the Correlations of Consciousness and Organization; Systematically Investigated and Applied to Philosophy, Mental Science and Practice*, 2d ed., rev., 2 vols. (London: Simpkin, Marshall, 1869), 1:iii–x, 1–4; Maudsley, *Body and Mind*, pp. vii–viii, 2–6, 12, 17–23, 40, 108–9; idem, *Responsibility in Mental Disease*, pp. 13–19; Bucknill and Tuke, *Manual of Psychological Medicine*, pp. 34–35, 47–48; Hack Tuke, "Progress of Psychological Medicine," pp. 324–31; and William Henry Octavius Sankey, *Lectures on Mental Diseases*, 2d ed., rev. (London: H. K. Lewis, 1884), pp. 1, 4. See also pp. 281–82 of this chap. and n. 50 below. For Laycock, see s.v. "Laycock, Thomas," in the *Dictionary of National Biography*, 11:744–45; and for Sankey, see s.v. "Sankey, William Henry Octavius," in *Munk's Roll*, 4:147–48.

26. Bynum, "Rationales for Therapy," chap. 2 of this book. Scull, *Museums of Madness*, pp. 125–63.

27. [Robert Ferguson], "Art. I. [Rev. of] *Isis Revelata* . . . By J. C. Colquhoun . . . Edinburgh, 1837. *Théorie des Somnambulismes*. Von J. U. Wirth. 1836. *A Treatise on Insanity*. By James Cowles Pritchard . . . London, 1835. *Rapports et Discussions de l'Académie Royale de Médecine sur le Magnétisme Animal, etc*. Par M. P. Foissac. Paris, 1833," in *Quarterly Review* 61 (January–April 1838): 298. Ferguson is not actually quoting, but rather succinctly and accurately paraphrasing Dugald Stewart's argument in his *Elements of the Philosophy of the Human Mind*, vol. 3, pt. 2, chap. 2, sec. 3 and 4. See Dugald Stewart, *The Collected Works of Dugald Stewart*, ed. Sir W. Hamilton, 11 vols. (Edinburgh: Thomas Constable, 1854–60), 4:147–53, 166–67. For Ferguson, see s.v. "Ferguson, Robert, M.D.," in the *Dictionary of National Biography*, 6:1217–18.

28. Ferguson, "*Isis Revelata* . . . ," p. 298.

29. Ibid., p. 299.

30. Ibid., p. 298.

31. J. Braid, *Neurypnology, or the Rationale of Nervous Sleep Considered in Relation to Animal Magnetism or Mesmerism*, ed. A. E. Waite (1843; reprint ed., London: George Redway, 1899), p. 86. For Braid, see Waite's "Biographical Introduction," ibid., pp. 1–66; and s.v. "Braid, James," in the *Dictionary of National Biography*, 2:1106–7.

32. Braid, *Neurypnology*, pp. 101–3, 112–13, 118, 126, 216–17. Braid himself did not actually employ the phrase "Expectant Attention" to describe the rationale of hypnotism in *Neurypnology*. His rather brief (and not altogether coherent) attempts to explain mesmeric or hypnotic phenomena in that work in fact place more emphasis on the physiological action of the nerves of "common sensation" and the "sympathetic" system and on associated local changes in the circulation in the induction of the phenomena than they do on the concurrent psychological processes involved. See Braid, *Neurypnology*, pp. 101–2, 164–67, 216–17, 219–21. However, this account underwent considerable elaboration and modification, both by Braid himself and by other contemporaries, and the term *Expectant Attention* came to be used somewhat imprecisely to denote the more finished (and psychologically more orthodox) version, popularized by Holland and Carpenter, of what was assumed to be Braid's preferred explanation. A certain confusion is often apparent in these later accounts (and, indeed, at times in Braid's own) between the attribution of phenomena to the kind of physiological mechanisms envisaged by Braid, on the one hand, and to the influence of "Imitation" and "Imagination" prompted by "Suggestion," on the other—the latter frequently being credited with direct and unmediated action of their own. These more purely psychological factors had long been routinely invoked by mental philosophers, physiologists, and psychologists seeking to give an orthodox psychological explanation for mesmeric phenomena, and the relation between "Imitation," "Imagination," "Expectant Attention," and associated physiological changes in the production of the phenomena was never very satisfactorily defined. See, for example, Dugald Stewart, *Collected Works*, 4:147–48, 150–59, 166–67; Ferguson, "*Isis Revelata*, . . ." pp. 294–95; Braid, *Neurypnology*, pp. 116–18, 135, 286–87, 337–38; W. B. Carpenter, *Principles of Human Physiology, with Their Chief Applications to Pathology, Hygiene and Forensic Medicine*, 5th

ed., rev. (London: Churchill, 1855), pp. 605–12, 619–29, 644–51; Holland, *Mental Physiology*, pp. 104–6; and Hack Tuke, *Influence of the Mind Upon the Body*, pp. 3–12, 18–20, 24–26, 353, 404–9, 415–17.

33. See Braid, *Neurypnology*, pp. 150–51, 157, 164–74, 210, 212–15; and Waite, "Biographical Introduction," ibid., pp. 19–29.

34. Braid, *Neurypnology*, pp. 164–67, 172–74.

35. Ibid., p. 150.

36. Thomas Wakley, reply to "C. C. C.," in *Lancet*, 29 October 1843, p. 192, quoted in Waite, "Biographical Introduction," p. 14, n. 2. For Wakley, see s.v. "Wakley, Thomas," in the *Dictionary of National Biography*, 20:461–65, and Samuel Squire Sprigge, *The Life and Times of Thomas Wakley, Founder and First Editor of the "Lancet"* . . . (London: Longmans, Green, 1897).

37. Waite, "Biographical Introduction," p. 14. For general accounts of the controversies surrounding Elliotson and the mesmerists, on the one hand, and Braid, his supporters, and critics, on the other, see Waite, "Biographical Introduction," pp. 4–19, 30–31, and T. M. Parssinen, "Professional Deviants and the History of Medicine: Medical Mesmerists in Victorian Britain," in *On the Margins of Science: The Social Construction of Rejected Knowledge*, ed. R. Wallis, Sociological Review Monographs No. 27 (Keele, Staffordshire: University of Keele Press, 1979), pp. 103–20. See also s.v. "Elliotson, John," in the *Dictionary of National Biography*, 6:682–84.

38. D. Hack Tuke, Editorial note to the report of the "Discussion of Sleep and Hypnotism" in the Psychological Section of the British Medical Association's Annual General Meeting at Cambridge, 1880, in *Journal of Mental Science* 26 (1880): 471.

39. Hack Tuke, *Influence of the Mind Upon the Body*, p. 404, footnote.

40. Ibid., p. 5, footnote.

41. Ibid., pp. 407–8.

42. Ibid., p. 407.

43. Ibid., p. ix.

44. Ibid.

45. A. T. Myers, "Hypnotism," in Hack Tuke, *Dictionary of Psychological Medicine*, pp. 604–6. For the Society for Psychical Research, see L. S. Hearnshaw, *A Short History of British Psychology, 1840–1940* (London: Methuen, 1964), pp. 157–60. For Myers, see s.v. "Myers, Arthur Thomas," in *Munk's Roll*, 4:365–66.

46. Myers, "Hypnotism," pp. 605–6. For Esdaile, see s.v. "Esdaile, James," in the *Dictionary of National Biography*, 6:865–67. For Milne Bramwell, see s.v. "Bramwell, John Milne," in *Who Was Who 1916–1928*, pp. 119–20.

47. See Ilza Veith, *Hysteria: The History of a Disease* (Chicago and London: University of Chicago Press, 1965), pp. 238–44.

48. Parssinen, "Professional Deviants," pp. 116–17; Hearnshaw, *British Psychology 1840–1940*, p. 17.

49. J. Milne Bramwell, "Hypnotism; and the Treatment of Insanity and Allied Disorders by Suggestion," in *A System of Medicine* . . . , ed. T. C. Allbutt and H. D. Rolleston, 2d ed., rev., 9 vols. (London: Macmillan, 1905–11), 8:1013–14.

50. J. A. Ormerod, "Hysteria," in *A System of Medicine,* ed. Allbutt and Rolleston, 8:693. For Ormerod, see s.v. "Ormerod, Joseph Arderne," in *Munk's Roll,* 4:304–5.

51. Ormerod, "Hysteria," p. 724.

52. See pp. 288–92 of this chapter.

53. See John Hughlings Jackson, *Selected Writings of John Hughlings Jackson,* ed. J. Taylor, G. Holmes, and F. M. R. Walshe, 2 vols. (London: Hodder and Stoughton, 1931–32), 1:41–42, 48–49, 169–70; 2:63, 72, 84–85, 95, 349–50; Sir Russell Brain, "Hughlings Jackson's Ideas of Consciousness in the Light of Today," in *The History and Philosophy of Knowledge of the Brain and Its Functions,* ed. F. N. L. Poynter (Oxford: Blackwell, 1958), pp. 83–87. For Jackson, see s.v. "Jackson, John Hughlings," in the *Dictionary of National Biography, 1901–1911,* pp. 356–58; and in *Munk's Roll,* 4:161–63. See also the memoirs of Jackson by James Taylor, Sir Jonathan Hutchinson, and Charles Mercier in John Hughlings Jackson, *Neurological Fragments,* ed. J. Taylor (London: Oxford Medical Publications, Oxford University Press, 1925), pp. 1–26, 27–39, 40–46.

54. See Jackson, *Selected Writings,* 2:24–25, 116, 211–12.

55. See ibid., 2:4–5, 90, 359–62, 412.

56. See, for example, ibid., 1:52, 366–67; 2:9, 84–85, 355; and H. Tristram Engelhardt, Jr., "John Hughlings Jackson and the Mind-Body Relation," *Bulletin of the History of Medicine* 49 (1975): 143–45.

57. See, for example, Jackson, *Selected Writings,* 1:330–31, 366–67; 2:342, 352.

58. Ibid., 1:452. See also 2:85, 355.

59. Ibid., 2:46–47, 50, 192, 297–99, 405–7, 414–16, 483–84.

60. C. Mercier, *A Text-Book of Insanity* (London: Swan, Sonnenschein, 1902), pp. 111–12. For Mercier's social, professional, and intellectual relations with Jackson, see C. Mercier, "Recollections," in Jackson, *Neurological Fragments,* pp. 40–46. For Mercier's own career, see s.v. "Mercier, Charles Arthur" in *Munk's Roll* 4:463–64, and in *Plarr's Lives,* 2:52.

61. See, for example, Jackson, *Selected Writings,* 2:17, 23–24, 46–47, 78, 189–90, 297–99, 405–6, 414–16, 417–18.

62. Mercier, *Text-Book of Insanity,* p. 69.

63. Maudsley, *Pathology of Mind,* p. 353.

64. Mercier, *Text-Book of Insanity,* pp. 111–12.

65. Jackson, *Selected Writings,* 2:17. See also 1:123; 2:16, 21, 192, 298.

66. Ibid., 1:41. See also 2:265.

67. Ibid., 1:418.

68. Following E. A. Burtt, Robert M. Young has argued more generally that the virtual exclusion of both normal and abnormal psychological phenomena from the domain of possible objects of scientific knowledge during the nineteenth century was the inevitable outcome of the essentially dualistic epistemology that has dominated scientific thought from the seventeenth century to the present. In this view, the hypothesis of strict psycho-physical parallelism was merely an unusually explicit (and rigid) recognition of the limitations that this epistemology imposed upon the possibilities for extending scientific knowledge into the domain of mind itself. See Robert M. Young, "The Functions

of the Brain; Gall to Ferrier (1808–1886)," *Isis* 59 (1968): 251–52, 261–62, 267–68; and idem, *Mind, Brain and Adaptation in the Nineteenth Century* (Oxford: Clarendon Press, 1970), pp. 1–2, 7–8.

69. See, for example, Maudsley, *Body and Mind,* pp. 83–87; idem, *Pathology of Mind,* pp. 389–91, 401–4, 427–28, 456–58; T. S. Clouston, *The Neuroses of Development* (Edinburgh: Oliver and Boyd, 1891), pp. 114–16, 123–24; idem, *The Hygiene of Mind,* pp. 168–73, 250; Bevan Lewis, *Mental Diseases,* pp. 286–90, 388–94, 398.

70. Mercier, *Text-Book of Insanity,* p. 111.

71. Clouston, *Clinical Lectures on Mental Diseases,* p. 295. See also ibid., pp. 285–87.

72. Mercier, *Text-Book of Insanity,* pp. 110, 111–12.

73. See, for example, Maudsley, *Pathology of Mind,* pp. 348–53; Bevan Lewis, *Mental Diseases,* pp. 152–53.

74. C. Mercier, "Vice, Crime and Insanity," in Allbutt and Rolleston, *A System of Medicine,* 8:872. See also ibid., pp. 870–71. Cf. Maudsley, *Responsibility in Mental Disease,* pp. 195, 202–3, 210–11, 216–17, 219–21.

75. Maudsley, *Body and Mind,* p. 41. Cf. Jackson, *Selected Writings,* 1:26, n. 1, 84; 2:4–5, 90, 398–99.

76. Maudsley, *Body and Mind,* pp. 67–68; idem, *Responsibility in Mental Disease,* pp. 40–45; idem, *Pathology of Mind,* pp. 19–20; C. Mercier, *Sanity and Insanity* (London: Walter Scott, 1890), pp. 191–92, 201–2, 298–99; Jackson, *Selected Writings,* 2:4–5. See also 1:26, n. 1, 84.

77. Maudsley, *Body and Will,* p. 122.

78. Jackson, *Selected Writings,* 1:417.

79. Ibid., 2:85. See also notes 58, 78 above.

80. Ibid., 2:12. See also 1:48–49, 169; 2:9, 85, 480.

81. Braid, *Neurypnology,* pp. 122–27, 327–28, n. 7.

82. Ibid., p. 125.

83. Ibid., p. 127, footnote (italics in the original).

84. Ibid., pp. 150–51, 169–70.

85. Ibid., pp. 150, 170–71.

86. D. Hack Tuke, Editor's note to S. Coupland, "A Case of Spontaneous Hypnotism," *Journal of Mental Science* 26 (1880–81): 54.

87. D. Hack Tuke, "On the Mental Condition in Hypnotism," *Journal of Mental Science* 29 (1883–84): 78.

88. D. Hack Tuke, "Hypnosis Redivivus," *Journal of Mental Science* 26 (1880–81): 537, 546; idem, "On the Mental Condition in Hypnotism," pp. 77–79.

89. See, for example, Hack Tuke, "Hypnosis Redivivus," pp. 537, 543, 546.

90. See the discussion of Hack Tuke's paper "On the Mental Condition in Hypnotism" in *Journal of Mental Science* 29 (1883–84): 124–26, especially the comments of Dr. Major and Dr. Savage.

91. Hack Tuke, "Hypnosis Redivivus," p. 531.

92. Holland, *Mental Physiology,* p. 102.

93. Ibid., p. 102, footnote.

94. Ibid., pp. 98–101, 105; Braid, *Neurypnology,* pp. 101–2, 112–18, 126, 127, footnote; Carpenter, *Human Physiology,* pp. 610–12, 618, 624–27, 644–51, 784–85.

95. Holland, *Mental Physiology,* pp. 104–5.

96. J. M. Charcot and G. La Tourette, "Hypnotism in the Hysterical," in Hack
    Tuke, *Dictionary of Psychological Medicine*, pp. 606–10; J. M. Charcot and P.
    Marie, "Hysteria," ibid., pp. 627–41. For Charcot and his collaborators' work
    on hysteria and hypnotism, see Georges Guillain, *J. M. Charcot, 1825–1893. His
    Life—His Work . . .* , ed. and trans. Pearce Bailey (London: Pitman Medical
    Publishing, 1959); and Alan Robert George Owen, *Hysteria, Hypnosis and Heal-
    ing; The Work of J. M. Charcot* (London: Dobson, 1971).
97. Horatio Donkin, "Hysteria," in Hack Tuke, *Dictionary of Psychological Medicine*,
    pp. 625–26. For Donkin, see s.v. "Donkin, Sir Horatio Bryan," in *Munk's Roll*,
    4:273.
98. Milne Bramwell, "Hypnotism and the Treatment of Insanity," p. 1016.
99. Ibid.
100. Ibid., pp. 1013–14.
101. Ibid., p. 1014.
102. Ibid.
103. Ibid., p. 1016.
104. Thomas Clifford Allbutt, "Neurasthenia," in *A System of Medicine*, ed. Allbutt
    and Rolleston, 8:736–37, 776. For Allbutt, see s.v. "Allbutt, the Right Honour-
    able Sir Thomas Clifford, K.C.B.," in *Munk's Roll*, 4:290–92, and in the *Dictio-
    nary of National Biography*, 1922–30, pp. 17–18. See also Sir Humphrey Davy
    Rolleston, *The Right Honourable Sir Thomas Clifford Allbutt . . . A Memoir* (Lon-
    don: Macmillan, 1929).
105. Ormerod, "Hysteria," p. 724.
106. See Veith, *Hysteria*, pp. 230, 237–38; Thomas S. Szasz, *The Myth of Mental Illness:
    Foundations of a Theory of Personal Conduct* (New York: Harper and Row, 1961),
    pp. 32–34.
107. See, for example, Conolly, *Construction and Government of Lunatic Asylums*, pp.
    139–44; idem, *Treatment of the Insane Without Mechanical Restraints*, pp. 73–74,
    76–81, 172–73; and W. A. F. Browne, "The Moral Treatment of the Insane; A
    Lecture," *Journal of Mental Science* 10 (1864): 335–36; idem, *Religio Psycho-Medici*
    (London: Baillière, Tindall and Cox, 1877), pp. 2–3, 4–5. See also Leigh, *Histori-
    cal Development of British Psychiatry*, pp. 224, 248. For Browne, see James Harper,
    "Dr. W. A. F. Browne (1805–1885)," *Proceedings of the Royal Society of Medicine* 48
    (1955): 590–93.
108. Robert Brudenell Carter, *On the Pathology and Treatment of Hysteria* (London:
    Churchill, 1853), p. 55. For Carter, see Veith, *Hysteria*, pp. 199–212; and *Plarr's
    Lives*, 1:201–3.
109. D. Noble, *Elements of Psychological Medicine; An Introduction to the Practical Study
    of Insanity*, 2d ed. (London: Churchill, 1855), p. 55 (italics in original).
110. Savage, *Insanity and Allied Neuroses*, p. 85.
111. See p. 294 of this chapter.
112. Donkin, "Hysteria," p. 620.
113. Ibid., pp. 623, 626. Cf. Carpenter, *Mental Physiology*, pp. 332–33; Maudsley, *Body
    and Mind*, p. 79.
114. Donkin, "Hysteria," pp. 620–21.
115. Ormerod, "Hysteria," p. 687.

116. Ibid., pp. 694–95 (italics mine).
117. See Szasz, *Myth of Mental Illness*, pp. 25–26, 32, 40–42, 45, 254, 294–95; Veith, *Hysteria*, pp. 209–12; and Carroll Smith-Rosenberg, "The Hysterical Woman; Sex Roles and Role Conflict in Nineteenth-Century America," *Social Research* 39 (1972): 662–66.
118. Carter, *Pathology and Treatment of Hysteria*, pp. 42–43, 55–56, 66–70, 93–94, 111–17, 129–30.
119. Ibid., p. 108.
120. Ibid., pp. 96, 108, 111–13, 129–30.
121. Ibid., pp. 92–93, 100, 104, 112–13.
122. Ibid., p. 94.
123. Ibid., pp. 108–9, 118, 120–21, 125–30.
124. Ormerod, "Hysteria," p. 716.
125. Donkin, "Hysteria," p. 626; Ormerod, "Hysteria," pp. 722, 724–25.
126. Donkin, "Hysteria," pp. 626–27.
127. Ormerod, "Hysteria," pp. 720–21.
128. Ibid., p. 721 (italics mine). According to Ormerod, the internal quotation is from S. Weir Mitchell, *Clinical Lessons on Nervous Diseases* (New York and Philadelphia: Lea Brothers, 1897), but I have been unable to trace the passage cited in this work.
129. See, for example, Clouston, *Neuroses of Development*, pp. 106–9; Mercier, *Sanity and Insanity*, pp. 210–19, 223–31; Donkin, "Hysteria," pp. 619–26; Maudsley, *Pathology of Mind*, pp. 135–37, 396–99; Ormerod, "Hysteria," pp. 687, 714–16.
130. Mercier, *Text-Book of Insanity*, p. 3.
131. Mercier, "Vice, Crime and Insanity," p. 874.
132. See, for example, Mercier, *Text-Book of Insanity*, p. 3; idem, "Vice, Crime and Insanity," p. 874; Allbutt, "Neurasthenia," pp. 759–60; and Sir James Crichton Browne, *What the Doctor Thought* (London: Ernest Benn, 1930), pp. 248–49.
133. Ormerod, "Hysteria," pp. 692–93.
134. Ibid., p. 693.
135. Allbutt, "Neurasthenia," pp. 759–60.
136. Ibid., p. 789.
137. Ibid., p. 759.
138. Ibid., p. 760.
139. Ibid., p. 788 (italics in the original).
140. Ibid., pp. 759–60.
141. Crichton Browne, *What the Doctor Thought*, pp. 227–28.
142. Ibid., p. 228.
143. See, for example, Brodie, *Psychological Inquiries*, 2:vi, 15–20, 86; Carpenter, *Mental Physiology*, pp. viii–xi.

ELAINE SHOWALTER

12 Victorian Women and Insanity

On Boxing Day 1851, Charles Dickens gave up an evening at the Pantomime to attend a very different kind of holiday celebration: the patients' Christmas dance at St. Luke's Hospital for the Insane. Describing his visit in an article for *Household Words,* he noted particularly the sex and the class from which St. Luke's drew its inmates: "The experience of this asylum did not differ, I found, from that of similar establishments, in proving that insanity is more prevalent among women than among men. Of the eighteen thousand seven hundred and fifty-nine inmates St. Luke's Hospital has received in the century of its existence, eleven thousand one hundred and sixty-two have been women. . . . Female servants are, as is well known, more frequently afflicted with lunacy than any other class of persons." He looked with particular interest at the female patients, the silent and withdrawn cases who sat in a long gallery, motionless except for one "scolding some imaginary person [and] . . . sewing a purposeless seam," and the mad women who attended the ball. "There was the brisk, vain, pippin-faced old lady, in a fantastic cap—proud of her foot and ankle; there was the old-young woman, with her dishevelled long light hair, spare figure, and weird gentility; there was the vacantly-laughing girl, requiring now and then a warning finger to admonish her; there was the quiet young woman, almost well, and soon going out."[1]

Despite the many gloomy reminders of asylum life which surrounded him and the "sad and touching spectacle" of the patients admiring the lighted Christmas tree, Dickens could not help but rejoice at the progress that had been made in the humane treatment of the insane, and his essay alternates between descriptions of the ball and an evocation of the brutal history of the eighteenth-century madhouse, when "nothing was too wildly extravagant, nothing too monstrously cruel to be prescribed by mad-doctors."[2] In the eighteenth century, visitors to Bedlam paid their pennies to see howling maniacs, naked and chained, alien creatures in

This essay was originally published in *Victorian Studies* (1980) and is reprinted by permission of the Trustees of Indiana University.

whom irrationality and filth had reached the extremes of the recognizably
human. As late as 1844, the Commissioners in Lunacy found lunatics
confined in dark and reeking cells, strapped down to their beds or to chairs.
William Thackeray, whose wife Isabella had become suicidal after the
birth of a third child, was unable to find an English asylum where he could
bear to leave her in the 1840s: "As for the poor little woman that's another
difficulty," he wrote to his mother in Paris. "Procter (who is a Lunacy
Commissioner and knows them all) took me to his favourite place which
makes me feel quite sick to think of even now. He shook his head about
other places."[3]

By the middle of the century, however, visitors to the Victorian asylum saw madness domesticated, released from restraint, and unnervingly
like the world outside the walls. Chiefly because of the pioneering work
of the Tuke family at the Quaker York Retreat, of Robert Gardiner Hill
at Lincoln, and of John Conolly at the Middlesex County Asylum at
Hanwell, instruments of physical restraint and the use of force were officially abolished in British asylums and replaced by the techniques of moral
management: classification, surveillance, and the creation of a homelike
therapeutic environment in which the kindly authority of the medical
superintendent was to encourage the patients to develop self-control, self-
respect, patience, and industry.

Many journalists besides Dickens were guests at social occasions that
were designed to display the reformed asylum at its best; if at first, as one
reporter noted, "the announcement of a ball in Bedlam seems . . . almost
as much an anomaly as a fancy fair in Pentonville Penitentiary," it soon
became a familiar and even conventional event.[4] Visitors to the Great
Exhibition of 1851 were invited to witness the splendors of Colney Hatch
Lunatic Asylum, and a special guidebook was prepared for them; in July
1853 nearly two thousand visitors enjoyed "games of a diverting character"
with the Colney Hatch patients at the annual outdoor fete.[5] Seen at such
close range and in such holiday or pastoral settings, madness was no longer
a gross and unmistakable inversion of appropriate conduct, but a collection
of disquieting gestures and postures. At the Bedlam Ball in 1859, a reporter
for the *Illustrated Times* noted a nagging sense of surface and charade, as
if the asylum had become a kind of pantomime in itself: "You feel in the
midst of the merriment that *there is something wanting*, that the wine is
corked, that the cake has a leaven of madness in it, . . . that there is a tile
off the roof of the ballroom."[6] Observers scrutinized the inmates for details
which betrayed their true identity; "with the exception of a slovenly
method of moving their feet," wrote one, "you might have fancied they
were so many country people dancing at a village wake or fair."[7] Were it
not for the adjectives Dickens selects to indicate his response to the St.
Luke's women—*fantastic, weird,* and *vacant*—we might not recognize them
as insane.

It is notable that the domestication of insanity, its assimilation by the Victorian institution, coincides with the period in which the predominance of women among the insane becomes a statistically verifiable phenomenon. English folklore reflects in "mad-songs" and ballads an ancient association of madness, confinement, and women; but until the middle of the century, records showed that men were far more likely to be confined as insane.

In the first half of the nineteenth century, there seemed to be evidence that women were indeed less susceptible to mental illness than men. A study by John Thurnam, medical superintendent of the York Retreat, published in 1845, indicated that in private asylums and provincial houses, male patients outnumbered women by about 30 percent. Thurnam concluded, "Having thus shown that in the principal hospitals for the insane in these kingdoms, the proportion of men admitted is nearly always higher, and in many instances much higher than that of women, and as we know that the proportion of men in the general population, particularly at those ages when insanity most usually occurs, is decidedly less than that of women, we can have no ground in doubting that men are actually more liable to disorders of the mind than women."[8]

In the same year that Thurnam wrote his report, however, Parliament passed legislation that totally transformed the institutional care of the insane. The Lunatics Act of 1845 required all counties to provide adequate asylum accommodation for pauper lunatics, who were defined as those persons whose maintenance came wholly or in part from public funds. Before the Lunatics Act was passed, paupers were usually sent to the workhouse, to public hospitals such as Bedlam, or to private madhouses in which conditions were appalling and treatment was notoriously cruel. Wealthy patients were often cared for at home or in the more luxurious private madhouses. One such case was Mary Lamb, who had killed her mother; when fits of mania came upon her, she was taken by her brother Charles to a private hospital, where "the good lady of the Madhouse, and her daughter, an elegant sweet behaved young lady, love her and are taken with her amazingly."[9] Unless they could obtain such expensive and affectionate care, many families may have been reluctant to commit their female members to asylums.

The construction of large public county asylums quickly changed this pattern. As rapidly as they were built, new asylums filled to overflowing and had to be expanded. Buildings designed to hold a few hundred patients, the maximum size if curative individual treatment could be provided, mushroomed into "lunatic colonies" of a thousand or more, too large to be anything but custodial.[10]

With this enormous expansion of the asylum population, sex ratios also changed. According to the census of 1871, for every 1,000 male lunatics, there were 1,182 female lunatics; for every 1,000 male pauper lunatics, 1,242 females.[11] By 1872, out of 58,640 certified lunatics in England and Wales, 31,822 were women. There were more female pauper inmates in county and borough asylums, in licensed houses, in workhouses, and in single care. Men still predominated among private patients of all categories and in registered hospitals, which were more expensive and selective than the asylums. This "large aggregation" of women could be explained partly, according to Edgar Sheppard, the medical superintendent of the male department at Colney Hatch, by the accumulation of female incurables, and the statistics indeed suggest that women stayed in the asylums for longer periods than men.[12] At Hanwell, for example, the average stay for a man was 3.7 years, for a woman 6 years.[13] Women in asylums also had lower death rates than men. By the 1890s, the accumulation or aggregation had spread to include all classes of patients and all types of institutions; female paupers and female private patients were in the majority in licensed houses, registered hospitals, and the county asylums.[14] The only remaining institutions with a majority of male patients were asylums for the criminally insane, military hospitals, and idiot schools. Looking outside the asylums to the surgical clinics, water-cure establishments, and rest-cure homes; to the new specialists in the "female illnesses" of hysteria and neurasthenia; and to the marginal therapies such as mesmeric healing, we find again that women were the primary clientele. Even in the novel, the madwoman, who starts out confined to the Gothic subplot—to the narrative and domestic space which Charlotte Brontë calls "the third story"— by the fin-de-siècle has taken up residence in the front room. Thus by the end of the century, women had decisively taken the lead in the career of psychiatric patient, a lead which they have retained ever since, and in ever-increasing numbers.

It can be observed readily that social class and income were major determinants of the individual's psychiatric career, and that the increase in female patients was related to the enormous expansion of asylum facilities for the poor. Pauper lunatics, whose numbers quadrupled between 1844 and 1890, formed the overwhelming majority of the total inmate population, and by 1890 they were indeed 91 percent of all mental patients. Simply being poor made them more likely to be labeled mad. According to Andrew Scull, "A wide range of contemporary observers commented on how much laxer were the standards for judging a poor person to be insane, and on how much readier both local poor law authorities and lower class families were to commit decrepit and troublesome people to the asylum; individuals who, had they come from the middle and upper classes, would never have been diagnosed as insane."[15]

The predominance of women showed up first among pauper lunatics, and it could be argued that this simply reflected the female majority of adult recipients of Poor Law relief, and of "the very much larger number of the very poor."[16] Poor Law administrators were increasingly reluctant throughout the century to grant outdoor relief ("a weekly subsistence dole upon which they could support themselves") to women deserted by their husbands, wives of prisoners, able-bodied widows with a single child, or mothers of illegitimate children; women applying for relief were judged according to their respectability rather than their need. As the percentage of Poor Law expenditure for outdoor relief was declining (especially between 1870 and 1890), the expenditure for the maintenance of lunatics in asylums was increasing.[17]

Doctors and reformers fully recognized the role of poverty and economic anxiety in causing madness. "The causation of insanity everywhere, specific disease apart," wrote Granville, "is an affair of three w's—worry, want and wickedness."[18] Some asylum cases were really suffering from malnutrition; "lactational insanity," for example, was chiefly encountered in mothers of large families who continued to nurse for long periods in order to save money and to prevent conception, and was caused by starvation and anemia. Asylum populations also included many women who were senile, tubercular, epileptic, physically handicapped, mentally retarded, or otherwise unable to care for themselves.

As Dickens had noted, servants were believed to be the largest occupational group of female lunatics, with the explanation that their economic status was so precarious. In 1859, in an article on women's employment, Harriet Martineau claimed this distinction for governesses, and ten years later a journalist visiting Bethlem Hospital was told that the majority of female patients were "governesses and the wives of badly-paid clerks."[19] Martineau believed that the financial insecurity of the governess trade made these women especially anxious and vulnerable; journalists offered more romantic explanations, ascribing the lunacy of the governess to over-study and the lunacy of the servant to religious hysteria and unrequited love.[20] Henry Maudsley, one of the most prominent Victorian psychiatric physicians, argued in 1879 that all of these assumptions were probably based on distorted statistics from a single hospital: the "common notion" that "governesses were victims of insanity out of all proportion to their numbers originated in the observation that a great number of governesses were received into Bethlem Hospital—as many as 110 in ten years; the reason of which was not that so many more of them than of other classes went mad, but that they were just the persons who fulfilled best the conditions of charitable admission into that hospital," that is, they were too poor to pay for care and treatment in private asylums, yet not poor enough to be paupers and thus suitable for admission into county asylums.[21] But the social isolation of aging governesses and their lack of family support systems would undoubtedly have contributed to their need for institutional care.

Finally, despite the well-publicized rise in the number of insane who were institutionalized and the efforts of doctors to make asylum treatment respectable, the stigma of certification remained powerful. The signatures of two doctors and a magistrate were required for commitment of a mental patient. Doctors such as John Arlidge and Charles Mercier were very sensitive to the disadvantages of certification for men needing to earn a living, and families seem to have been more resistant to incarcerating mildly disturbed or potentially curable male members. The primary occupational risk of the "certified" woman was marriage, and Thomas Bakewell suggested that a term in an asylum could even be an attraction in a prospective wife, for "humility is a quality which men wish for in a wife. This complaint cannot so properly be said to teach humility, as to implant it in the very nature."[22]

In a given institution, the sex ratio also reflected many nonmedical factors, such as the sex of the asylum proprietor and the layout of the asylum premises. Asylums maintained strict segregation of the sexes, extending even to the kitchens and in some cases to the mortuaries; thus quotas for male and female patients had to be part of the building plans. St. Luke's, for example, had remodeled its dormitories in the 1830s on the assumption that the number of women patients would always exceed the number of men.[23]

In private licensed houses, too, there were more places for female patients by the end of the century, and the reasons for this are somewhat complicated. In the eighteenth century, and up to the 1840s, women were often the licensed proprietors of private madhouses or inherited their supervision from a father or husband. But the lunacy reform movement, by advocating a medical monopoly of the treatment of the insane, forced women into marginal, secondary, or charitable roles, much as the rising profession of obstetrics demoted midwifery. "If insanity is a disease requiring medical treatment," insisted John Charles Bucknill, editor of the *Asylum Journal of Mental Science*, in 1857, "ladies cannot legally or properly undertake the treatment. . . . If private interests are to override public ones, the widow of a clergyman ought on the same principle to hold the rectory of her departed husband, and manage the parochial duties by means of curates."[24] Such arguments led the Commissioners of Lunacy to announce in their 1859 report that they were considering granting new licenses only to medical men, and women applicants were thereafter discouraged, although not always refused. Because they wanted asylum inmates to have "free intercourse within doors, and a ready access to the open air," the commissioners further stipulated that the proprietors of small private asylums should admit only one sex.[25] Nearly all female licensees chose to limit their admissions to women, probably because as a less qualified group they might have had difficulty attracting male patients. Many prominent doctors, too, including Hill, Conolly, and Maudsley, owned private female asylums. In 1872, eighteen metropolitan licensed houses were restricted to women, and six to men. Among provincial houses, fifteen served women, while only two were for men.

In their effort to upgrade the status of the psychiatric profession, some doctors denigrated the work done by women in asylum management and administration. Bucknill campaigned to have the position of matron in the county asylums abolished, and his sarcastic suggestion that matrons, if absolutely required, should be selected by weight, was interpreted as an insult to the stout Charlotte Walker, whose maternal concern for patients had been praised by Dickens at St. Luke's. In the end, Bucknill was forced to apologize in the *Journal of Mental Science.* [26] Matrons, female nurses, and attendants were paid on a much lower scale than male workers, were regarded as less reliable, and were subject to more rules and restrictions.[27] Any effort to equalize their status encountered intense opposition, as when Arlidge indignantly protested that in one asylum the matron was as well paid as the medical officers.[28] By law, any establishment that was licensed to receive lunatics had to be visited regularly by a physician, who would of course be male. Not until 1927 were state mental hospitals in England legally allowed to employ women doctors; actual appointments did not occur at many hospitals until after World War II. Thus it was gradually established that the role of the patient would be filled by a woman and the role of physician by a man.

Within the asylums the women's experience would vary enormously. In single-sex private asylums, ladies encountered a decor and a regime designed to remind them of home or school. The bedrooms, according to an observer in 1850, "would be very much after the fashion of a ladies' boarding-school, with white dimity curtains and chintz hangings at the windows."[29] Inverness Lodge, Brentford, to which the novelist Edward Bulwer-Lytton committed his wife in 1858, was "a very fine house in fine grounds, which had formerly belonged to the Duke of Cumberland." Lady Lytton, however, perfectly sane and furious at her husband's action, was neither pacified nor deceived by her surroundings, as she related in her memoir. Looking through her window, she saw between thirty and forty women walking in the grounds. " 'Are all those unfortunates incarcerated here?' I asked of the little keeper. 'Those,' she said, rather evasively, 'are our ladies. They are out gathering strawberries.' "[30]

In mixed asylums, the sexes were separate but not quite equal. Dietary allotments were substantially lower for women. All asylum patients were subject to surveillance, or "careful watching," as the Victorians called it; but women were more carefully watched than men. At the 1859 hearings of the House of Commons Select Committee on Lunatics, representatives of the Alleged Lunatics' Friend Society protested the censorship of patients' mail, except for that of ladies, who, they agreed, *needed* to be protected against possible indecorous self-revelation.[31] Women patients also had to be protected against rape and seduction. In the first half of the century, Hill reported, "there are many instances on record of the female patients being with child by the keepers and the male patients."[32] After 1845, the commissioners took particular note of security arrangements for women; at Colney Hatch, only doctors and the chaplains had keys to the female ward. When, despite all these precautions, an unmarried woman bore a child in the asylum, the infant was turned over to the guardians of the mother's home parish or, in the case of vagrants, to the local workhouse.[33]

Within the asylums, female patients often shocked both doctors and male patients by their rowdiness, restlessness, and use of obscene language. "Female lunatics are less susceptible to control than males," declared one male inmate of the Glasgow Royal Asylum. "They are more troublesome, more noisy, and more abusive in their language. . . ."[34] A gentleman patient trying to converse with one of the "poor women" in his private asylum returned dazed to his room when she accosted him in the public road "with one of the worst words in the English language."[35] Bucknill was equally scandalized by the "extraordinary amount of obscenity in thought and language" he had observed in "well-nurtured" patients suffering from manias. "Religious and moral principles alone give strength to the female mind," he pronounced. "When these are weakened or removed by disease, the subterranean fires become active, and the crater gives forth smoke and flame."[36] The commissioners visiting Colney Hatch "regularly remarked that the female department, as is usually the case in all Asylums, was the most noisy."[37]

Such reports primarily reflect the expectations and wishes of male observers that women should be quiet, virtuous, and immobile. Granville, for example, who carried out a conscientious inspection of several institutions for his 1877 report for the *Lancet* Commission on Lunatic Asylums, was also disturbed by the talkativeness of female patients. If idle, they are "chattering about their grievances"; at Colney Hatch he sees in the female wards "an excess of vehement declaration and quarreling."[38] Granville recommended that work for women be found that would keep them too busy to talk.

Asylum routine was designed to encourage normative behavior, with the result that the women were obliged to live according to the narrowest of Victorian sex stereotypes. Inmate labor played an important role in the economy as well as in the therapeutic ideology of the public asylum, but sex roles determined the division of labor even more rigidly than outside the walls. Male patients worked at a variety of jobs in workshops, in the gardens, and on the asylum farms. Women's employment offered much less choice, took place indoors, and in many cases was meaningless make-work. Cleaning, laundry, and needlework were the primary tasks; in 1891 female patients supplied one asylum with clothing, making 2,378 dresses, 1,530 shirts, and 396 pairs of drawers.[39] In Conolly's scheme for a model asylum, the traits he thought appropriate for women patients were projected onto his optimistic vision of their happy hours making puddings in "the busy and cheerful and scrupulously clean kitchen," like so many lunatic Ruth Pinches.[40] At Bethlem in the 1860s, female inmates were allowed to exhibit their fancywork to charitable ladies who visited the wards.[41] These occupations were still a considerable step above those reported by Granville at Bethnal House, where women had spent their days sorting colored beans into separate piles which were dumped back together again at night.[42]

One of the reasons female asylum patients may have seemed excited and restless was that they had fewer opportunities than men for outdoor activity, active recreation, or even movement within the building. In one large asylum, it was reported in 1862, only 50 out of 886 female patients ever went from their ward to the dayroom.[43] At Colney Hatch, women left the asylum for fewer walks or outings than male patients. Dr. D. F. Tyerman, who headed the male department, believed physical exercise was essential to mental health and so had a "properly-prepared and level Cricket-ground" constructed in the 1850s where male patients could play. In the 1870s, there were annual matches against visiting teams of medical students, which the female patients were allowed to witness from "a specially fenced-off enclosure."[44] In contrast, five times as many women as men patients in this asylum were punished by seclusion in padded cells in the period 1865–74. Turkish baths and sedatives were also used to keep women patients calm.[45]

And yet, one of the most striking ironies of women's experience in the Victorian asylum was that despite its limitations, the asylum probably offered a more tolerant and more interesting life than some women could expect outside. T. S. Clouston advised medical superintendents not to keep hysterical cases in the asylum too long after convalescence, because "they sometimes get too fond of the place, preferring the dances, amusements and general liveliness of asylum life . . . to the humdrum and hard work of poor homes."[46] Even to middle-class women, the asylum could be an acceptable environment; for as the Victorian asylum became more overtly benign, protective, and custodial, it also became an environment grotesquely like the one in which women normally functioned. Such factors of asylum life as strict chaperonage, restriction of movement, limited occupation, enforced sexlessness, and constant subjugation to authority were closer to the "normal" lives of women than of men. The theory of asylum management was, according to one progressive spokesman, to treat inmates "as children under a perpetual personal guardianship."[47] Michel Foucault sees in this Victorian equation of insanity and childhood a revival of patriarchal power which would later be codified by the mythologies of psychoanalysis. For the crude external force of the eighteenth-century madhouse, the nineteenth-century asylum substituted the moral force of paternal authority; the keeper becomes the omniscient father, a figure women were accustomed to believing.[48]

Although the afflictions of pauper patients in the asylums were loosely diagnosed in such terms as *mania* and *melancholia*, Victorian psychiatric textbooks focused on more ideologically complex analyses of middle-class women and their disorders. From the theoretical perspective, female psychiatric symptoms were interpreted according to a biological model of sex differences and associated with disorders of the uterus and the reproductive system. While physicians might pay attention to the contexts of the female complaint, such as poverty, the death of a relative, or physical complications, they were totally indifferent to content. Expressions of unhappiness, low self-esteem, helplessness, anxiety, and fear were not connected to the realities of women's lives, while expressions of sexual desire, anger, and aggression were taken as morbid deviations from the normal female personality. The female life cycle, linked to reproduction, was seen as fraught with biological crises during which these morbid emotions were more likely to appear. Woman, wrote one authority, is "the victim of periodicity; her life is one perpetual change and these changes even are still again subdivided."[49] Given so unstable a constitution, it seemed a wonder that any woman could hope for a lifetime of sanity, and psychiatric experts often expressed their surprise that female insanity was not more frequent. As Clouston summed up the case, "The risks to the mental functions of the brain from the exhausting calls of menstruation, maternity, and lactation, from the nervous reflex influences of ovulation, conception and parturition, are often enormous if there is much original predisposition to derangement, and the normally profound influences on all the brain functions of the great eras of puberty and the climacteric period are too apt, in these circumstances, to upset the brain stability."[50]

A "predisposition to derangement" meant an inherited mental structure, a tyranny of nerve organization that was almost inescapable. Such predisposition was more readily recognized in women than in men; in one startling example, Furneaux Jordan analyzed the "bodily conformation" and "congenital impulses of character" of battered wives, noting interesting differences of complexion, spinal curve, and personality between those who were merely assaulted and those who were actually killed.[51]

At every stage of their lives, women had to take great care not to upset their precarious brain stability. Thus female adolescence was discussed in terms of menstrual management. The menstrual discharge in itself predis-

posed women to insanity, since it was widely believed that madness was
a disease of the blood. Either a morbid quantity, quality, or deficiency of
the blood, according to this theory, could affect the brain; thus psychiatric
physicians attempted to control the blood by diet, leeching, and venesec-
tion.[52] Late, irregular, or "suppressed" menstruation was regarded as a
dangerous condition and was treated with purgatives, forcing medicines,
hip baths, and leeches applied to the thighs.[53] A totally opposite view,
however, was advanced by Edward Tilt in his 1851 study, *On the Preservation
of the Health of Women at the Critical Periods of Life.* Tilt believed that menstruation itself was so disrupting to the female brain that it should be
retarded as long as possible, and he advised mothers to prevent menarche
by ensuring that their teen-age daughters remain in the nursery, take cold
shower baths, avoid featherbeds and novels, eat low-protein diets, and
wear drawers. This nursery regime, he insisted, was "the principal cause
of the pre-eminence of English women, in vigour of constitution, soundness of judgement, and . . . rectitude of moral principle."[54]

Having survived puberty, women still faced mental shipwreck in
pregnancy and childbirth. Puerperal insanity, ranging from the mild and
short-term symptoms of postpartum depression to incurable psychosis and
suicide, accounted for about 10 percent of female asylum admissions,
and was widely accepted as a legitimate criminal defense, especially in
cases of infanticide. Such social causes of the disorder as poverty, inadequate obstetrical care, and the stigma of bearing illegitimate children were
sometimes cited as contributing factors; but doctors, lawyers, and judges
preferred to deal with the depression and violence of puerperal mania as
an isolated, individual, and biologically determined phenomenon.[55]

The end of women's reproductive life was as profound a mental
upheaval as the beginning. "The death of the reproductive faculty," wrote
one physician, "is accompanied . . . by struggles which implicate every
organ and every function of body."[56] Doctors spoke in violent metaphors
of "revolution" in the female economy, of "climacteric paroxysms" creating a "distinct shock to the brain," and "attacks of ovario-uterine excitement approaching to nymphomania."[57] Although men, too, were thought
to be subject to climacteric insanity, the menopausal form far predominated; in the Royal Edinburgh Asylum, for example, 196 out of 228 cases
were women.[58] This designation may have been a convenient way for
asylums to label their elderly female patients. In psychiatric literature,
menopausal women were more harshly discussed, more openly ridiculed,
and more punitively treated than any other female group, particularly if
they were unmarried. One standard subheading in medical textbooks was
"Ovarian Insanity," or "Old Maid's Mania," the deluded passion of a
spinster "for some casual acquaintance of the opposite sex whom the
victim believes to be deeply in love with her."[59] The ovarian maniac was

alleged to pick her clergyman as the usual object of these fantasies, and might even claim he had seduced her. Such immodest expressions of sexual appetite were regarded as ludicrous in spinsters and tragic in married women. Husbands of menopausal women were advised to withhold the desired "sexual stimulus." Treatments suggested for the erotic and nervous symptoms of menopause were so unpleasant that one can easily imagine their deterrent effectiveness. W. Tyler Smith, for example, recommended a course of injections of ice water into the rectum, introduction of ice into the vagina, and leeching of the labia and the cervix. "The suddenness with which leeches applied to this part fill themselves," he writes admiringly, "considerably increases the good effects of their application, and for some hours after their removal there is an oozing of blood from the leech-bites."[60]

In presenting textbook cases of female insanity, doctors usually described women who were disobedient, rebellious, or in open protest against the female role. Tilt writes that female adolescence is a state of "miniature insanity," when girls previously well behaved become "snappish, fretful . . . full of deceit and mischief."[61] In his lecture series on hysteria, F. C. Skey warned his audience that the typical hysteric was not a person of weak mind but "a female member of a family exhibiting more than usual force and decision of character, of strong resolution, fearless of danger, bold riders, having plenty of what is termed *nerve.*"[62] It was not uncommon for women in asylums to have delusions of being male; Miss J. V., for example, described herself as "a mixture of a nymph and half-man, half-woman and a boy."[63] Doctors were unsympathetic to all of these behaviors and attitudes. Clouston reminisces gloomily about one "young lady patient . . . so excitable and lively, so reckless in speech and conduct" that he was reluctant to release her, even though her relatives assured him that this was her normal condition. Although she married and had children, "her surplus stock of nervous energy finding its natural outlet, and her organic cravings their physiological satisfaction," he predicted that she would pass her madness on to the next generation.[64]

Unconventional sexual behavior in women—premarital intercourse, erotic fantasies, seductiveness, obscene language, and orgasmic excitement —was clinically described as nymphomania. In its final and rarely seen stages, the nymphomaniac allegedly attempted to throw herself into the arms of the first man she met and became furious if he tried to resist her.

Because nymphomaniac symptoms appeared so frequently in asylums —John Millar, the proprietor of Bethnal House, said they were "constantly present when young females are insane"—doctors sought to trace them to organic causes ranging from uterine furor to "enlarged nymphae."[65] William Moseley pleaded for understanding of the nymphomaniac's plight:

This disease is unjustly attributed to a worse nature and a more corrupt heart: to a class of human passions of a demoralizing tendency; to the want of a good education; and to the absence of good moral and religious feelings. But the reverse of this is true and has been so fully and frequently demonstrated to us, by facts in our practice, as to teach us to *pity*, sympathise and *not to blame*. Yes! it is an *organic disease*, against the tide of which neither the firm resolutions, nor good principles, nor frequent fervid prayers of Miss A—, nor of Miss S—, the daughter of a clergyman, nor of Mrs.—, a married lady, with children, could make sufficient head to stifle these feelings, or keep their distressed minds in a state of self-approval.[66]

Since overt sexuality was a symptom of many supposed categories of female insanity, its manifestation at any stage of the female life cycle could lead to incarceration even when no other symptoms were present. Many case histories of female patients cite sexual immorality as the reason for psychiatric intervention. One such case involved Miss C. G., a seventeen-year-old girl committed to the Royal Edinburgh Asylum because "without showing any previous sign of insanity, except conduct that was called wayward and disobedient, she left her home, wandered to where some workmen lived, a lonely place many miles off, and spent the night with them."[67] It was easy for fathers, brothers, and husbands to find doctors willing to certify that sexually rebellious women were lunatics; Forbes Winslow, editor of the *Journal of Psychological Medicine*, was one who had a lucrative practice in such cases. As late as 1895, Edith Lanchester, a socialist convert living in Battersea with her lover, a mechanic, was kidnapped by her father and brother and committed to an asylum on the authority of Dr. G. Fielding Blandford, who judged her insane "because he believed her opposition to conventional matrimony made her unfit to take care of herself."[68]

Books by Georgiana Weldon (*The History of My Orphanage; or The Outpourings of an Alleged Lunatic* [1878]) and Louisa Lowe (*The Bastilles of England; or The Lunacy Laws at Work* [1883]) drew attention to the abuses of the system, and especially to the power that could be exerted by vengeful husbands over erring wives. An independent will could be regarded as a form of female deviance that was dangerously close to mental illness and nearly as subversive as adultery. Writing to an old friend about the annulment of his marriage to Effie Gray on the grounds of incurable impotence, John Ruskin defended himself (with unintentionally embarrassing double entendres) by accusing his strong-willed ex-wife of "literal nervous affection of the brain—brought on chiefly I believe by finding that she could not entirely bend me to all her purposes."[69]

At the same time, some doctors recognized that the intellectual and sexual constraints of the female role, especially in the middle classes, were more maddening than its opportunities and expansions. As early as 1838, Moseley suggested that the life of the middle-class woman lacked sufficient mental occupation. Later in the century, Andrew Wynter linked alcoholism and drug use among middle-class women to boredom, isolation, and want of intellectual training.[70] Florence Nightingale made the same point more passionately in "Cassandra" when she described women deprived of meaningful work, so frantic with unused energy that they feel "every night when they go to bed, as if they were going mad."[71] If we see insanity as a point along a spectrum of emotions and behviors, a reflection of tensions within a society, then it is interesting to note that fantasies of being male also emerge in women's literature in the 1880s, when feminist writers such as Olive Schreiner, Mary Coleridge, and Ethel Voynich were struggling with the conflicts between the professional and the traditional pressures of womanhood.[72]

If we examine the content of female madness, the symbolic behavior of patients, the themes of delusions and fantasies, and the ways in which novelists made use of insanity, we see that mental breakdown was often an expression of resolution of conflicts in the claustrophobic middle-class feminine role, and that Victorian psychiatric labeling and incarceration was an efficient agency of sociosexual control. In the sensation novels of the 1860s and 1870s, for which Mary Braddon's *Lady Audley's Secret* is a prototype, madness, usually hereditary in the female line, is the standard explanation for any act of feminine passion, self-assertion, or violence.

Yet it is important to see how thoroughly many middle-class women themselves colluded in this process, how eagerly they embraced insanity as an explanation of their unfeminine impulses, and welcomed the cures that would extinguish the forbidden throb of sexuality or ambition. At the conclusion of *Mary Barton* (1848), for example, Mrs. Gaskell has involved her heroine in a series of extraordinary events that have forced her to act aggressively in a man's defense. Mary has taken a long journey alone, commandeered a boat in order to pursue a witness at sea, and testified in court that she loves Jem rather than Harry Carson. Having so clearly demonstrated her competence, how can she be folded up small enough to be packed back into the little case of wife? Mary goes mad, and when she recovers she has regressed to a more pliant and familiar level: "Her mind was in the tender state of a lately-born infant's. . . . She smiled gently as a baby does . . . and continued her innocent infantine gaze into his face, as if the sight gave her such unconscious pleasure."[73] This is not the spiritual rebirth of a Rochester or a Pip or an Arthur Clennam into new wisdom. It is the infantilization and reprogramming of a woman who has so far outgrown her role that she must be broken down to fit back into it.

The widening sphere of middle-class female experience and opportunity after 1850 brought new problems of role definition and management, and psychiatric physicians established themselves rapidly, along with gynecologists, as the privileged confidants of troubled women. As their status became more secure, specialists in hysteria, neurasthenia, nymphomania, and nerve disorders became increasingly powerful. Charles Reade satirized the trend in *Hard Cash* (1863) when a series of doctors called in to analyze the problem of the lovelorn Julia Dodd give mutually contradictory and extravagant diagnoses. When Julia explains to one physician that she does not have the symptoms he lists, "Dr. Short looked a little surprised; his female patients rarely contradicted him. Was it for them to disown things he was so good as to assign them?" By the 1880s, gynecologists and psychologists ascribed nearly all female diseases to uterine malfunction, for which belts, injections, and internal appliances were prescribed. Lecturing to the Royal College of Physicians, Dr. T. Clifford Allbutt lamented the plight of the woman patient: "She is entangled in the net of the gynaecologist, who finds her uterus, like her nose, a little on one side, or again like that organ is running a little, or it is as flabby as her biceps, so that the unhappy viscus is impaled on a stem or perched on a prop, or is painted with carbolic acid every week in the year except, during the long vacation when the gynaecologist is grouse shooting or salmon catching."[74]

Many of the power issues latent in the relationship of the woman patient and the gynecologist were raised in a famous case in 1866–67, the expulsion of Isaac Baker Brown from the Obstetrical Society of London for practicing clitoridectomy (surgical removal of the clitoris) as a cure for female insanity. Brown was convinced that masturbation was the primary cause of madness. In his own writing and in his testimony to the Obstetrical Society, he explained that all cases of female insanity, with the exceptions of alcoholism and hereditary disease, were "failures of nervous power" produced by "peripheral irritation, arising originally in the branches of the pudic nerve, more particularly the incident nerve supplying the clitoris."[75] The disease progressed through eight stages: hysteria, spinal irritation, hysterical epilepsy, catalepsy, epilepsy proper, idiocy, mania, and death.

Brown believed that the symptoms of female insanity manifested themselves at puberty. Girls became "restless and excited . . . and indifferent to the social influences of domestic life." There might be loss of appetite and depression, "a quivering of the eyelids, and an inability to look one in the face." One clue was that such girls often wanted to work, to escape from home and become "a nurse in hospitals, '*sœur de charité*,' or other pursuits of like nature . . . according to station or opportunities."[76] One can easily imagine what he would have recommended for Florence Nightingale.

Brown performed his first operation in 1859, excising the clitoris of a twenty-six-year-old unmarried dressmaker who suffered from digestive problems. Other operations quickly followed, with many patients referred by their families or by other physicians. A twenty-year-old girl had symptoms of disobedience to her mother's wishes and enjoyed "serious reading"; a Miss E. R. had never had an offer of marriage, would not be polite to callers, took long solitary walks, was "forward and open" to gentlemen, and said "people's faces were masks."[77] As he became more confident, Brown operated on patients as young as ten years old, on idiots, epileptics, paralytics, depressives, and even women with eye problems. Proceeding on the assumption that masturbation made women unwilling to fulfill their conjugal obligations, Brown urged clitoridectomy for women seeking divorce and believed that the operation would make them more contented, and certainly more manageable wives. He had successfully performed such operations on recalcitrant wives five times.[78]

The fifty beds at his private clinic, the London Surgical Home, were always filled, and patients came from all social classes. In the 1860s, Brown's sexual surgery often went beyond clitoridectomy to the removal of the labia. In most cases, he claimed total cure: a patient with backache who showed no improvement was accused of malingering and discharged as "a regular imposter."[79] And in no case, Brown claimed, was he so certain of a cure as with acute nymphomania, for he had never seen a recurrence of the disease after surgery.[80]

It was not primarily because they disagreed with Brown's diagnosis or the effectiveness of his method that the Obstetrical Society originally met on the case, but because patients had complained of being tricked and coerced into the treatment. Some had been threatened that they would become insane if they did not have surgery. Dr. Tyler Smith told the society that "there are a number of young women upon whom this operation has been performed without the . . . perfect knowledge of themselves and their relatives. . . . If they are honourable, and any proposal of marriage comes to them, the young women or their parents are obliged to tell the parties proposing that they are mutilated, and thus they are obliged to expose themselves to the possibility of being treated as imperfect persons."[81]

In defense, Brown argued that many members of the society had performed the operation themselves, and some came forward. Dr. Charles Routh, an eminent gynecologist, knew of an idiot girl who improved so much after clitoridectomy that she was able to read the Bible, converse, and go into domestic service.[82] Dr. T. Hawkes Tanner, however, who had performed three operations, was disappointed at his results, and both Maudsley and Forbes Winslow testified that in their experience masturbation "was not a cause but a consequence of insanity."[83] Others, granting the grave danger of masturbation, wondered if less extreme remedies could be found for it. One such contribution came from Dr. Wynn Williams: "It is true, we are ordered, if a member offend us, to cut it off; and he thought that the clitoris was not the offending member, but the arms and hands. These, then, were the members that should be cut off. Of course, he did not seriously recommend the amputation of the arms; but there could be no reason why they should not be put back by restraint behind the back."[84]

The final decision to expel Brown was made after a speech by Seymour Haden, secretary of the society, who appealed to the manly honor of his brother physicians. As Haden explained to them, the issues of the case had to do with misuse of male authority. As "a body who practise among women," he declared, "we have constituted ourselves, as it were the guardians of their interests, and in many cases, . . . the custodians of their honour *(hear, hear)*. We are in fact, the stronger, and they the weaker. They are obliged to believe all that we tell them. They are not in a position to dispute anything we say to them, and we therefore, may be said to have them at our mercy. . . . Under these circumstances, if we should depart from the strictest principles of honour, if we should cheat or victimize them in any shape or way, we would be unworthy of the profession of which we are members."[85] *(Loud cheers).*

Isaac Baker Brown died two years after the Obstetrical Society's hearing, his surgical career, as some thought, tragically cut short (a medical historian, writing in 1965 about the case, comments that Brown was obsessed with "the removal of the clitoris, a *minor appendage* of the female genitalia").[86] Probably because of his unfortunate obsession, sexual surgery was ultimately less frequently practiced in nineteenth-century England than in France, Germany, or the United States, where the last recorded clitoridectomy took place in 1924, and where the more drastic operation of "oophorectomy," or removal of the ovaries, was performed as a psychological remedy as late as 1946.[87] Today, however, "the dominance of a medical model of insanity in England leads to a focus on physical symptoms in women which are accessible to the armoury of drugs and shock treatments so often administered, notably for postpartum depressions, or at menopause."[88] Even Brown's surgery may strike us as mild and well intentioned in comparison to the psychosurgery of the 1970s—such as the recommendation in one current textbook that lobotomies be performed for women who are depressed because they are married to psychopathic men.[89]

We learn from the study of Victorian women and insanity that definitions of both insanity and femininity are culturally constructed, and that the relationship between them must be considered within the cultural frame. Insanity is intricately connected with a host of social and economic factors: with the availability of custodial care, with the rates of unemployment and migration, with urbanization and loneliness, and with changes in family size and cohesiveness. We must ask, nonetheless, whether women were indeed more susceptible to the stresses of all of these variables than men, or whether the relationship of femininity and insanity was culturally constructed in such a way that women bore the brunt of social transformation. The traditional beliefs that women were more emotionally volatile, more nervous, and more ruled by their reproductive and sexual economy than men inspired Victorian psychiatric theories of femininity as a kind of mental illness in itself. As the neurologist S. Weir Mitchell remarked, "The man who does not know sick women does not know women."[90] In the first half of the century, when doctors advocated the strenuous exercise of individual will in combating lunacy, women were seen as more vulnerable since they were uneducated and untrained; later in the century, when theories of hereditary predisposition came to the fore, educated women were criticized as carriers of psychological disease.

By the end of the century, psychiatric physicians had begun to explore the shadowy "borderlands of insanity" for new patients and had established themselves as experts in the nearly invisible signs of "unsoundness of mind." Women, particularly if they were disobedient, aggressive, or unattractive, were often perceived as displaying these signs and were usually so guilt ridden about their deviation that they could be readily persuaded to accept psychiatric labels for their emotions and desires. Well before Freud and psychoanalysis declared that women were physically deficient and emotionally masochistic beings, Victorian psychiatric theory had evolved to explain mental breakdown in women (or the working class) as evidence of innate inferiority. As Mercier wrote, "Insanity does not occur in people who are of sound mental constitution. It does not, like small pox and malaria, attack indifferently the weak and the strong. It occurs chiefly in those whose mental constitution is originally defective, and whose defect is manifested in lack of the power of self-control and of forgoing immediate indulgence."[91]

Some of the disorders for which women were committed to asylums in the nineteenth century no longer exist. Hysteria has virtually disappeared; nymphomania, puerperal mania, and ovarian madness no longer present acute symptoms. But new "female" diseases such as *anorexia nervosa* and agoraphobia have taken their place; and in England and the United States, women's use of outpatient, private, and community-based psychiatric services greatly exceeds that of men.[92] In literature, the madwoman who made fleeting and ominous appearances in the Victorian novel has become the heroine; tensions and anxieties that were at the edge of female experience in the nineteenth century have moved to the center, and the visit to the psychiatrist, or the nervous breakdown, has become a standard, even obligatory, episode in the fictional life of women in the twentieth century. If Dickens could visit an asylum today, he would be confirmed in his assumption that insanity is more prevalent among women than among men; he might also understand how not only the social circumstances, but the social services available to women can make them ill, and how the asylum, like the Marshalsea, creates its own population.

Notes

1. Charles Dickens, "A Curious Dance Round a Curious Tree," *Household Words*, 17 January 1852, in *Charles Dickens' Uncollected Writings from "Household Words," 1850–1859*, ed. Harry Stone, 2 vols. (Bloomington: Indiana University Press, 1968), 2:387–88. Dickens wrote the article in collaboration with W. H. Wills.
2. Ibid., pp. 390, 382–83.
3. William Makepeace Thackeray to his mother, September 1842, *The Letters and Private Papers of William Makepeace Thackeray*, ed. Gordon N. Ray, 4 vols. (London: Oxford University Press, 1945), 2:81. Mrs. Thackeray had been treated in Esquirol's clinic in Paris and at a water-cure establishment in Graeffenberg. Thackeray visited the York Retreat with Procter but finally made private arrangements for his wife with a Mrs. Bakewell who lived in Camberwell.
4. *Illustrated Times*, 29 December 1859, quoted in Anthony Masters, *Bedlam* (London: Michael Joseph, 1977), p. 163.
5. Richard Hunter and Ida MacAlpine, *Psychiatry for the Poor: 1851 Colney Hatch Asylum—Friern Hospital 1973* (London: Dawsons, 1974), pp. 30, 41.
6. Quoted in Masters, *Bedlam*, p. 164.
7. "New Year's Eve in a Pauper Lunatic Asylum," *Athenaeum* (1842), pp. 65–66.
8. John Thurnam, *Observations and Essays on the Statistics of Lunacy*, quoted in William Parry-Jones, *The Trade in Lunacy* (London: Routledge and Kegan Paul, 1972), pp. 49–50.
9. Charles Lamb to Samuel Taylor Coleridge, 3 October 1796, *The Letters of Charles and Mary Anne Lamb*, ed. Edwin W. Marrs, Jr. (Ithaca, N.Y.: Cornell University Press, 1975), 1:49.
10. John Arlidge, *On the State of Lunacy and the Legal Provision for the Insane* (London: Churchill, 1859), p. 102.
11. J. Mortimer Granville, *The Care and Cure of the Insane* (London: Hardwicke and Bogne, 1877), 2:230. In the general population, there were 1,056 women for every 1,000 men.
12. Edgar Sheppard, *Lectures on Madness in Its Medical, Legal, and Social Aspects* (London: Churchill, 1873), pp. 3–5, quoted in George Rosen, *Madness in Society: Chapters in the Historical Sociology of Mental Illness* (New York: Harper and Row, 1968), pp. 189–90.
13. Granville, *Care and Cure*, 1:142.
14. Parry-Jones, *The Trade in Lunacy*, p. 50.
15. Andrew Scull, "Museums of Madness" (Ph.D. diss., Princeton University, 1974), p. 602.
16. Pat Thane, "Women and the Poor Law in Victorian and Edwardian England," *History Workshop Journal* 6 (1979): 29.

17. Geoffrey Best, *Mid-Victorian Britain, 1851–75* (London: Panther, 1973), p. 161.

18. Granville, *Care and Cure*, 1:48.

19. Harriet Martineau, "Female Industry," *Edinburgh Review* 110 (1859): 307; and "Inside Bedlam," *Tinsley's Magazine* 3 (1869): 462.

20. *Illustrated London News*, 24 March 1860, quoted in Masters, *Bedlam*, p. 166.

21. Henry Maudsley, *The Pathology of Mind* (London: Macmillan, 1879), quoted in Vieda Skultans, *Madness and Morals: Ideas on Insanity in the Nineteenth Century* (London: Routledge and Kegan Paul, 1975), p. 69.

22. Thomas Bakewell, *The Domestic Guide in Cases of Insanity* (London: T. Allbutt, 1805), p. 54.

23. See C. N. French, *The Story of St. Luke's Hospital* (London: William Heineman, 1951), p. 43.

24. John Charles Bucknill, "Tenth Report of the Commissioners in Lunacy to the Lord Chancellor," *Asylum Journal of Mental Science* 3 (1857): 19–20, quoted in Parry-Jones, *The Trade in Lunacy*, p. 81.

25. See Lyttleton Winslow, *Manual of Lunacy* (London: Smith, Elder, 1874), pp. 77–81. *Small* is not defined, but in practice single-sex asylums were licensed for up to 50 patients. A few private asylums were very large; Grove Hall, Bow, for example, accommodated 450 patients. Generally, asylums with more than 40 patients admitted both sexes, and mixed asylums considerably outnumbered single-sex asylums.

26. French, *St. Luke's Hospital*, p. 79. Many matrons were the wives of asylum superintendents and were automatically assumed to be unqualified for their jobs.

27. At Colney Hatch in 1852, for example, female attendants were paid £15 a year, with board, lodging, and laundry; male attendants received £25 plus the same benefits (Hunter and MacAlpine, *Psychiatry for the Poor*, p. 93). Asylum nursing was not regarded as a respectable occupation for women, although there were efforts to upgrade it. "A Sane Patient," describing his female warders, writes: "From what ranks they are recruited I do not know, and have no special wish to ask" (*My Experiences in a Lunatic Asylum* [London: Chatto and Windus, 1879]).

28. Arlidge, *On the State of Lunacy*, p. 113.

29. [John Conolly], *Familiar Views of Lunacy and Lunatic Life* (1850), quoted in Parry-Jones, *The Trade in Lunacy*, p. 101.

30. Louisa Devey, *Life of Rosina, Lady Lytton*, 2d ed. (London: Swan Sonnenschein, Lowrey, 1887), pp. 298–99. Lady Lytton's novel about her experiences, *A Blighted Life*, was published in 1880.

31. Select Committee Report, "Care and Treatment of Lunatics," 1859, 156th sess., vol. 2, *British Parliamentary Papers* (Shannon: Irish University Press, 1968), 4: 20–21. The Alleged Lunatics' Friend Society, formed in 1845, was a small organization chiefly concerned with abuses in the private asylums. J. T. Perceval, the author of an account of his own stay in several madhouses, recently republished as *Perceval's Narrative*, was the honorary secretary.

32. Robert Gardiner Hill, *Lunacy: Its Past and Present* (London: Longmans, Green, Reader, and Dyer, 1870), p. 4.

33. Pregnancies which occurred while a patient was under asylum care were carefully investigated to establish paternity. See C. T. Andrews, *The Dark*

Awakening: A History of St. Lawrence's Hospital (London: Cox and Wyman, 1978), pp. 77–78; and Hunter and MacAlpine, *Psychiatry for the Poor*, pp. 98–99.

34. *The Philosophy of Insanity*, written by a late inmate of the Glasgow Royal Asylum for Lunatics at Gartnavel, ed. Frieda Fromm-Reichmann (1860; reprint ed., London: Fireside, 1947), p. 84.

35. "A Sane Patient," *My Experiences*, p. 149.

36. John Charles Bucknill, *Manual of Psychological Medicine*, p. 273, quoted in Horatio Storer, *The Causation, Course, and Treatment of Reflex Insanity in Women* (1871; reprint ed., New York: Arno, 1972), p. 109.

37. Hunter and MacAlpine, *Psychiatry for the Poor*, p. 113.

38. Granville, *Care and Cure*, 1:180. Before lunacy reform, noisy women were muzzled with the brank, or "scold's bridle." See D. H. Tuke, *Chapters of the History of the Insane in the British Isles* (1882; reprint ed., Amsterdam: E. J. B. Bunset, 1968), p. 22. At Bethlem, women patients could be sent to the worst ward in the basement for using "bad language." See testimony of Dr. W. Wood, 7 July 1851, Select Committee of Commissioners in Lunacy on Bethlem Hospital, *British Parliamentary Papers*, 6:271.

39. Hunter and MacAlpine, *Psychiatry for the Poor*, p. 133.

40. John Conolly, *Treatment of the Insane without Mechanical Restraints* (1856; reprint ed., London: Dawsons, 1975), p. 58.

41. "Inside Bedlam," *Tinsley's Magazine*, p. 459.

42. Granville, *Care and Cure*, 2:177.

43. Andrew Scull, "Museums of Madness," p. 425.

44. Hunter and MacAlpine, *Psychiatry for the Poor*, pp. 45, 76, 88.

45. Granville, *Care and Cure*, 1:184. At the Hanwell Asylum, however, Mr. Peeke Richards successfully calmed excitable women patients by allowing them to move around and to visit other wards (ibid., 2:231).

46. T. S. Clouston, *Clinical Lectures on Mental Diseases*, 5th ed. (London: J. and A. Churchill, 1898), pp. 530–31.

47. Granville, *Care and Cure*, 1:21.

48. Michel Foucault, *Madness and Civilization* (London: Tavistock, 1967), pp. 253–55.

49. Bucknill, *Manual of Psychological Medicine*, p. 78.

50. Clouston, *Clinical Lectures*, pp. 581–82.

51. Furneaux Jordan, *Character as Seen in Body and Parentage* (London: Kegan Paul, Trench, Trubner, 1886), in Skultans, *Madness and Morals*, pp. 237–40.

52. See Skultans, *Madness and Morals*, p. 12; James Sheppard, *Observations of the Proximate Causes of Insanity* (London: Longman, Brown, Green, and Longmans, 1844), in Skultans, *Madness and Morals*, pp. 52–53; and Parry-Jones, *The Trade in Lunacy*, p. 196.

53. See John Millar, *Hints on Insanity* (London: Henry Renshaw, 1861), in Skultans, *Madness and Morals*, p. 230; Henry Maudsley, *Body and Mind* (London: Macmillan, 1873), in Skultans, pp. 230–31; Forbes Winslow, *On the Obscure Diseases of the Brain and Disorders of the Mind*, 4th ed. (London: Churchill, 1868), p. 510.

54. Edward J. Tilt, *On the Preservation of the Health of Women at the Critical Periods of Life* (London: Churchill, 1851), p. 31.

55. See Roger Smith, "Medicine and Murderous Women in the Mid-Nineteenth

Century," *Society for the Social History of Medicine Newsletter* 2 (1977): 7. I am indebted to Roger Smith, Department of History, University of Lancaster, for letting me see his work on this topic. A female reply to the medicolegal view of puerperal insanity may be found in *Maternity: Letters from Working Women,* ed. Margaret Llewelyn Davies (London: Virago, 1978). First published in 1915, these accounts of maternal breakdown cite "lack of rest and economic stress" in case after case.

56. W. Tyler Smith, "The Climacteric Disease in Women," *London Medical Journal* 1 (1848): 601.

57. See Maudsley, *Body and Mind,* in Skultans, *Madness and Morals,* p. 232; W. T. Smith, "Climacteric Disease," pp. 604, 606.

58. Clouston, *Clinical Lectures,* p. 621. This was for the period 1874–82.

59. Ibid., p. 527. See also Forbes Winslow, *Mad Humanity: Its Forms Apparent and Obscure* (London: C. A. Pearson, 1878), p. 228; and Geoffrey Mortimer, *Chapters on Human Love,* quoted in Peter T. Cominos, "Innocent Femina Sensualis in Unconscious Conflict," in *Suffer and Be Still,* ed. Martha Vicinus (Bloomington: Indiana University Press, 1971), p. 164.

60. Smith, "Climacteric Disease," p. 607.

61. Edward J. Tilt, *The Change of Life in Health and Disease,* 2d ed. (London: John Churchill, 1857), p. 265.

62. F. C. Skey, *Hysteria* (London: Longmans, Green, Reader, and Dyer, 1867), p. 55.

63. Clouston, *Clinical Lectures,* p. 531.

64. Ibid., pp. 189–90.

65. Millar, *Hints on Insanity,* in Skultans, *Madness and Morals,* p. 59.

66. William Moseley, *Eleven Chapters on Nervous and Mental Complaints* (London: Simpkin, Marshall, 1838), in Skultans, *Madness and Morals,* p. 48.

67. Clouston, *Clinical Lectures,* p. 562.

68. Hal D. Sears, *The Sex Radicals: Free Love in Victorian America* (Lawrence, Kans.: Regents Press of Kansas, 1977), p. 87. I am indebted to Sally Mitchell for this reference. Among the more notorious early cases is that of Miss A. Nottidge, who was confined at Moorcraft House in London from 1846 to 1848 because she had joined a religious commune called the "Agepemone" or "Abode of Love." See Lyttleton Winslow, *Manual of Lunacy,* p. 164. Parry-Jones believes the evidence in this case shows Nottidge to have been properly confined (*Trade in Lunacy,* p. 236).

69. Jeffrey L. Spear, "Ruskin on His Marriage: The Acland Letter," *Times Literary Supplement,* 10 February 1978, p. 163.

70. William Moseley, *Chapters,* in Skultans, *Madness and Morals,* pp. 41–50; Andrew Wynter, *The Borderlands of Insanity* (London: Robert Hardwicke, 1875), in Skultans, pp. 236–37.

71. Florence Nightingale, "Cassandra" (1852) in Ray [Rachel] Strachey, *The Cause* (London: Virago, 1978), p. 408. When she worked as director of the London Institution for the Care of Sick Gentlewomen in Distressed Circumstances, Nightingale's feminist interpretation of female mental illness was strengthened. She wrote to a physician: "The patients were chiefly governesses, and

the cases, while I was there, were almost invariably hysteria or cancer. . . . I had more than one lunatic. I think the deep feeling I have of the miserable position of educated women in England was gained while there" (Cecil Wood-ham Smith, *Florence Nightingale, 1820–1910* [New York: McGraw-Hill, 1951], p. 124).

72. See Elaine Showalter, *A Literature of Their Own: British Women Novelists from Brontë to Lessing* (Princeton: Princeton University Press, 1977), pp. 182ff.

73. *Mary Barton*, chap. 34.

74. Sir Humphrey Davy Rolleston, *The Right Honourable Sir Thomas Clifford Allbutt: A Memoir* (London: Macmillan, 1929), p. 87.

75. Isaac Baker Brown, *On the Curability of Certain Forms of Insanity, Epilepsy, Catalepsy, and Hysteria in Females* (London: Robert Hardwicke, 1866), p. 7.

76. Ibid., pp. 14–15.

77. Ibid., pp. 37, 72–73.

78. Ibid., p. 84.

79. Ibid., pp. 24–25.

80. Ibid., p. 70.

81. "The Obstetrical Society Meeting to Consider the Proposition of the Council for the Removal of Mr. I. B. Brown," *British Medical Journal* (1867): 407.

82. *British Medical Journal* (1866), p. 673.

83. T. Hawkes Tanner, "On Excision of the Clitoris as a Cure for Hysteria," *British Medical Journal* (1866), p. 672; see also pp. 705–6.

84. *British Medical Journal* (1866), p. 673.

85. "Obstetrical Society Meeting," p. 396.

86. John A. Shepherd, *Spencer Wells: The Life and Work of a Victorian Surgeon* (Edinburgh: E. and S. Livingstone, 1965), p. 82 (italics mine).

87. See G. J. Barker-Benfield, *The Horrors of the Half-Known Life* (New York: Harper and Row, 1976), pp. 120–21.

88. Susan Lipshitz, "Women and Psychiatry," in *The Sex Role System: Psychological and Sociological Perspectives,* ed. Jane Chetwynd and Oonagh Hartnett (London: Routledge and Kegan Paul, 1978), p. 104.

89. See Anthony Clare, *Psychiatry in Dissent* (London: Tavistock, 1976), pp. 300–301; and Desmond Curran, Maurice Partridge, and Peter Storey, *Psychological Medicine: An Introduction to Psychiatry,* 8th ed. (Edinburgh: Churchill Livingstone, 1976), p. 346.

90. S. Weir Mitchell, *Doctor and Patient* (Philadelphia: Lippincott, 1888), quoted in Ilza Veith, *Hysteria: The History of a Disease* (Chicago: University of Chicago Press, 1965), pp. 219–20.

91. Charles Arthur Mercier, *A Textbook of Insanity,* 2d ed. (London: Allen and Unwin, 1914), p. 17.

92. As of 1969, women resident patients in mental hospitals in England and Wales outnumbered male patients, but the imbalance was due to the preponderance of female patients in the old age groups (sixty-five and over). See *On the State of the Public Health: The Annual Report of the Chief Medical Officer of the Department of Health and Social Security for the Year 1970* (London: Her Majesty's Stationery Office, 1971), pp. 121–22.

PART FOUR
Psychiatry and the Law

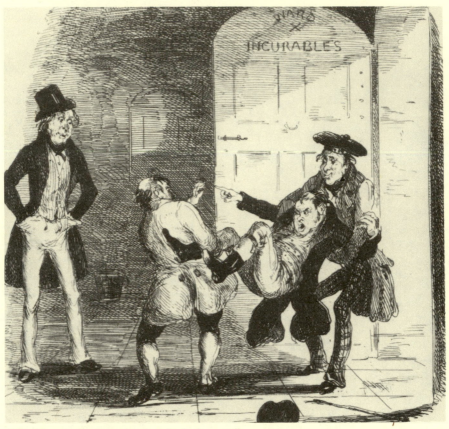

"Sir, I'm not the Lunatic, that is the Lunatic"

This drawing by Phiz illustrates a doubtless apochryphal story satirizing the ingenuousness and pretensions of asylum superintendents.

A lunatic, learning that his relatives planned to have a keeper convey him to a nearby asylum, slipped away unnoticed and presented himself at the asylum gates. He secured an interview with the superintendent, and, posing as the keeper, said he would return later with a client for the madhouse. He warned the superintendent that the lunatic was very clever and would try to convince him that he was committing the wrong man. After being assured by the superintendent that such a deception would not work, the lunatic returned home and then allowed himself to be decoyed back to the asylum.

Back in the superintendent's presence once more, it went as planned, and when the innocent keeper protested that there must be some mistake, he was seized and carted off to the ward for incurables. Phiz's picture captures his last despairing attempt to convince his captors that they had got hold of the wrong man.

(Source: Adapted from James Grant, *Sketches in London*, 2d ed. [London: Tegg, 1840] pp. 268–72.)

338

P E T E R   M c C A N D L E S S

13 Liberty and Lunacy: The Victorians and Wrongful Confinement

In 1863 Charles Reade published *Hard Cash,* a melodramatic novel depicting the ease with which sane persons could be committed to English asylums. The book's readers doubtless shared the hero's terror when he found himself confined as a lunatic: "At the fatal word 'asylum,' Alfred uttered a cry of horror and despair, and his eyes roved round the room in search of escape."[1] The fear of wrongful confinement conveyed by this passage has haunted the public mind as long as asylums have been prevalent. Today, hardly a year goes by without some frightful revelation about sane persons rotting in mental hospitals.[2] In early eighteenth-century England, when the number of private madhouses was rapidly increasing, Daniel Defoe charged that men often disposed of unwanted wives by committing them to these establishments. He demanded that private madhouses be suppressed or at least brought under effective regulation and inspection.[3] Parliament did nothing at the time, but continuing concern about the possibility of improper confinement led to the appointment in 1763 of a select committee to investigate private madhouses, and to the passage, eleven years later, of an act to regulate them. The "Madhouse Act" tried to prevent wrongful confinement by licensing and inspecting private madhouses, and by the certification and registration of patients.[4] Neither this act (which left great room for abuse) nor further reforms of the nineteenth century relieved the public of its anxiety, and the Victorian era was marked by periodic outbursts of rage against the "mad-doctors" and the commitment laws. Two such lunacy panics, in 1858–59 and 1876–77, led to the appointment of important select committees of the House of Commons.[5]

This essay was originally published in the *Journal of Social History,* 11, and is reprinted by permission.

It is ironic that the more Parliament did to allay the fear of wrongful confinement, the more the public became concerned about its possibility. Ironic, but not difficult to understand. The number of persons committed to asylums rapidly increased during the nineteenth century, especially after 1845, when Parliament established a system of public asylums for the insane poor.[6] This fact alone created some apprehension. But the tactics of those who campaigned for lunacy reform also played a part. For many years they relentlessly exposed asylum abuses in an attempt to attract popular support for reform. The distrust of asylums they unwittingly helped to foster remained after reform had been achieved. It is likely that the growth of the reading public in the nineteenth century helped feed this distrust. The spread of literacy and the availability of cheap magazines and newspapers meant that tales of wrongful confinement could reach a wider audience than before.[7] Such stories made good melodrama, and it is not surprising that many editors were not loath to print them.

Perhaps because of this melodramatic aspect, some historians have assumed that the fear of improper confinement was largely illusory, a bogey raised by sensationalist writers, self-seeking politicians, and editors who were anxious to sell newspapers.[8] It is true that few cases of wrongful confinement can be substantiated. The Lunacy Commissioners, the men responsible for detecting and remedying such cases, did not believe that they occurred.[9]

Yet there is reason to believe that the public's anxiety was not entirely groundless. Doctors, knowing little about the pathology of insanity, often relied on subjectively determined symptoms, and sometimes the reasons they advanced as proof of mental derangement were patently absurd. Frequently, too, they confused insanity with immorality, especially sexual, and with other forms of nonconformist behavior. Because of these diagnostic tendencies, it is likely that some persons, perhaps many, were wrongly confined.

The Victorians' attitudes toward wrongful confinement, like so many of their views, were paradoxical. While they were horrified by the prospect of lunatics at large, and fervently supported involuntary confinement for the insane, they were equally terrified by the thought of sane persons languishing in madhouses, and often viciously attacked those responsible for the confinement of mental patients. One possible explanation for this paradox lies in the widely held assumption that it was a relatively simple matter to determine who was sane and who was not. Few Victorians doubted that there was an essential distinction between the sane and the insane, or that most of the latter properly belonged in an asylum. This was one of the verities of the age; even a strident critic of the commitment laws like Thomas Mulock[10] could write that "the number of really and unmistakeably insane persons is very great, and, of course, there must be institutions fitted to receive them." People certainly differed over where to draw the line between the sane and the insane, but few disputed that such a line could be drawn without a great deal of difficulty.

These attitudes help explain why, when a case of alleged wrongful confinement arose, the public rage was almost always directed against the individuals who operated the asylum system, almost never against the system itself. Most Victorians could not or would not see any contradiction between their concern for the liberty of the sane and their insistence on the incarceration of the insane. And, if one accepts their belief that distinguishing between the two was an easy matter, the contradiction largely disappears. From their perspective, if a sane person were confined, it could only be because the greed, stupidity, or malevolence of those responsible for his commitment had perverted the asylum system from its true purpose.[11]

Of course, in practice, the matter of distinguishing between the sane and the insane did not prove so simple. One can sympathize with the doctors who were responsible for making such distinctions, handicapped as they were by insufficient knowledge and faced with the certainty of public ridicule should they err. But one's sympathies are tempered by the doctors' general refusal to acknowledge the limitations they labored under, for they, too, largely accepted the popular concept of clear-cut boundaries between the sane and insane worlds. But they differed with the popular view in one important sense. They rejected the idea that diagnosing insanity was basically a commonsense matter, something any rational person could do. They contended that it required a degree of expertise which only a medical man (preferably an alienist, or specialist in mental diseases) could provide. The law, which gave medical men the power of certification, essentially accepted this contention. The English public never wholly accepted it, however, and many people remained suspicious of the doctors' abilities and intentions even as reliance on them increased.

These suspicions were aroused, it seems, by two things. One, the doctors themselves frequently differed sharply over the mental state of a particular individual. This could hardly inspire confidence in their judgment. Two, many doctors seemed to be constantly trying to enlarge the boundaries of insanity, constantly adding to the symptoms that indicated mental derangement. This certainly inspired fear and, periodically, rage. The Victorian alienists tried to establish themselves as the arbiters of mental normalcy, and in so doing, they showed an alarming tendency to equate sanity with behavioral acceptability. For many doctors, the extent to which an individual deviated from the Victorian social and moral codes, from what we call Victorianism, often became the measurement of his mental state. Considering the supposed strength of Victorianism, one might suspect that the public would have supported and applauded the doctors' efforts. Of course, many people probably did. What is surprising is the number of those who fought against this tendency. Whether these people demurred out of a simple concern for individual liberty, or because they themselves felt stifled by the rigidities of Victorianism, is difficult to say. The latter possibility, if correct, would indicate a widespread, if oblique, attack on the accepted code of behavior. The resistance to the doctors' efforts may have been an attempt to scuttle what would undoubtedly have been a very effective means of enforcing adherence to the code.

All medical men could sign certificates of insanity, but those who specialized in mental diseases bore the brunt of the public outrage in cases of alleged wrongful commitment. These alienists (as they called themselves) or "mad-doctors" (as their detractors called them), were variously described as hypocrites, frauds, sadists, knaves, and moneygrubbers.[12] The violence with which these men were attacked is difficult to understand unless we realize that to be unjustly confined as a lunatic was popularly regarded as one of the greatest indignities an individual could suffer. As the *Spectator* expressed it in 1839, "A lunatic, in law language, is *civilitus mortuus.* . . . If committed unduly, he receives in his single person nearly all the civil injuries that can be inflicted; for not only is his liberty thereby taken away and his property removed from his control but he suffers an imputation which operates with all the force of a libel. . . . A party detained on a charge of insanity may be acquitted and restored to liberty; but we all know that this is a question of such a nature that it cannot even be raised without attaching suspicion ever after to the individual to whom it relates."[13]

This is not to say that the Victorians were constantly concerned about the problem of wrongful confinement. Periodically, some real or imagined injustice aroused public opinion to a high pitch of excitement. During these lunacy panics, newspapers and magazines often printed articles demanding inquiries and suggesting reforms. But the uproar seldom lasted beyond a few months; gradually people lost interest and shifted their attention elsewhere. Most of the time the work of criticizing the commitment laws rested in the hands of a tiny group of activists. These persons, mainly former mental patients or relatives of patients, wrote books and pamphlets, investigated alleged abuses, and campaigned for changes in the law. Like good Victorians they also founded organizations to pursue their objects: to them we owe the curiously named Alleged Lunatic's Friend Society (founded in 1845) and its successor, the Lunacy Law Reform Association (founded in 1873). Often these people were ignored or ridiculed, but occasionally they found many of their charges echoed by respectable newspapers and journals, such as the *Times, Daily Telegraph,* and *Lancet.* Sometimes, too, their exposures reached a wide audience through the medium of popular fiction. Henry Cockton in *Valentine Vox* (1840) and Charles Reade in *Hard Cash* (1863) constructed novels around the theme of wrongful confinement, drawing liberally on newspaper accounts and the works of former asylum inmates.

Although it is by no means certain, it seems that the problem of wrongful confinement was basically a middle- and upper-class concern. The most outspoken critics of the commitment laws—persons like Thomas Mulock, Richard Paternoster, John Perceval, and Richard Saumarez— came from the middle and upper classes; so did most of the individuals whose cases excited public attention.[14] A working-class person seldom became the focus of concern over wrongful confinement. Moreover, the critics tended to concentrate their attack on the private asylums, which catered mainly to the comfortable classes, and largely (though not wholly) ignored the public asylums, which basically served the working classes. The realities of Victorian society partially explain this class distinction. A well-educated middle- or upper-class person who believed himself (or her-self) wrongfully confined was more likely to know how to make his case known and where to seek help than an ill-educated working-class person; he was also more likely to have professional acquaintances who could help him: journalists, doctors, and lawyers.

Another factor which probably helped direct public attention toward the cases of the well-to-do was the common belief that the rich were much more likely victims of wrongful confinement than the poor. In the minds of many Victorians money was at the root of the problem of wrongful confinement. No one was likely to commit a working-class person to get his money; wealthy persons, however, did not have this safeguard. This seemed so obvious that it hardly needed to be stated; and it seldom was, at least explicitly. Nonetheless, the assumption is evident in many discus-sions of the problem of wrongful confinement, and the fact that many of the more sensational cases revolved around money disputes helped confirm the popular view.

The belief that human greed was a major factor in producing cases of wrongful confinement also helps explain why the critics of the lunacy laws singled out the private asylums for particular condemnation. The rationale for discriminating between private and public asylums was simple and obvious: private asylums, unlike public, were operated for profit, and therefore presented a much greater threat to personal liberty. The officers of public asylums, so the argument ran, had nothing to gain from crowding their institutions with patients. If anything, the pressure was the other way around; it was in their interest to release patients at the earliest opportunity, so as to relieve the ratepayers of a financial burden.[15] Private asylums, however, had to make a profit to survive. Many persons argued that the profit motive tempted the proprietors of these establishments to keep them filled in any way they could, and that even the basically honest might be blinded by their own self-interest.

Dr. John Conolly, an eminent alienist, conceded that the "great profit" proprietors could make from the confinement of patients might sometimes "operate against proper caution."[16] Richard Paternoster, a former asylum inmate, was less charitable; in his view, the proprietors were concerned with nothing but profit. Mulock, who also spent some time in an asylum, sarcastically described a typical proprietor in the following terms: " 'Mr. Holdfast, Dove Park Retreat, whose Christian benevolence, disinterested kindness to the afflicted, and pious suavity of mind and manner, render him eminently qualified for the position he so usefully fulfills.' Upon nearer acquaintance, this landed individual is discovered to have the two-fold aspect of a butcher and a swellmobsman, with the mixed manners of a cab-driver and a bailiff's follower—in fact, a ruffian of all works whose vocation is unmistakeable." Paternoster and Mulock, like most critics of the lunacy laws, implied that collusion between moneygrubbing asylum keepers and designing relatives to shut up sane individuals was a regular occurrence.[17]

Most critics of the commitment law believed that it made wrongful confinement possible by not adequately protecting the civil rights of the alleged lunatic. They considered it scandalous that the law entrusted to "a chance pair of medical men . . . the power of sending any man or woman to a madhouse." They regarded the medical certificates required for the confinement of patients as a screen for abuse rather than as a protection against it.[18] Paternoster referred to the certificates as *lettres de cachet*, while Mulock charged that they placed an "irresponsible power" in the hands of men "assailable on the side of sordidness." Both claimed that doctors often received a fee from proprietors to send patients to particular asylums.[19]

Arrangements of this sort did exist, although how widespread they were is difficult to determine. George Bodington, proprietor of Driffold Asylum, complained to the Home Office in 1859 that proprietors often bribed family doctors to send patients to their asylums. Some proprietors, he claimed, had even placed advertisements in the medical journals "offering to pay two or three percent out of the monies paid for the board and care of the patients, to the Medical Men thro' whose interest they may obtain them." A couple of years earlier another proprietor, Dr. Forbes Winslow, had criticized the practice of advertising for patients in an address he delivered to the Association of Medical Officers of Asylums and Hospitals for the Insane. Bodington conceded that open advertising seemed to have ceased, but he was certain that "accommodations" between proprietors and family doctors were "still carried on secretly to a considerable extent."[20]

Such arrangements certainly seem unethical. But, before 1862, there was some doubt whether they were illegal as well. The Lunacy Act of 1845 prohibited any medical man interested in or attending a licensed house from signing a certificate for the admission of a patient into that house.[21] But what constituted interest in or attendance at a licensed house was not entirely clear—at least not to some doctors who were responsible for signing certificates. The confusion was illustrated in 1858 during a commission of lunacy concerning Lawrence Ruck. The commission of lunacy was a chancery procedure ostensibly intended to protect a lunatic's person and property, although its real purpose was to prevent the dissipation of family fortunes by incompetent heirs. The proceeding was usually initiated by the alleged lunatic's relatives, who had to prove that he was "of unsound mind" and "incapable of managing his own affairs."[22]

Ruck's commission had been brought by his wife, who several months before had had him committed to Moorcroft House, a private asylum owned by Dr. Arthur Stillwell. One of the certificates on which Ruck had been confined had been signed by John Conolly, who received fees as a consulting physician to the asylum. Conolly acknowledged that the law prohibited a medical man connected with a particular house to certify patients to be sent to that asylum. But he was satisfied that he had done nothing wrong; he did not "consider himself" to be "connected with the establishment, as I only send male patients to it." The lunacy commissioners, however, considered Conolly's arrangement with Moorcroft House illegal; and Ruck later brought a successful action for false imprisonment against Conolly and Stillwell.[23] But the fact that an eminent and respected alienist like Conolly could interpret the law in the way he did apparently convinced the commissioners that the law was too vague. Following a suggestion of George Bodington, they inserted a clause specifically prohibiting all such arrangements into an act of 1862.[24]

There is not much reason to believe that doctors often violated the commitment laws. Their critics claimed that they did, but could offer very little proof. Accusations of wrongdoing sometimes took the form of anonymous letters to the newspapers, such as one sent to the *Times* in which the writer stated that he "knew" of two doctors who had examined a suspected lunatic together and "signed, after [a] fifteen-minute conversation with him, certificates of separate visits." The law required separate examinations.[25] During the commission on Ruck, the doctor who had signed the second certificate confessed that he and Conolly had examined the patient together. Conolly, however, insisted that he had seen Ruck alone.[26]

Occasionally doctors filled out certificates in an illegal or improper fashion. In at least one case, the courts ordered the release of a patient because the certificate on which he was committed did not state the required information; it did not include the address at which he was examined.[27] Evidence of more serious irregularities was reported in 1851 by the visiting magistrate of Gloucestershire. According to the *Lancet,* the justices had discovered in one year fifty illegal certificates. On sixteen of these all the information except the signature, profession, and address of the certifying medical man had been completed by the proprietor. The *Lancet* pointed out, accurately enough, that "if signed in blank such certificates might be made available to any patient at any time."[28]

But if proprietors sometimes illegally filled out a certificate, the action was not necessarily part of a plot to deprive a sane person of his freedom. Many doctors simply did not know how to fill out such a document properly. They were ignorant of the types of facts required to demonstrate that the person they certified was indeed insane. Hoping to remedy this deficiency, the author of *Hints on Insanity* included in his book examples of satisfactory and unsatisfactory certificates.[29] To what extent such medical ignorance led to situations like that discovered by the Gloucestershire justices is difficult to say. The lunacy commissioners claimed that they rarely found certificates which did not meet the statutory requirements.[30]

But critics of the commitment laws were convinced that all the legal formalities might be observed and wrongful confinement could still occur.[31] Reade made this point most dramatically in *Hard Cash.* The hero, Alfred Hardie, discovers that his father has committed a terrible crime. Fearing Alfred will expose him, the father arranges his son's confinement in a private asylum. Alfred is brought to the asylum (on his wedding day, no less!), and after he unsuccessfully attempts to escape, complains to the matron that his confinement is illegal. She replies that it is perfectly legal; a relation has signed the order and two "first-rate lunacy doctors" have signed the certificates. "What on earth has that to do with it, madam, when I am as sane as you are?" Alfred inquires. "It has everything to do with it," the woman answers. "Mr. Baker [the asylum proprietor] could be punished for confining a madman in this house without an order, and two certificates; but he can't for confining a sane person under an order and two certificates."[32]

The public was horrified by Alfred's predicament. But did conspiracies of the type imagined by Reade actually occur? The evidence is inconclusive. Persons were sometimes committed under suspicious circumstances. Richard Paternoster claimed that he was confined as a punishment for his conduct toward his family. Paternoster, a former employee of the East India Company, was committed in August 1838 to Kensington House on his father's order. The alleged reason for his confinement was a threatening letter he had written after a disagreement with his family over money he had been promised. The metropolitan commissioners concluded that he was detained without cause and released him after he had been confined six weeks. His release was by no means a foregone conclusion; the commissioners had argued among themselves as to his sanity, and the decision to discharge was by a six to four vote.[33] After his liberation, Paternoster brought an action against his father, the proprietor William Finch, and seven others who had taken part in his commitment. Among the many witnesses who testified on Paternoster's behalf was Edward Seymour, one of the commissioners. On the urging of the jury and his counsel, and "to prevent an exposure of the most painful description," Paternoster consented to an "arrangement." The defendants agreed to pay all legal costs and to purchase him a life annuity of £150.[34]

Lewis Phillips, a glass and lamp manufacturer, was committed in March 1838 to Bethnal Green Asylum.[35] Phillips's confinement was ordered by his brothers, his partners in the family firm. He claimed that they put him away to get his share in the enterprise and that the officers of the asylum had "assisted in this nefarious scheme." When he had been in the asylum for some months, one of his brothers visited him and informed him that he might be released and allowed to leave the country in the company of a keeper if he signed a dissolution of partnership. After hesitating for a few days, he signed and was immediately taken to Antwerp. Within two weeks he had escaped and returned to England. He then indicted the parties involved for conspiracy, but "his solicitor was paid £170 to compromise the matter rather than it should come before the public." Thomas Duncombe told Phillips's story to the House of Commons in 1845 during a debate on the Lunacy Act. No one disputed his account.[36]

Phillips and Paternoster may have been victims of conspiracies. But the available evidence does not support the claim that conspiracies occurred frequently. In most cases of alleged unjust confinement, there was no proof of collusion or malicious intent. The law, as doctors often pointed out, made collusion, at most, extremely improbable. It was just barely credible that the proprietor or superintendent of an asylum, two medical men, and one relative or friend could all be so base as to enter into a plot to deprive someone of his freedom.[37] Conspiracies might occur, but the conspiratorial theory of wrongful confinement was naïve; it implied that if honest men could be found to sign certificates, the threat to liberty would disappear.[38]

The greatest danger to civil liberty arose not from an unlikely collection of evildoers, but from ignorance, arrogance, and narrow-mindedness. Critics of the commitment laws occasionally perceived this. "Fools are more to be feared than the wicked," Richard Saumarez observed, "and . . . nothing is more dangerous than the quackery of those who have not given their undivided study to this complaint, and yet pretend to give an opinion which permanently consigns a fellow-creature to be treated as an animal."[39] Another critic pointed out that even honest and experienced men could commit errors of judgment. In difficult cases many doctors called to certify would be likely to accept the relatives' diagnosis, "thinking of two evils, it is better to risk the confinement of an eccentric person improperly, than to leave him at liberty to become a disgrace to himself and his family."[40]

The case of Richard Hall is a perfect illustration of how this could happen. Hall, a china dealer, was committed in July 1862 to Munster House, Fulham, on an order signed by his wife and two medical certificates. He was examined by the commissioners a few days later and released as sane. He subsequently brought an action against Dr. Semple, who had signed one of the certificates. Hall charged Semple with having signed the certificate maliciously and without sufficient grounds, and with having induced another doctor to sign the second certificate. Semple admitted to the court that the only evidence he had of Hall's insanity were certain "facts" communicated by Hall's wife. Since 1853, the law had prohibited doctors from signing certificates based solely on secondhand information.[41] Semple founded his defense not on the premise that the "facts" provided by Mrs. Hall were true, but on the feeble excuse "that he really believed them to be so." Dr. Stone, the medical superintendent at Munster House, conceded that he had been unable to find any signs of insanity in Hall but added, "Still, I considered him so seeing the certificate of Dr. Semple." There was no evidence that either Semple or Stone had acted maliciously, although the motives of Hall's wife are another matter. The jury accordingly brought in a verdict of negligence against Semple and awarded Hall £150 damages.[42] The *Times* significantly claimed that the most alarming aspect of the case was "that there has been no conspiracy, and that two medical men, not in league with one another, have been guilty of such reckless misconduct."[43]

The *Times*'s assessment may have been justified, but in a sense it was also unfair. Doctors pointed out in their defense that they were faced with a dilemma when called upon to certify or confine an alleged lunatic. If they declared him insane and confined him, and a jury later disagreed with the diagnosis, people would accuse them of nefarious behavior; if they pronounced him sane and left him at large, and he later committed an outrage, the public would condemn them as incompetent. "Want of judgment in a case of this kind may result in a loss of reputation," the author of the fictional *Diary of a London Physician* explained.[44]

The public, for its part, was understandably disturbed by the evidence upon which some doctors based a diagnosis of insanity. Dr. George Burrows claimed that maniacs emitted a particular smell, a "symptom so unerring, that if detected in any person, I should not hesitate to pronounce him insane, even though I had no other proof of it."[45] The *Lancet* observed of Burrows's uncanny olfactory ability that it removed "other practitioners, not similarly gifted, to a distance truly humiliating."[46]

The public's low opinion of medical judgment in cases of insanity was largely derived from records of lunacy trials that had been published in newspapers. Some of these trials, like *Hall* v. *Semple,* were actions for false imprisonment. More often they took the form of commissions of lunacy. Usually these commissions were routine and rather unremarkable affairs uncontested by the alleged lunatic. But if he chose to contest the proceeding, the case might drag on for days or even weeks before a verdict was reached. Such commissions attracted considerable public attention. Doctors were frequently called upon by both sides to comment on the alleged lunatic's state of mind, and they often came to remarkably different conclusions. These men placed themselves in a difficult position, for the spectacle of two or more prominent medical men arguing respectively for the sanity and insanity of an individual could hardly increase public confidence in their pronouncements. The *Lancet* asserted that doctors in these cases were often "misunderstood, ridiculed . . . and abused because their opinions were misrepresented."[47] But in fact they did not always distinguish themselves in their testimony.

Edward Davies, a tea dealer, was the subject of a celebrated commission held in 1829. The proceedings had been instituted by Davies's mother, who appears to have closely controlled her son's life. When he showed signs of rebellion, she had him committed to George Burrows's Clapham Retreat, and then took out a commission to protect his property. She engaged several doctors to testify before the tribunal. These men included Sir George Tuthill, physician at Bethlem Hospital; John Haslam, former apothecary at the same asylum, now a physician; another physician named Frampton; and Burrows. They argued that Davies was suffering delusions in regard to his mother's conduct. Tuthill declared as one of the reasons for his belief in Davies's lunacy the "fact" that Davies had given important papers to a person he hardly knew. The source of this "fact" was Davies's mother. Tuthill cited as further evidence of Davies's madness "the insanity of his paternal uncles," "his learning to box," and "his saying that he could weep over his little rabbits, which he had not seen for six weeks." Frampton told the jury that he considered Davies insane "on the seventh of December because he would not admit himself to have been insane on the eighth of August." The same doctor stated that Davies was incapable of managing his tea business, but admitted that he "never inquired" into the way Davies had actually handled it. Davies's purchase of a country estate Frampton called an act of insanity, "considering his circumstances." Questioned further, the good doctor conceded that he knew "nothing of Davies's circumstances." Burrows claimed that Davies was the victim of a delusion because he believed that these physicians, "men of honour and character who could have no interest in the case, would state of him that which they knew to be untrue."

When the jury heard this evidence they stopped the case without hearing Davies's witnesses and returned a unanimous verdict in his favor. The spectators greeted the decision with "loud and general applause."[48] In Davies's hometown of Newton, Montgomeryshire, the citizens held a public demonstration to celebrate this "triumph over cruelty and oppression." Sheep were roasted in the marketplace for the benefit of the poor; the respectable held a supper at the Castle Inn; and the evening was brought to a close with the burning of Davies's mother in effigy.[49]

The doctor's testimony in the Davies case was critically analyzed in an article in the *Quarterly Review*. The author confessed incredulity at the proceedings and sought for an explanation of how "eminent" physicians of "good educations, good moral character, and no evil intentions whatever" could make such absurd statements. He believed that one mistake doctors made in lunacy cases was to disregard the way the alleged madman had actually behaved. Instead they stuck to "what they call 'examining his mind.'" If they discovered "any feeling which they consider disproportionate to its cause—any singularity of mood or manner, which they believe to be morbid, they pronounce the patient to be of *unsound mind*, and then infer, *as a necessary consequence*, that he ought to be confined." Another error doctors often made was to judge the alleged lunatic's state of mind by reference to what they knew of their own minds.[50]

Doctors often adopted a subjective standard of sanity, declaring persons sane or insane according to the "rightness" of their opinions and thoughts. John Haslam even advocated that they do so. In one of his many books on insanity, he argued that the "practitioner's own mind must be the criterion, by which he infers the insanity of any other person."[51] The results of proceeding in this way could be ridiculous, Dr. J. G. Davey, medical officer at the Middlesex County Asylum at Colney Hatch, firmly believed in mesmerism and clairvoyance, and thought everyone should. He told a commission on lunacy concerning a Mrs. Cumming that an "assertion that clairvoyance is nonsense" implied insanity "to a certain degree" and that "all right-thinking men" believed in mesmerism. Dr. W. V. Pettigrew, medical superintendent at Effra Hall Asylum, informed the same commission that a superstitious person was an insane person. Asked if this meant "our forefathers were all mad," he replied, "It may have been, there are very few who are not mad."[52] Dr. Matthew Allen, proprietor of High Beach Asylum, told a commission on a Mr. Campbell that one of the symptoms of Campbell's insanity was that he objected to woolen trousers, and preferred corduroy because they were better for walking.[53]

If doctors could base a diagnosis of insanity even partly on judgments as value laden as these, it can hardly be surprising that they frequently confused insanity with immorality and other forms of nonconformity. The inclination to do so has not been confined to the Victorians (E. H. Hare, a modern psychiatrist, has called this tendency "the besetting sin of psychiatrists").[54] But nineteenth-century doctors were probably more prone to it than their predecessors or successors, because of the strictness of the Victorian moral code. Between 1780 and 1850, England underwent what Harold Perkin has called a "Moral Revolution," in which the traditional puritan moral code of the middle ranks was imposed on the rest of society. Although its causes are a matter of debate, its general results are not: there was a considerable stiffening of the standards of behavior, speech, writing, and dress.[55] Of course, not everyone lived by the code, or even tried to. Recent research has shown the fallacy of judging the Victorians' morality by their moral pronouncements.[56] But Victorianism exerted considerable pressure on people to conform outwardly at least. Unless one were a great aristocrat, one had to be respectable to be acceptable.[57]

The greater adherence to respectable behavior the new moral code demanded paved the way for a broadened definition of insanity. Actions that eighteenth-century society would have considered merely boorish or eccentric became totally unacceptable in the more refined social setting of the nineteenth century.[58] There was a tendency to equate the respectable with the reasonable, the unrespectable with the irrational. Restraint—of the passions, for example—was reasonable; indulgence of them was not. The person who seriously overstepped the bounds of acceptable conduct —through drunkenness, license, gluttony, or extravagance—courted an accusation of madness. As Mill pointed out in *On Liberty*, individuals who indulged too much in "what nobody does" or failed too glaringly to do "what everybody does" ran the risk "of a commission *de lunatico*, and of having their property taken away from them and given to their relations."[59]

The evidence given at such commissions bears this out. A witness told a commission concerning the Rev. Edward Frank that Frank must be insane because "the extreme profligacy of his conduct" was inconsistent with his position as a clergyman. Frank's maid thought him insane because he refused to sleep with his wife. He was accused of allowing another man to live in adulterous relations with his wife, and of having committed adultery himself. The solicitor general summed up the case as follows: "What did they think of the mind of such a man? He would not say that because a man was profligate he was therefore mad. . . . But here they saw a man conducting himself . . . in a manner totally unbecoming the character of a man, a Christian, and a clergyman—in fact, in a manner proving himself to be deranged."

In another case, that of a Mr. J. Taylor, the alleged lunatic was accused of having asked several women to marry him and of several other peca-

dilloes. The following dialogue took place between Taylor and the head
of the commission:

> *Mr. Winslow*—Don't you think you are a rather old gentleman to think
> of marrying? [He was in his late eighties.]
> *Mr. Taylor*—I don't know. Suppose I was 999, what has that got to do
> with it? I suppose you will ask me next how many hairs I have
> got on my eyebrows. . . .
> *Mr. Winslow*—Do you sleep well at night?
> *Mr. Taylor*—I did not sleep very well last night.
> *Mr. Winslow*—What do you do when you lay awake?
> *Mr. Taylor*—Oh, I can't tell you that. What do you do? Where do you
> live? What do you do when you lay awake? My turn is come now;
> let us have fair play (much laughter).
> *Mr. Winslow*—You shall have your turn by-and-by; now, do you sing
> at night?
> *Mr. Taylor*—Yes, sometimes; I believe there is no Act of Parliament
> against singing. . . .
> *Mr. Winslow*—But you sing at night!
> *Mr. Taylor*—So do the nightingales.

After further questioning, Taylor understandably protested that "this is
all nonsense, it is an affront to the commission of gentlemen here." In both
his case and Frank's the commissions returned a verdict of insanity.[60]

In these cases the accusations issued from nonmedical persons. But
doctors, particularly alienists, gave such proceedings an air of scientific
authority. By ascribing unconventional ideas and actions to insanity, they
set themselves up as the guardians of the respectable code, and of the social
system it buttressed.[61] Merely challenging the existing scheme of social
relationships might qualify one for an accusation of madness. The relatives
of the Rev. W. J. J. Leach had him confined and subjected to a commission
ostensibly because his relations with his servants were not those of a
gentleman. A scandalized Dr. Forbes Winslow told the commission that
Leach had said that servants "ought to be treated . . . more as equals, and
that he dined and took his meals with his servants and kissed them in the
morning, and allowed them to sit on his knee. He had also said that after
family prayers he had his servants in the drawing room and played cards
with them until 3:00 in the morning, and between deals he read chapters
out of the Bible to them. I told him that such proceedings as those were
contrary to views entertained by gentlemen and persons in his position."

Winslow said that he had been called into the case by Leach's family
after the clergyman had proposed marriage to his housemaid. The alienist
had declared Leach insane and recommended that he be confined. Leach
had then been committed to Winslow's private asylum.[62] Leach was ultimately declared sane, but it was with cases like his in mind that J. S. Mill

wrote that there was "something both contemptible and frightful in the sort of evidence on which, of late years, any person can be judicially declared unfit for the management of his affairs. . . . In former days, when it was proposed to burn atheists, charitable people used to suggest putting them in a madhouse instead; it would be nothing surprising now-a-days were we to see this done, and the doers applauding themselves, because, instead of persecuting for religion, they had adopted so humane and Christian a mode of treating these unfortunates."[63]

The tendency to diagnose insanity from antisocial behavior was most marked in relation to immorality, particularly sexual. This is not surprising. To the Victorians, as Walter Houghton has observed, sexual license was "the blackest of sins," for it threatened the most sacred of nineteenth-century institutions, the family. They harbored a fear of license similar to their fear of insanity, and for some of the same reasons: the fact that it was prevalent and "seemed to be increasing." Despite, or perhaps because of, the rigors of the moral code, many Victorians were convinced that sexual vice was more widespread than ever before. Many believed that insanity was also rampant.[64] In order to account for this disturbing situation, some doctors posited a connection between the two: they argued that sexual immorality was one of the causes of insanity, or alternatively, that unrestrained license was a symptom or even a type of madness. Whichever explanation they chose, the conclusion was inescapable: insanity and immorality marched together.

Adherents to such theories included some of the most eminent alienists of the century. Forbes Winslow asserted that the moral "well-being of the individual" was necessary for the "regulation" of his mind. The consequences of deficient or improper moral training could be grasped fully only in asylum wards. Winslow estimated that five-sixths of all cases of insanity, exclusive of congenital disorders, was the result of "the excessive indulgence of those passions which God has given us as necessary stimulants for the support and propagation of our animal nature."[65]

Although some doctors warned that all forms of sexual misconduct could lead to insanity, they placed particular emphasis on the "solitary vice" of masturbation. The indulgence of this habit, they claimed, led to a loss of mental power, then to idiocy mixed perhaps with epilepsy, and, if persisted in, to death.[66] The adherents of what E. H. Hare calls the masturbatory hypothesis had little solid evidence to support their case, beyond the fact that many asylum patients had been observed to indulge in "self-abuse." Nevertheless, before the end of the nineteenth century, few doctors criticized the theory. Fear of social ostracism may have held some skeptics back. Masturbation had long been condemned by Christianity as sinful. In the eighteenth century some physicians had begun claiming that it was harmful as well, thus underpinning its prohibition on moral grounds. The physician who questioned the hypothesis courted attack as a subverter of morality.[67] It is significant that one doctor who did reject the orthodox view, Sir James Paget, added regretfully that he wished "he could say something worse of so nasty a practice; an uncleanliness, a filthiness forbidden by GOD, an unmanliness despised by men."[68]

But the doctors did not simply refrain from criticizing the masturbatory hypothesis; many of them actively promoted it. Explaining why they did so is not easy, but recently two historians have put forward intriguing interpretations. R. P. Neuman, writing from a sociohistorical perspective, argues that many nineteenth-century doctors shared a widespread fear that the practice of masturbation was increasing, and aided the efforts of anxious parents by condemning it as physically harmful. He believes that many doctors endorsed the masturbatory hypothesis because they accepted the respectable sexual code and wished to defend it at a time when its religious basis was being challenged. In effect, they used their medical authority to give a scientific foundation to their own moral values.[69] A. N. Gilbert explains the doctors' enthusiasm for the theory medically. He argues that most doctors accepted it willingly because it was valuable as an explanation for otherwise inexplicable illnesses. "Self-abuse" provided an all-purpose "cause-all," for it was widely practiced, especially among the young whose high mortality rates most needed explaining. Indeed, it was cited as a cause of everything from acne to insanity to venereal disease. The value of the theory was enhanced by the fact that it came with a built-in excuse for medical failure: if the patient worsened or died, it was because he persisted in his pernicious habit.[70]

But the doctors not only claimed that masturbation and other immoral acts were a frequent cause of insanity. Many of them alleged that these acts might be the result of insanity, or even that madness and vice were identical. Dr. John Cheyne contended that "various immoral and vicious practices ought to be ascribed to insanity." Writing of masturbation among the insane, Sir William Ellis stated that it was "often the consequence, as well as the cause of the disease."[71] Winslow compared madness to lust and avarice and declared them similar in origins, characteristics, and development.[72] In the view of Dr. Henry Maudsley the relationship between insanity and immorality was deterministic. "Moral peculiarities," he proclaimed, were "constitutional." They were the signs of a type of what he called the "insane temperament." For him, as for many other doctors, bad and insane were virtually the same.[73]

The doctors' tendency to confuse immorality and insanity was undoubtedly encouraged by the introduction into medical vocabulary of the term *moral insanity*. Dr. James Prichard first employed it in the 1830s to denote forms of insanity marked by little or no intellectual derangement, in which the malady showed itself "in the state of the feelings, temper, or habits." A person suffering from moral insanity, Prichard alleged, acted in a perverted fashion, and was incapable "of conducting himself with decency and propriety in the business of life."[74] The cases Prichard used to illustrate moral insanity were rather heterogeneous. According to modern psychiatrists they included manic depressives, obsessionals, schizophrenics, and alcoholics. Denis Leigh refers to Prichard's thinking in reference to moral insanity as "muddled." Yet the concept found wide acceptance among nineteenth-century alienists. Leigh thinks this popularity may be accounted for by the use of the word *moral*. Prichard never clearly defined his use of the term, and employed it to mean both ethical and emotional. Confusion as to exactly what he meant was inevitable, and in a society as concerned with morality as was Victorian England, a theory which seemed to ascribe moral perversity to insanity was bound to have a strong appeal.[75]

By confusing immorality and other forms of nonconformity with insanity, doctors threatened to turn the asylum into a reformatory. Many alienists, convinced that the morally depraved would eventually become insane if they were not already, recommended that they be treated as insane and confined. Winslow contended that persons addicted to lust and avarice were infected by the "maniacal taint" and asked, "Ought not St. Luke's and Bedlam to be the proper hiding place of each?"[76] John Conolly included among those persons requiring the "protection, seclusion, and order" of an asylum "young men, whose entire idleness, whose grossness of habits . . . or general irregularity of conduct, brought disgrace and wretchedness on their relatives"; young women who lacked "that restraint over the passions without which the female character is lost"; men of good family who associated with "the lowest profligates and frequent[ed] the vilest abodes of vice without shame"; and women with high social standing who "would drink to excess and expose themselves to every possible degradation."[77] Henry Landor, proprietor of Heigham Retreat, described similar cases with the hope, he said, that doctors would recognize them as insane, "and take the earliest steps to control them, and save them from the consequences of indulgence in their propensities."[78] Obviously, the consequences were as much social as medical; what was to be prevented by confinement was as much a loss of respectability—both for the patient and his family—as the ravages of disease. Doctors pointed to the asylum as a place where the moral lunatic could be cured of his vices, or at least prevented from indulging them and so bringing shame on himself and his family.

To what extent such recommendations were carried out in practice is impossible to tell. Certainly a large segment of the public was not enthusiastic about the doctors' efforts "to protect men from the consequences of their own vices," as was evidenced by the journalistic comment on the Windham lunacy inquiry of 1861–62.[79] William Frederick Windham, descendant of Pitt's ally William Windham, and heir to the Windham estates in Norfolk, was the subject of the longest and costliest commission in lunacy in history. His relatives, who brought the commission, contended that young Windham was an imbecile. All they proved was that he was a profligate and a prodigal. He was accused of masturbation, associating with prostitutes and other low persons, paying engineers to let him drive their trains, and generally wasting his fortune. The jury—after thirty-four days and 140 witnesses—found him sane and competent. About the latter, there should have been some doubt. Windham subsequently threw away his entire estate, and ended his days as a coachman—quite happily, if the stories are to be believed.[80]

The press, although not sympathetic toward Windham personally, generally agreed that a verdict of insanity in his case would have constituted a danger to individual liberty. The *Lancet* significantly declared that the "error running through this lamentable case seems to be a blind or perverse confounding of vice with insanity," while the *Daily Telegraph* warned against the "dangerous precedent" of pronouncing someone mad "because he is wicked, or debauched, or a spendthrift." The *Times* and *British Medical Journal* made similar comments.[81]

There is not much one can say with confidence about the controversy over wrongful confinement. The civil libertarians could not prove their rather sweeping charges, which the alienists wrote off as the products of overactive imaginations. "The sane people confined in lunatic asylums," Dr. J. C. Bucknill declared, "are ghosts of newspaper raising. They cannot be brought to the bar as tangible realities."[82] But the line that divided the sane from the insane was so uncertain, and the symptoms of insanity were often so subjectively determined, that charges of improper confinement were seldom open to proof. Persons who had been confined were sometimes declared sane by commissions of lunacy, or by the commissioners, and critics of the lunacy laws pointed to such decisions as proof that liberty was endangered. Very few of these cases were as clear-cut as the juries' verdicts made them appear. The law, as Lord Chancellor Westbury told the House of Lords in 1862, considered insanity a "fact" to be proved "in like manner as any other fact."[83] A verdict of sanity simply meant that a charge of insanity could not be upheld. Yet, as Bucknill lamented, the public was convinced that these decisions demonstrated "that the boasted liberty of the subject is at the mercy of a knot of 'mad doctors.' "[84]

Yet if the libertarians' charges were incapable of proof, there remained sufficient reason for concern. The utter ignorance of many medical men regarding insanity; the occasional arrangements between doctors and asylum proprietors for the procurement of patients; the dubious and subjective evidence doctors often advanced in favor of a diagnosis of insanity; and their tendency to confuse insanity with immorality and other forms of nonconformity all placed individual liberty in a potentially precarious position. The danger to liberty was real enough, but it did not emanate primarily from corrupt or malicious motives. For the most part, the men who certified and confined lunatics did so because they believed that it was in the best interests of society and the individuals concerned. Lacking pathological indicators of insanity, doctors had to depend on less reliable symptomatic evidence. They could hardly be faulted for that, and probably in many cases no one would have disagreed with their diagnosis. But the confidence, even arrogance, they sometimes displayed in deciding the fate of their fellow citizens justifiably disturbed some observers. As the *Daily Telegraph* noted apprehensively in 1863, "Dr. Forbes Winslow would divide the human race into those who are mad and those who are sane— an easy division, a happy distinction, if we knew the limits of reason or insanity, but dangerous and deplorable under the present state of our knowledge."[85]

The *Telegraph*'s condemnation of Winslow showed a rare appreciation of the thorny nature of the problem of dividing the sane from the insane. But its editorial failed to mention one uncomfortable fact. Someone had to make such a division; the system of involuntary confinement demanded it. Winslow and his colleagues were the agents of a society determined to banish the mentally disturbed from its midst. The doctors made the immediate decision to confine, but ultimately the responsibility rested with the society that gave them the power to do so. The Victorian public tended to overlook its responsibility by treating the asylum as something apart, at once indispensable and disreputable. (Perhaps in this sense the asylum had something in common with another important Victorian institution, the brothel.) Few persons questioned the desirability of asylums, yet they inspired fear and loathing in a large percentage of the population. The lunacy panics of the period may represent one way in which the public tried to reconcile its fears and its desires. The outbursts reflected the anguish of a society convinced of the need for a system of involuntary confinement yet uncomfortable with the implications of its existence, and suspicious of the abilities and intentions of those charged with its operation. The attacks on the doctors and others connected with the system were often irrational, hysterical, and misdirected. Yet occasionally, as with the opposition to the doctors' attempts to turn nonconformity into insanity, the attackers showed a keen sense of the danger to individual freedom. Their resistance on this point may also indicate a rebellion against some of the more rigid aspects of the Victorian code of respectability. If some of the doctors had gotten their way, enforcement of Victorianism would have been greatly strengthened. Those who discount such a possibility might well ponder the fate of the dissidents who are currently languishing in the mental hospitals of the Soviet Union.

Notes

The writing of this essay was made possible by a stipend from the College of Charleston Faculty Research fund.

1. Charles Reade, *Hard Cash*, 2d ed. (New York: Harper, 1889), p. 230.
2. E. Fuller Torrey, *The Death of Psychiatry* (Radnor, Pa.: Chilton, 1974), p. 88; Bruce Ennis, *Prisoners of Psychiatry* (New York: Harcourt, Brace, Jovanovich, 1972), pass.; Thomas Szasz, ed., *The Age of Madness* (New York: Aronson, 1973), pp. 198–202.
3. Daniel Defoe, "Demand for Public Control of Madhouses (1728)," in *Three Hundred Years of Psychiatry, 1535–1860*, ed. R. Hunter and I. MacAlpine (London: Oxford University Press, 1963), pp. 266–67.
4. "A Case Humbly Offered," *Gentleman's Magazine* 33 (1763): 25–26; Report of the Select Committee of the House of Commons on the State of Private Madhouses, House of Commons Journals, 22 February 1763, pp. 486–89; 14 Geo. III c. 49. For the story of private madhouses in England, see William L. Parry-Jones, *The Trade in Lunacy* (London: Routledge and Kegan Paul, 1972).
5. Select Committee on the Care and Treatment of Lunatics, appointed February 1859, and the Select Committee on the Operation of the Lunacy Law, appointed February 1877. *Parliamentary Debates*, 152, 3d ser. (15 February 1859), p. 411; 232, 3d ser. (12 February 1877), p. 247.
6. In 1844 the number of patients in English and Welsh asylums was about eleven thousand. By 1854 it had increased to almost twenty thousand, and by 1866 to over thirty thousand. *Report of the Metropolitan Commissioners in Lunacy, 1844* (London, 1844), p. 184; Eighth Report of the Commissioners in Lunacy, *Parliamentary Papers* (hereafter cited as *PP*), 29 (1854): 11; Twentieth Report, *PP*, 32 (1866): 9–13. Most of the increase was in the public asylums.
7. Richard D. Altick, *The English Common Reader* (Chicago: University of Chicago Press, 1957), pass.
8. Kathleen Jones, *Mental Health and Social Policy* (London: Routledge and Kegan Paul, 1960), pp. 2–3, 11; G. F. A. Best, *Shaftesbury* (London: Batsford, 1964), pp. 49–50; Georgina Battiscombe, *Shaftesbury* (London: Constable, 1974), pp. 258–59, 318–20, 329–31.
9. Select Committee on the Care and Treatment of Lunatics, *PP*, sess. 1, 3 (1859): 104; ibid., 22 (1860): ix.
10. Mulock was a journalist and former Baptist minister who spent some time as an inmate of Stafford Asylum because, he claimed, he had offended a local magistrate. His daughter, Dinah Maria, was the novelist Mrs. Craik, author

of *John Halifax, Gentleman.* There is an excellent short summary of Mulock's
life in John Prebble, *The Highland Clearances* (London: Secker and Warburg,
1963), chap. 6.

11. Thomas Mulock, *British Lunatic Asylums* (Stafford: n.p., 1858), p. 13; "The World
at Large," *Chamber's Edinburgh Journal* 15 (1851): 353; W. L. Burn, *The Age of
Equipoise* (London: Allen and Unwin, 1964), p. 289.

12. Mulock, *Asylums,* pp. 12–13, 25–26; Richard Paternoster, *The Madhouse System*
(London: Paternoster, 1841), p. 33.

13. *Spectator,* 1839, p. 156.

14. Paternoster was a civil servant in the East India Company. Mulock was a
minister and later a journalist. Perceval, secretary of the Alleged Lunatics'
Friend Society, was the son of Spencer Perceval, prime minister from 1809 to
1812. Saumarez, at one time chairman of the ALFS, came from a distinguished
Jersey family, and rose to the rank of admiral in the navy. For Paternoster,
see *The Madhouse System,* pass.; for Mulock, see above, n. 11; for Perceval, see
Perceval's Narrative: A Patient's Account of His Psychosis (London: Hogarth, 1962),
introduction by Gregory Bateson; for Saumarez, see *Dictionary of National
Biography,* "Saumarez."

15. *Times,* 24 August 1858, 7 January 1862; Select Committee on Lunatics, 1859, sess.
2, p. 542.

16. John Conolly, *Inquiry Concerning Insanity* (London: Taylor, 1830), pp. 3–4. Some
years later, Conolly became a proprietor himself and changed his views.

17. Paternoster, *Madhouse System,* p. 33; Mulock, *Asylums,* p. 5; Henry Cockton, *The
Life and Adventures of Valentine Vox, the Ventriloquist* (London: Tyas, 1840), p. xiii;
Reade, *Hard Cash,* p. 187.

18. One certificate was required for the confinement of a pauper; two for private
patients.

19. Mulock, *Asylums,* pp. 10–11; Paternoster, *Madhouse System,* pp. 11–12.

20. Bodington to Home Office, 22 February 1859, PRO/HO/45–6686; Forbes Winslow, "The Mission of the Psychologist," *Journal of Psychological Medicine* 10
(1857): 615–17.

21. 8 & 9 Vict. c. 100 s. 49. This prohibition was amplified somewhat in an amend-
ing act of 1853, but the law remained unclear. See 16 and 17 Vict. c. 96 s. 12.

22. The commission first received statutory recognition in 1833, and in a series of
succeeding acts the procedure was simplified and made less expensive. See 3
and 4 Wm. IV c. 36, 5 & 6 Vict. c. 84, 16 and 17 Vict. c. 70, 25 and 26 Vict. c. 86.

23. "Commission of Lunacy on Mr. Ruck," *Journal of Mental Science* 4 (1858): 131;
Fourteenth Report of the Commissioners in Lunacy, *PP,* 1860, 18:51; *Daily
Telegraph,* "Ruck v. Stillwell and others," 22 June 1859.

24. Bodington to Home Office, 22 February 1859, Commissioners in Lunacy to
Home Office, 5 March 1859, PRO/HO/45–6686; 25 and 26 Vict. c. 111 s. 24.

25. *Times,* letter to editor from "Vigil," 5 October 1844. Separate examinations had
been required since 1828. See 9 Geo. IV c. 41 s. 30.

26. "Commission of Lunacy on Mr. Ruck," pp. 130–31.

27. *Queen* v. *Pinder,* Court of Queen's Bench, Hilary Term, 1855, *Law Journal* (1855),
pp. 148–53.

28. *Lancet,* 1852, p. 410.
29. John Millar, *Hints on Insanity* (London: Renshaw, 1861), pp. 78–81.
30. Select Committee on Lunatics, 1859, sess. 1, p. 102.
31. Paternoster, *Madhouse System,* p. 11.
32. Reade, *Hard Cash,* p. 236.
33. Paternoster, *Madhouse System,* pp. 50–51; Edwin Hodder, *The Life and Work of the Seventh Earl of Shaftesbury,* 3 vols. (London: Cassell, 1886), 1:234.
34. *Times, Paternoster* v. *Finch* and others, 8 February 1840.
35. The proprietor of Bethnal Green Asylum was at this time Dr. John Warburton, son of the infamous Thomas Warburton.
36. *Parliamentary Debates,* 82, 3d ser. (1845), pp. 410–13.
37. Winslow, "The Lord Chief Baron and the Nottidge Case," *Journal of Psychological Medicine* 2 (1849): 574–75; "The Lord Chief Baron's Law of Lunacy," *Fraser's Magazine* 40 (1849): 364–65; *Times,* letter to editor from "M.D.," 2 October 1855.
38. See, for example, the evidence of Gilbert Bolden before the Select Committee on Lunatics, 1859, sess. 1, p. 302.
39. Richard Saumarez, *Second Address to the Committee of the Rev. Paul Saumarez* (n.p., 1839), pp. 5–6.
40. *Times,* letter to editor from "Vigil," 5 October 1844.
41. See 16 and 17 Vict. c. 96 s. 10.
42. *Times, Hall* v. *Semple,* 6 December 1862. Dr. Stone seems to have provided Charles Reade with the inspiration for the foolish Dr. Bailey in *Hard Cash,* which appeared the following year. Bailey, the medical attendant where Alfred is confined, considers the young man insane simply because two eminent doctors have signed certificates to that effect. See *Hard Cash,* p. 239.
43. *Times,* 10 December 1862.
44. John B. Steward, *Practical Notes on Insanity* (London: Churchill, 1845), pp. 20–22; Conolly, *Inquiry into Insanity,* fn. 7, p. 9; Joseph Staples, *Diary of a London Physician* (London: Berger, 1863), p. 196.
45. George M. Burrows, *Commentaries on the Forms, Symptoms, and Treatment, Moral and Medical, of Insanity* (London: Underwood, 1828), p. 297.
46. *Lancet,* 1830, p. 138.
47. *Lancet,* 1852, pp. 292–93.
48. *Times,* "Commission of Lunacy on Edward Davies," 19–28 December 1829.
49. *Times,* "Note on Davies Case," 30 January 1830.
50. "Insanity," *Quarterly Review* 42 (1830): 355–56, 372–73.
51. John Haslam, *Observations on Madness and Melancholy* (London: Callow, 1809), p. 37.
52. "The Case of Catherine Cumming," *Journal of Psychological Medicine* 5 (1852), Appendix 53:62.
53. *Times,* "Commission of Lunacy on Thomas Telford Campbell," 23 September 1844. On Allen, see Margaret C. Barnet, "Matthew Allen, M. D. (Aberdeen) 1783–1845," *Medical History* 9 (1965): 16, 28.
54. E. H. Hare, "Masturbation and Insanity," *Journal of Mental Science* 108 (1962): 21, n. 16; see also Torrey, *Death of Psychiatry,* pp. 64, 94.
55. Harold Perkin, *The Origins of Modern English Society, 1780–1880* (Toronto: University of Toronto Press, 1969), pp. 280–88; Maurice J. Quinlan, *Victorian Prelude* (New York: Columbia University Press, 1941), pp. 42–54, 122–23; Walter Hough-

ton, *The Victorian Frame of Mind* (New Haven, Conn.: Yale University Press, 1957), p. 359; Gertrude Himmelfarb, *Victorian Minds* (New York: Knopf, 1968), pp. 282–83, 289–90.

56. Peter Cominos, "Late Victorian Sexual Respectability and the Social System," *International Review of Social History* 8 (1963): 33, 44–45, 228–30; Steven Marcus, *The Other Victorians* (New York: Basic, 1966); Brian Harrison, "Underneath the Victorians," *Victorian Studies* 10 (1967): 239–62.

57. Cominos, "Sexual Respectability," pp. 42, 225–26; Geoffrey Best, *Mid-Victorian Britain* (New York: Schocken, 1972), pp. 260–61.

58. Best, *Shaftesbury*, pp. 43–44; Muriel Jaeger, *Before Victoria* (London: Chatto and Windus, 1965), pp. 14–16.

59. John Stuart Mill, *On Liberty* (Chicago: University of Chicago Press, 1955), pp. 99–100.

60. *Times*, 4 August 1825, 14 January 1839.

61. Cominos, "Sexual Respectability," pp. 31, 36, 239–40, 247.

62. "Case of the Rev. W. J. J. Leach," *Journal of Psychological Medicine* 11 (1858): 668–70.

63. Mill, *On Liberty*, fn., p. 100.

64. Houghton, *Victorian Frame of Mind*, pp. 356, 359, 364–65; Cominos, "Sexual Respectability," p. 33; J. C. Bucknill, "The Accumulation of Chronic Lunatics in Asylums," *Journal of Mental Science* 1 (1855): 195; "The Increase of Lunacy," *North British Review* 50 (1869): 128; *Times*, 8 February 1853.

65. Winslow, "Moral State of Society," *Journal of Psychological Medicine* 3 (1850): 187–88, and "Crime, Education, and Insanity," *Journal of Psychological Medicine* 5 (1852): 187. See also George Moore, *The Use of the Body in Relation to the Mind* (London: Longman, 1846), p. 335; *The Power of the Soul over the Body Considered in Relation to Health and Morals*, 2d ed. (New York: Harper, 1848), pp. 195, 217.

66. Millar, *Hints on Insanity*, pp. 37–38; Henry Maudsley, *Body and Mind*, 2d ed. (London: Macmillan, 1873), pp. 86–87; Sir William Ellis, *A Treatise on the Nature, Symptoms, Causes, and Treatment of Insanity* (London: Holdsworth, 1838), fn., pp. 96–97, 335, 338–39; Burrows, *Commentaries on Insanity*, p. 22; Robert P. Ritchie, "An Inquiry into a Frequent Cause of Insanity in Young Men," *Lancet*, 1861, pp. 159, 185, 234, 284.

67. Hare, "Masturbatory Insanity," p. 16; H. Tristram Englehart, "The Disease of Masturbation: Values and the Concept of Disease," *Bulletin of the History of Medicine* 48 (1974): 239–48; Robert Macdonald, "The Frightful Consequences of Onanism: Notes on the History of a Delusion," *Journal of the History of Ideas* 28 (1967): 423–31.

68. Sir James Paget, *Clinical Lectures and Essays* (New York: Appleton, 1875), pp. 284–85. Paget was Queen Victoria's personal physician.

69. R. P. Neuman, "Masturbation, Madness, and the Modern Concepts of Childhood and Adolescence," *Journal of Social History* (Spring 1975): 1–27.

70. A. N. Gilbert, "Doctor, Patient, and Onanist Diseases in the Nineteenth Century," *Journal of the History of Medicine* (July 1975): 217–34; Thomas Szasz, *The Manufacture of Madness* (New York: Dell, 1970), pp. 180–206; Alex Comfort, *The Anxiety Makers*, 2d ed. (New York: Dell, 1970), pp. 69–113.

71. John Cheyne, *Essays on Partial Derangement of the Mind* (Dublin: Curry, 1843), p. 85; Ellis, *Treatise on Insanity*, fn., p. 335.

72. Winslow, "Moral State of Society," p. 192; see also, "Mad Folk," *Belgravia* 10 (1869): 210; "Insanity and Its Treatment," *Belgravia* 10 (1870): 462; Edward P. Rowsell, "Who Is Sane?" *New Monthly Magazine* 114 (1858): 196–97.

73. Maudsley, *Body and Mind*, pp. 128, 136, 137. This material did not appear in the first (1870) edition of the book.

74. James C. Prichard, *A Treatise on Insanity* (London: Sherwood, Gilbert, and Piper, 1835), pp. 4–5.

75. Denis Leigh, *The Historical Development of British Psychiatry* (Oxford: Pergamon, 1961), pp. 169–89; Alexander Walk, "Some Aspects of the Moral Treatment of the Insane up to 1854," *Journal of Mental Science* 100 (1954): 809.

76. Winslow, "Moral State of Society," p. 192.

77. Conolly, *A Remonstrance with the Lord Chief Baron, Touching the Case of Nottidge v. Ripley,* 3d ed. (London: Churchill, 1849), pp. 9–10.

78. Henry Landor, "Cases of Moral Insanity," *British Medical Journal* (1857): 543; see also Winslow, "Moral State of Society," p. 192.

79. *Times,* 31 January 1862.

80. *Daily Telegraph,* "Commission of Lunacy on W. F. Windham," 17 December 1861–31 January 1862; "A Solicitor," *The Great Lunacy Case of W. F. Windham* (London: Harrison, 1862); *An Inquiry into the State of Mind of W. F. Windham* (London: Oliver, 1862). For a short biography of Windham, see R. W. Ketton-Cremer, *Felbrigg: The Story of a House* (London: Hart-Davis, 1962).

81. *Lancet,* 1862, p. 126; *Daily Telegraph,* 7 January 1862; *Times,* 7, 21, 31 January 1862; *British Medical Journal,* 11 January, 8 February 1862.

82. Bucknill, "The Newspaper Attack on Private Lunatic Asylums," *Journal of Mental Science* 4 (1858): 152.

83. *Parliamentary Debates,* 165, 3d ser. (1862), p. 1297.

84. Bucknill, "The Newspaper Attack," pp. 148–51.

85. *Daily Telegraph,* 14 December 1863.

Roger Smith

14 The Boundary Between Insanity and Criminal Responsibility in Nineteenth-Century England

Medicolegal History and the Insanity Defense

Medicolegal studies can make an important contribution to a new look at the history of insanity. The formalized nature of the law as a social process and its representation of commonplace or lay values both heighten the symbolic content of medicolegal decisions. Since the early nineteenth century, psychiatry and the law have increasingly interacted in relation to certification, decisions as to the capacity to administer business and property, testamentary capacity, and culpability in criminal law.[1] The law has required sharp boundaries to be drawn between the presence or absence of insanity (or of types of insanity), and this boundary-drawing process has left a full but largely unresearched historical record. This record is about administrative procedures only at one level; in addition, such procedures embody an evaluative and symbolic content.

In this essay, I will outline some general ideas as well as some specific cases resulting from a study of medical knowledge and a defense of insanity in nineteenth-century British criminal trials.[2] The decision to find insanity in such circumstances was a dramatic event, often fraught with controversy. These trials have an intrinsic human interest. At the same time, the history of the insanity defense contributes to the resolution of at least three questions:

1. It examines the historical thesis that since the 1750 to 1850 period individual and social problems have been increasingly described and managed in terms of medical concepts and therapies. It is widely accepted that the professionalization of psychiatry and the establishment of medical definitions of deviance have had a marked effect on the modern social order. This "medicalization" thesis has in part been produced by a new historical sociology of medicine which, in its turn, is often motivated by

disquiet about recent medical dominance. Whatever its origins may be, this work has encouraged a new examination of historical records, particularly as regards asylums, and a long overdue concern with the social context of the differentiation of insanity as a major social problem.[3] One would initially expect a study of the insanity defense to support a picture of medicalization, to demonstrate the increasing acceptance of medical accounts of criminality, and to add to an understanding of how medical dominance came about. However, two factors inhibit any straightforward utilization of the historical materials. First, the available evidence suggests that though the insanity defense became more common, it did not become much more successful in the nineteenth century.[4] Medicalization, if it exists, is therefore a twentieth-century phenomenon in this area. Second, owing to a lack of research, we know very little about medicolegal relations before the early nineteenth century. It is therefore somewhat difficult to erect a convincing thesis (of any kind) about *change* occurring in the nineteenth century. Forensic medicine became a recognized specialty at this time,[5] but it is not possible to say with any confidence what this might mean, or whether there was even much novelty in the fact that medicine was seen as an adjunct of administrative social control.[6] This second reservation should, I think, be generalized in relation to the broad medicalization of insanity thesis.

2. The second topic is linked with the first (though it is a linkage that has tended to be ignored), and it concerns the spread of public acceptability that "scientific" pronouncements have a unique truth content. The development of the scientific world view has ancient roots, but its penetration into the area of human and social action is largely correlated with modern social and intellectual developments. The unique status of scientific knowledge in our century has encouraged general historians and sociologists to avoid the issue, since it is supposed that the study of "truth" must be very different from the study of contingent circumstances. It has also encouraged medical historians to see the history of their area as unproblematic: the progress of medicine is the progress of scientific knowledge. Since the nineteenth century, medical evidence regarding insanity has been put forward as part of a scientific contribution to problem-solving.[7] From what has been said, it follows that a full historical account of the insanity defense will describe aspects of the social process accompanying the encroachment of a scientific world view in the human disciplines. The insanity defense exemplifies the way in which scientific statements about a human being convey meanings and evaluations regardless of the putatively neutral descriptive content of such statements. The extent to which a history of the medicolegal area can contribute to an explanation of the growth of both the content and the public acceptability of the human science disciplines remains an open question; I will not explore it further here.[8]

3. Argument about the proper relations of psychiatry and the law, in general, and the operation of the insanity defense, in particular, continues to preoccupy medicolegal practitioners. The reasons for this are complex (and some reasons will be suggested later), but the insanity defense has always aroused discussion out of proportion to its numerical significance in the administration of the law. Given the directionalist historical structure of Anglo-American common law, and given the medical directionalist interpretation of psychiatric history, medicolegal writers frequently include substantial historical references.[9] The majority of writers, however, have had in mind immediate practical issues in the administration of deviance. As a result, the complexity and contingency of historical events have rarely been given their due, and cases and points have been selected without regard to their original context.[10] This is done with utilitarian intent; but even if one accepts the value of that intent, it is at least arguable that a more serious historical study would have greater long-term utility.[11] This point is over and above any desire to have medicolegal history exhibit the ordinary standards of historical scholarship.[12] There is, therefore, some point in looking more closely at the historical use and evaluation of the insanity defense, particularly when such work associates the administrative framework, the content of beliefs, and the process of mediation between the individual and society.

The insanity defense has its origins in medieval law which required the presence of certain states of mind as a necessary condition of guilt (the mens rea requirement).[13] The relevant point at this time is that the insanity defense did not either arouse much controversy or become linked with medical accounts of insanity until the first half of the nineteenth century. It is possible to discern several correlates of these two changes in Britain:

1. The defense came into wider use, it was perceived to be in much wider use, and it became especially visible in several cases involving attacks on the sovereign or on political leaders (Hadfield, in 1800, Bellingham, in 1812, Oxford, in 1840, and M'Naghten, in 1843).[14] As I have indicated, this did not mean that the defense became more successful, although there was public fear and judicial apprehension about the dangers of its success. The insanity defense was involved with debates about a perceived increase in crime,[15] and especially about capital punishment. The insanity defense was associated in people's minds with murder trials. Indefinite custody, which was held to be worse than a conviction for noncapital crimes, followed a successful acquittal in insanity cases; consequently, the defense was for the most part resorted to only when there was a danger of conviction on a capital charge.[16] Thus to understand the increased use and visibility of the defense, it is necessary to examine changes in criminal law procedure and sentencing, and the effect upon it

of social indecision between fear of crime and the spread of humanitarian sentiment.

2. The complex social significance attached to the defense was self-reinforcing, particularly when the grounds on which the defense could be sustained were relatively formalized (in a manner unusual in English law) in the "M'Naghten Rules" in 1843. These rules, formulated by the judges for the House of Lords, were the result of an attempt to dilute criticism of one particular trial and to reassure critics that there were rigorous legal controls over the "spread" of the practice of acquitting murderers.[17] The rules immediately became the focal point of controversy, although it is important to see that they were a reflection and not a cause of the controversy. The rules embodied the traditional legal view that the accused's inability to have formed a criminal intent was to be evidenced by a defect of reason. As I will discuss, the rules failed to regularize the law, and apparently contradictory verdicts continued to be reached.

3. This period experienced the high tide of lunacy reform, with the entrenchment of the institutional response to insanity. This concentrated attention on all the social implications of insanity, and legislation relating to the criminally insane was passed along with that relating to the private and pauper insane in general.[18] The London charity institution, Bethlem, financed for the purpose by the government, received many of the criminally insane in the first half of the century. Like all other penal and medical institutions, it experienced overcrowding. There was further special accommodation at Fisherton House, Salisbury, from 1849, but many of the criminally insane remained in a variety of other institutions across the country. The construction of Broadmoor was decided on in the 1850s, an indication in itself of the special meaning attached to the category of "criminal insanity."[19] Asylum construction of all kinds created new career opportunities, and both asylums and careers involved new economic commitments and a moral campaign on behalf of the insane and their humane treatment.[20] Nowhere were these values more clearly embodied and publicized than in arguments for the treatment as opposed to the punishment of the insane who had been arraigned for crimes. Alienists expressed a persistent concern about the insanity defense: giving evidence in a public trial, or merely criticizing its procedures, was an important way for the alienists' claims to expertise and status to be ventured and tested. In addition, the need to administer the criminally insane accompanied the integration of the medical view of the insanity defense into a branch of government.

4. There was an extended attempt to integrate the medical experience of insanity with mainstream experimental science, which was represented by the rapidly expanding body of neurophysiological research. Alienists continued to use nosological and etiological schemes based on a mass of

crosscutting environmental, hereditary, psychological, and physiological variables. Nevertheless, an abstract ideal of insanity acquired definite meaning in terms of physical abnormality in the nervous tissue, surrounding membranes, or neural blood circulation.[21] This "ideal" type of knowledge enabled alienists to claim that their practice was scientific. They transferred the objective ethos of science to the results of their decisions, in court as well as in private examination. It was hoped that the adoption of a physicalist view of mental disorder would provide objectively definable criteria of insanity and also vindicate a medical response to criminal insanity. The Victorian understanding of physicalist explanation invoked crude determinism at the level of causal events; this meant that crimes produced by insanity could not entail responsibility. Given these beliefs, the medical view of the insanity defense inevitably collided with legal and lay suppositions about the likelihood of evil intent.

These four considerations (visibility of the defense, legal formalization, lunacy reform, and medical physicalism) give a broad framework for considering the use of the insanity defense. Yet, in spite of such generalizations, it is striking that the examination of individual trials shows that a great variety of other factors were involved. It is not possible to understand any single verdict or the commentaries on it without considering special variables which may have been present. To assume that the success or failure of an insanity defense represents the triumph of medicine or the enforcement of legalism is to reify medical and legal elements as if they transcended social circumstances. There was something peculiarly difficult and interesting about the insanity defense; such difficulty and interest were not circumscribed by medicine and law. Yet medicolegal writing has been insensitive to the host of symbolic social mediations enacted in the insanity defense. Why, it may be asked, has the insanity defense been the focus of so much attention? Some illustrative cases will help us formulate an answer.

The Controversial Use of the Insanity Defense: Four Cases

The best-known Victorian insanity trials are those which, it is believed, helped advance psychiatric medicine or established a point of law or led to new legislation. Thus Lord Denman's summing-up in the trial of Edward Oxford, who was accused of shooting at the Queen's carriage in 1840, can be read as sympathetic to the causal attribution of his crime to mental disease.[22] M'Naghten's trial, of course, led to the rules, while the administrative embarrassment following the trial of George Victor Townley in 1863 (for killing his ex-fiancée) led to new legislation.[23] However, I will consider four less well known trials, all from the middle years of the 1850s. These trials illustrate the complexity of conditions, belief, symbolism, and evaluation coming to a head in the insanity defense. Such trials were, after all, the most public and dramatic occasions on which society decided to locate insanity.

Luigi Buranelli was an Italian immigrant who lived an unremarkable life until the death of his wife. "From that time, the prisoner laboured under melancholia and delusions; he became violent and ungovernable, and bent upon suicide."[24] Evidence as to his insanity was given in court by his landlady and others, who described his wildness of manner and incoherence of speech. More importantly, Buranelli had been hospitalized for an anal fistula, and medical witnesses described how he magnified his experience regarding the effects of the fistula and interwove it with delusions of urine flowing from the wound. According to the *Lancet*'s editorial writer, Buranelli was a man "who was not to be convinced by any appeal to his senses or to his reason."[25]

The crime occurred in 1855 when Buranelli's mistress, who was pregnant by him, broke away. His landlord insisted that he leave the house, where his mistress was another tenant, because of his intolerable conduct. Buranelli later returned with specially prepared pistols, shot the landlord dead, and rushed upstairs with the apparent intention of shooting his mistress and then himself. These last two killings were prevented. It was easy to reconstruct a history of his psychological state leading up to the crime which emphasized normal motives and a consciousness of the nature and quality of the crime. He had quarreled with the man he killed and with the woman he tried to kill; the jury, therefore, had good grounds for returning a guilty verdict. The prosecution case was also supported by medical witnesses, particularly by the prestigious London physician, Thomas Mayo, who minimized the extent of Buranelli's mental disorder. Mayo had written widely on insanity; he saw hypochondriacal illusions as evidence of a weakness of mind and, more importantly, as evidence of a weakness of character which had allowed the kind of unfolding toward crime in Buranelli's case which a deterrent law was designed to guard against. Mayo viewed Buranelli from within the dominant Victorian discourse of the responsibility of the individual for his character. The judiciary and the Home Secretary agreed, and Buranelli was hanged.

This result was at the expense of Buranelli's defense of insanity, which was in its turn supported by reputable medical witnesses. The first editor of the alienists' new specialist journal, J. C. Bucknill, observed regretfully that "this trial has presented the painful and humiliating spectacle of mental pathologists differing entirely in their judgement."[26] The defense argued that Buranelli's crime had been insanely impulsive. Its principal witness was Dr. John Conolly who, for many alienists and social reformers, was a figurehead for modern values of humanity, modern practice of quality institutional care, and modern commitment to the revelations of scientific knowledge. According to reformist opinion, Dr Mayo, the jury, and then the Home Secretary were being both ignorant and vindictive in rejecting Conolly's evidence: the verdict "was a violent and monstrous outrage upon decency and truth."[27]

It was possible for the observer to choose either a discourse of normal psychology, linking motive and crime under a weakness of character exaggerated by circumstance (and Italian racial inheritance), or a discourse of medical psychology, linking growing delusions and mental incoherence with a tendency to impulsive violence. Each discourse reconstructed the case history in the light of its purposes. The purposes at stake were high: life and death for the individual being the symbol for the establishment of responsive care or armed deterrence. At a less significant level, interests within the medical world itself were at odds, with asylum alienists ending up as the hurt outsiders. The commentaries on Buranelli's case illustrate the reciprocity of the values of science and the values of reform. Scientific alienism attempted to transfer the ascription of responsibility away from the level of the individual and on to the level of society. The transference involved a conceptual transition from a psychology of the individual mind to the physiology of nature, which required a new collective attitude toward science.

The difficulties and emotive implications of this transition were well illustrated in the case of Charles Westron, in 1856. Westron murdered his solicitor, Mr. Waugh, in broad daylight on a respectable London street. It was an offensive murder to the public since Mr. Waugh had previously shown kindness and patience in relation to Westron's financial affairs. Westron was a cripple, and the defense produced a long history of symptoms of insanity that supported the acceptance of a hereditary incapacity in both mind and body. The jury seems to have been perplexed as to how to reconcile a belief in mental abnormality in the defendant with a desire to see retributive justice for the dead man. The jury therefore brought in a verdict that was greeted with laughter from the public gallery because of its contradictoriness: "We find the prisoner guilty of wilful murder. We do not think he ought to be acquitted on the ground of insanity, but we recommend him to mercy because in his case there were strong dispositions to insanity."[28] The *Times* described this as "a mockery of the solemnities of justice."[29]

The contradictoriness was not actually with the jury but with the ordering imposed on reality. The jury was dealing with events of marginal intelligibility given existing ways of thinking. While Westron showed symptoms of insanity, he also killed out of revenge for supposed injuries.

Mr. Justice Wightman acknowledged this marginality by exercising his power to record rather than to pronounce sentence of death, which ensured its commutation by the Home Secretary. After the trial, Westron was committed to Millbank Prison in conformity with the view that he had an unsound mind, which required the exercise of mercy, but that he would nevertheless benefit from convict punishment, such punishment also acting as a deterrent to "idle habits and ill-regulated minds."[30] The real point of difficulty was to know how much responsibility to exact when heredity and indulgence together led to uncontrolled, or perhaps uncontrollable, crime. Available ways of seeing either attributed responsibility or excluded it, and in finding a practical way through this, the jury showed that society's cognitive schemes were incoherent at this point.

Once at Millbank, Westron's mental unsoundness became more apparent, and he was transferred on a Home Secretary's warrant to Bethlem, where he would have been already had he been found not guilty on the ground of insanity; he died of apoplexy in 1863.[31] Some commentators apparently felt that the recorded sentence enabled Westron to "escape" his just deserts, and this view was reinforced by the transfer to Bethlem. Alienists, in contrast, saw the law as twisting and turning in the face of an indubitable case of an inherited disposition to insanity which logically necessitated the exercise of mercy, and which should properly have followed from recognition of the medical viewpoint in court.

The margin between crime and insanity had to be fixed not just between individuals but within the individual's own life history. This is a complex question. In all the cases that are discussed here, most commentators found defendants partly responsible for their insanity or weakness of mind; this was general in Victorian theories concerning the causation of insanity. In the circumstances, it was, then, problematic to express the behavioral products of the insanity in terms of a determinist discourse. The issue was perhaps most acute when someone gave every appearance of being congenitally deviant, in the sense that he or she had never acquired the basis of moral conduct.

This was the problem in the trial of William Dove, in 1856, who was accused of murdering his wife with strychnine over an extended period of time. The prosecution produced a strong account of intentional action, with evidence about the bad relations between husband and wife, the defendant's procuring of the poison, and his references to its effects and to the course of his wife's "illness." The defense case rested on the argument "that Dove was insane, and was thus either prevented from mental disease from knowing that the act was wrong, or constrained by an irresistible impulse to do it."[32] The evidence produced to substantiate insanity did not relate to the crime, which showed foresight and intention, but to the accused's life history. This history revealed an individual who had always been difficult, irrationally violent, restless, and sometimes physically dangerous. His conversation and conduct had often been extravagant and incoherent; while in jail he wrote a letter to the devil in his own blood, a Faustian compact encouraging a popular view that he was simulating insanity.[33] The resident physician and the surgeon at the Quaker Retreat, Dr. Caleb Williams and Mr. Kitching, gave evidence that Dove had been morally insane from birth: he suffered from a "perverted state of the moral feelings from infancy" and demonstrated a "general inability to comprehend or take his share in transacting the common affairs of life."[34] In the view of another alienist, however, these were words describing "a wilful, passionate, mischievous and cruel boy" as much as words describing insanity.[35] It was a fine decision to know which discourse the words belonged to. In the society of the 1850s, it was not surprising that the popular judgment was that some alienists were twisting the meaning of words in pursuit of a misplaced and self-interested sentimentality. The jury returned a verdict of guilty, to the satisfaction of Mr. Baron Bramwell, and Dove was hanged.

In his evidence, Dr. Williams argued that Dove's crime had been irresistible because "a man by nourishing an idea may become diseased in his mind, and then he cannot control it. This is moral insanity."[36] His manner of phrasing his argument was extremely badly chosen since, according to the discourse to which most of his listeners perceived his words as belonging, it sounded as if he were countenancing all vice if only it was carried on long enough: "If the jury would support that theory, gone was the security of every hearth in the country."[37] Dr. Williams complained that, under the restrictive conditions of the court, he had not been allowed to explain what he meant. He did mean to draw a line between vice and insanity (he was, after all, an officer in a religious foundation), and this line was the boundary of mind and body: the mind was inalienable, but where its instrument was disordered, then there was insanity and a lack of accountability. When he described Dove's moral feelings as "perverted," he was using a discourse where "perversion" was a disorder produced by (unknown) material changes occurring in the nervous system. The circularity of the doctor's point of view, that deviance pointed to insanity, that insanity by definition meant physical disorder, and that physical disorder produced deviance, was merely the circularity common to the interrelations of all parts within any particular discourse. But the trial exposed this way of seeing as unconvincing because the "objective" basis in the world of physical existence remained hidden and unspecified, while the medical statements were easily assimilated by a voluntarist discourse where Dove was "objectively" evil if ever anyone was.

The same problem of the substitution of alternative languages to describe a single crime was evident in the last case I will cite. One night in June 1854, Mrs. Mary Ann Brough (who briefly had been a wet nurse to the Prince of Wales) cut the throats of her six children who were still at home and attempted to cut her own. Her defense of insanity was successful, and yet she was with equal justification described as bad as well as mad. I will first describe the madwoman.

Mrs. Brough, in her own account of the murders, described how she had been tired and low in spirits, and how her mind had been oppressed by a "black cloud" that affected her vision but had lifted when she came round from the effects of her own injury.[38] She had suffered from partial paralysis and her speech had been impaired, both since her last confinement. She also had had severe headaches, and she had been warned by her doctor to avoid overexcitement. Medical opinion at her trial argued that there was a general syndrome in which brain disease led to an inability to control movements, and Mrs. Brough was classified as belonging to this general pathological class. Under the influence of emotional excitement, she might well not have been in a position to know or to control what she was doing. The autopsy, conducted in Bethlem when she died nine years later, was understood by doctors to vindicate this view by demonstrating a physical lesion in nervous tissue.[39] The "black-cloud" description used by Mrs. Brough occurred in other cases in which a person apparently became overwhelmed by violent movements.

An entirely different description of Mrs. Brough was possible. For many years she had carried on a clandestine adulterous relationship with a man from a nearby village in Surrey; they had met at intervals in London. The week before the murders, Mr. Brough had his wife followed to London where conclusive evidence of her disloyalty was obtained. Consequently, he left his house and began legal proceedings to effect a separation from his wife. He was due to return with a legal document the morning following the night of the murders. Mrs. Brough also wrote a note to the eldest child, who was living away from home, to the effect that she didn't want her husband to get her few possessions should she die. It was natural for Victorians to suggest that she had every rational reason to have been depressed and anxious. Faced by the consequences of her own immorality, namely, the removal of her children, she reacted with the violent egotism that was possible only after one had indulged in vice for a long period of time. It seemed to be irrefutable that the murders would not have occurred if she had controlled herself at an earlier date. "If she were insane, her mental derangement was the result of the immoral life she had led for years, and as her insanity was *self-created*, the gallows ought to have claimed her for its victim."[40]

There were grounds for considering both descriptions of Mrs. Brough as appropriate. The choice as to which discourse was to prevail was dependent on identification with the values that were associated with one of the discourses. This way of putting the issue contrasts with the alienists' view that the division between sane and insane corresponded to something in nature external to society. That Mrs. Brough had a nervous weakness meant, to an alienist, that the voluntarist approach to her crime was excluded a priori. Yet it must not be assumed that the jury, in using the medical label for Mrs. Brough, deferred in any simple sense to the medical way of seeing. As Dr. Bucknill commented, it was more probable that it was the extreme and exceptional nature of the crime, coupled with awe and humanitarian sentiment toward a mother who had killed her children, that led to the acquittal.[41] From a commonsense point of view, the criminal effect was so out of proportion to the cause, even a cause in which vice featured prominently, that the language of pathology acquired utility as a receptacle for gross abnormality. It was socially contingent, however, that medicine provided the category that was accepted as describing gross abnormality.

The Boundary of Incompatible Medical and Legal Discourses

Medicolegal writers tend to comment on cases of the use of the insanity defense with an eye on whether the resulting verdict was "correct." This disguises the way the alienists and the legal system worked with different theoretical representations of the nature of human movements, and that the reaching of a verdict was a question of deciding which discourse to use. A decision to use one discourse rather than the other could have been made only in terms of the values that discourse realized. Yet, in contrast, the alienists contended that they had privileged access to empirical facts which validated their location of insanity. In reality, because of their prior assumption of the medical discourse, the validation was evaluative, as critics pointed out. Many Victorians objected to the way in which advocates of the human sciences (including the alienists) were propagating the values of determinism (including criminal nonresponsibility) under the slogan of "the truth." Consequently, medical evidence of insanity advanced in status only with the social phenomenon of the increasing acceptability of the determinist discourse. In the future, the exploration of the reasons for this change will integrate medicolegal history with the general social history of science and medicine.

The law considered responsibility for crime in terms of the presence or absence of certain states of mind, evidence about which, it was argued, could be assessed through the normal process of cross-examining witnesses.[42] This was complementary to the lay view that most conduct is willed, that it therefore entails responsibility, and that such conduct is preceded by knowledge, motive, and intention, evidence for which is present in a person's circumstances, expression, and conduct. Alienists argued that it was the presence or absence of disease causally influencing a crime which should decide the issue of responsibility. It was very difficult to produce convincing evidence for such a causal relationship, and in court, alienists were criticized for making vague rather than precise statements. Alienists and their critics took what was ostensibly the same evidence, someone's crime and conduct, but assigned it connotations that were derived from incompatible discourses. This meant that statements by alienists could look perverse and dangerous to the public, while alienists could accuse the public of being prejudiced and vindictive. Opponents talked as if there were an empirical foundation to their arguments, whereas the divide between them was of cognitive possibility and associated evaluative commitment.[43]

An analysis of medicolegal controversy at the level of the discourses in which it was expressed leads to a suggestion about why this controversy has been endemic, and why various administrative fixes proposed have never proved to be either emotionally or intellectually satisfying. The discourse of crime and the discourse of insanity had boundaries which necessarily overlapped, since they were alternative representations of human nature. The area of overlap, even semantically encapsulated in the term *criminal insanity*, was the area in which a decision regarding which discourse to use had to be made afresh on each occasion. The overlap was also a space into which local variables, such as public reaction to the crime or sympathy with the defendant, could enter.[44]

Thus one would expect the effect of a plea of insanity to have been extremely variable; that this was the case was widely accepted at the time, but responses differed. The legal systematist, Fitzjames Stephen, tried to develop a coherent formula that would standardize the administration of the defense.[45] The leading forensic expert, Professor A. S. Taylor, concluded that "the great defect of the English law is . . . the *uncertainty of its application*. The cases referred to show that an acquittal on the plea of insanity is on some occasions a mere matter of accident."[46] He looked for an answer in terms of an improvement in the presentation and utilization of expert evidence, by having it introduced in a neutral capacity by the court.[47] Alienists accused the law of conducting a lottery with a person's life.[48] They didn't see how scientific truth, as they construed it, could be a way of seeing, among other ways, that could be accepted or rejected as it was "arbitrarily" deemed to have value or not by a lay jury. From the alienists' viewpoint, the vagaries of the law stood as a bigoted denial of the potentiality of scientific objectivity.

The commitment to each discourse had its evaluative content and sectional interest. It is a natural extension of sociological work on professionalization to suggest that there was a correlation between the interests of the new and socially rather exposed alienists and their advocacy of physicalist theories of insanity. It can be argued that alienists hoped that physicalist theories would create a body of expert and esoteric knowledge, the possession of which would vindicate their claim to status and autonomy. In the institutional setting of the court, however, this would-be expertise was in competition with the entrenched legal discourse, and the users of this discourse were unwilling to relinquish the power and influence which their fluency in it gave them.

Yet the correlation of a physicalist and determinist discourse with alienists and a voluntarist discourse with lawyers (and the laity) does not go very far. This is because the existence of determinist and voluntarist discourses was endemic, as it still is, in the culture as a whole. Taking the existence of *both* discourses as the interesting social phenomenon suggests that the medicolegal issue was part of a much wider process of classification. The relevant classification is the distribution of significance between the individual and the group. In modern Western individualist society, this is a perpetual problem, both in terms of intellectual abstractions and everyday politics. The flexible and indecisive pattern of utilization of the insanity defense follows where there is no settled representation of the spheres of individual and group action.

The use of a voluntarist or of a determinist way of thought, or the expectation that control of individual movements would be exercised from within or without (as our language metaphorically expresses it), has reached a consensus in many areas at particular times. But controversy has been rife at the boundary areas, where the intelligibility of using one discourse rather than another has not been obvious to participants, or where the type of thought has been legislated by a group with an interest in its own version of classification.

The striking social reality was the coexistence of alternative descriptions which, logically speaking, were mutually exclusive. It was a frequent criticism of the medical argument for a rephrasing of the Rules, so that a lack of responsibility followed from an inability to control movements rather than an inability to know the nature and quality of a crime, that logical consistency meant that alienists were invoking the determinism of all human actions.[49] Emphatically, however, alienists did not intend this consequence: like everybody else, they drew boundaries in time and space around the legitimacy of determinist scientific thought. They often assigned responsibility for the acquisition of illness, as when they credited overindulgence in the individual or in his or her ancestors, while they denied it for movements in illness. They discussed crimes as lacking in responsibility, and then argued that the perpetrators of such crimes should be placed in medical institutions whose original rationale lay in provoking responsible actions. The debate concerned when to switch discourses and, correspondingly, when to expect people to control themselves or the doctor to control them on behalf of society. Alienists, lawyers, and the public were in conflict over the point of switching. Put this way, the medicolegal debate becomes a dramatic and emotive example of the broader question of the organization of a society based on individualist values. The medicolegal debate about the margin between the two discourses was the representation of a basic tension between the power of the individual and the power of the collective.

The problematic boundary-drawing which alienists themselves conducted is illustrated in two striking ways. First, they drew a spatial boundary within the nervous system between higher brain levels which were the locus of mind, and lower levels which functioned automatically (following a reflex-action model). The higher levels were described as inhibiting the automaticity of the lower levels, and insanity, par excellence of the impulsive kind, was envisaged as producing determinist consequences because disorder had affected the controlling action of the higher levels. For a period of time, the problem of the boundary between discourses was translated into a neurophysiological problem concerning the integration of levels within the nervous system.[50] Second, alienists drew a temporal boundary between discourses in a person's life, separating the voluntary choice of an action and the repetition of an action so that it became a habit mediated by the lower automatic nervous structures. This division enabled them simultaneously to write in a moralistic way about the responsibility of everyone for their character, while believing that mercy and care were the proper responses to insanity, which was in effect a habit out of control.[51] Difficulty emerged only when society, as in the criminal trial, focused attention on the transition from choice to habit.

The boundary of expectation between willed action and movements produced by physical events or controlled by social institutions thus had both synchronic and diachronic dimensions. The latter increasingly became a focus of attention in the nineteenth century. The most precise illustration of the problem created by the temporal boundary between discourses is given by crimes committed by individuals who are under the influence of drink. Once again, the law permitted a flexible response since, though a person was held responsible for getting drunk, it was accepted that he or she might perform movements when drunk which would not have been intended when sober.[52] In a more general way, the systematization of hereditarian theories of physical, mental, and criminal disorder (especially within the theoretical framework of "degeneration" through subsequent generations) tended to shift the onus of controlling deviant actions more and more on to the collective and away from the individual.[53]

The history of controversy over the insanity defense can be generalized, therefore, and while it has involved a good deal of professional self-interest, it needs to be seen as part of the way in which Victorians tried to make human action intelligible with a dualistic outlook and with individualist values. The people known collectively as the criminally insane were of interest and difficulty because they were anomalies not easily assimilated by either of the developed discourses. The law was necessarily vague, since each occasion on which the insanity defense was used provoked reconsideration of a fundamental division in ways of seeing and corresponding ways of distributing power.

Notes

Earlier versions of this essay were read at a symposium on "History and Mental Disorder" at the Wellcome Institute, London, in April 1978, and at a medical sociology conference of the British Sociological Association at York, in September 1979. Another version appeared in *Psychological Medicine* 9 (1979). Research for this essay was supported by a grant from the Wellcome Trust.

1. For legal compendiums, see Danby P. Fry, *The Lunacy Acts* (London: Charles Knight, 1854; rev. eds. 1864, 1877); Charles P. Phillips, *The Law Concerning Lunatics, Idiots, & Persons of Unsound Mind* (London: Butterworths, 1858); George Pitt-Lewis, R. Percy Smith, and J. A. Hawke, *The Insane and the Law* (London: J. and A. Churchill, 1895). The history of certification in relation to the French medical profession is discussed in Robert Castel, *L'ordre psychiatrique: l'âge d'or de l'aliénisme* (Paris: Les éditions de minuit, 1976). The question of "false" confinement is examined in Peter McCandless, "Liberty and Lunacy: The Victorians and Wrongful Confinement," chap. 13 in this volume; and the most famous Victorian "lunacy inquiry" into the capacity of a person to administer his affairs is discussed in Kingsley Jones, "The Windham Case: The Enquiry Held in London in 1861 into the State of Mind of William Frederick Windham, Heir to the Felbrigg Estate," *British Journal of Psychiatry* 119 (1971): 425–33.

2. Roger Smith, *Trial by Medicine: Insanity and Responsibility in Victorian Trials* (Edinburgh: Edinburgh University Press, 1981); idem, "Mental Disorder, Criminal Responsibility and the Social History of Theories of Volition," *Psychological Medicine* 9 (1979): 13–19; idem, "Scientific Thought and the Boundary of Insanity and Responsibility," *Psychological Medicine* 10 (1980): 15–23.

3. This work is given cogent form in Andrew T. Scull, *Museums of Madness: The Social Organization of Insanity in Nineteenth-Century England* (London and New York: Allen Lane, St. Martin's Press, 1979); see also the other essays in this volume and Geoffrey Pearson, *The Deviant Imagination, Psychiatry, Social Work and Social Change* (London: Macmillan, 1975), pp. 48–78.

4. Nigel Walker, *Crime and Insanity in England. Vol. 1. The Historical Perspective* (Edinburgh: Edinburgh University Press, 1968), pp. 85–88, 264–67. A similar conclusion was reached in William A. Guy, "On Insanity and Crime; and on the Plea of Insanity in Criminal Cases," *Journal of the Statistical Society* 32 (1869): 159–91.

5. Cf. J. Nemec, *International Bibliography of Medicolegal Serials, 1736–1967* (Bethesda, Md.: National Library of Medicine, 1969); idem, *International Bibliography of the History of Legal Medicine* (Bethesda, Md.: National Library of Medicine, 1973);

Giovanni Bass, *Die Gerichtsmedizin als Spezialfach in Paris von 1800 bis 1850,* Zürcher medizingeschichtliche Abhandlungen, n.s. no. 22 (Zurich: Juris-Verlag, 1964).

6. George Rosen traced the administrative concept of "medical police" back into seventeenth- and eighteenth-century mercantilist policies: "Cameralism and the Concept of Medical Police," *Bulletin of the History of Medicine* 27 (1953): 21–42. Ludmilla Jordanova has revised Rosen's work and suggested implications of the early incorporation of medicine into the French administration in "Medical Police," Wellcome Unit for the History of Medicine, Oxford, 1979. For the earlier psychiatric literature: Heinrich Laehr, *Die Literatur der Psychiatrie im XVIII. Jahrhundert* (Berlin: Verlag von Georg Reimer, 1892).

7. E.g., John Charles Bucknill, *Unsoundness of Mind in Relation to Criminal Acts,* 2d ed. (London: Longman, Brown, Green, Longmans and Roberts, 1857); Henry Maudsley, *Responsibility in Mental Disease* (London: Henry S. King, 1874); Isaac Ray, *A Treatise on the Medical Jurisprudence of Insanity* (1838; reprint ed., Cambridge, Mass.: Belknap Press of Harvard University Press, 1962).

8. Such explanations have been attempted especially for the social sciences: e.g., Terry N. Clark, *Prophets and Patrons: The French University and the Emergence of the Social Sciences* (Cambridge, Mass.: Harvard University Press, 1973); Thomas L. Haskell, *The Emergence of Professional Social Science: The American Social Science Association and the Nineteenth-Century Crisis of Authority* (Urbana: University of Illinois Press, 1977); Robert A. Nye, *The Origins of Crowd Psychology: Gustave Le Bon and the Crisis of Mass Democracy in the Third Republic* (London and Beverly Hills: Sage Publications, 1975); J. D. Y. Peel, *Herbert Spencer: The Evolution of a Sociologist* (London: Heinemann, 1971).

9. Walker's *Crime and Insanity* supplants much less systematic studies of the administration of English law. For the United States (sharing a common legal background with England, especially in the nineteenth century), see Stephen R. Lewinstein, "The Historical Development of Insanity as a Defense in Criminal Actions," *Journal of Forensic Science* 14 (1969): 275–93, 469–500; Anthony M. Platt and Bernard L. Diamond, "The Origins of the 'Right and Wrong' Test of Criminal Responsibility and Its Subsequent Development in the United States: An Historical Survey," *California Law Review* 54 (1966): 1227–60; Abraham S. Goldstein and Martin Marcus, "The McNaughton Rules in the United States," in *Daniel McNaughton: His Trial and the Aftermath,* ed. Donald J. West and Alexander Walk (Ashford, Kent: Headley Brothers for British Journal of Psychiatry, 1977), pp. 153–69. For a worldwide comparison of the insanity defense, see Heinrich Oppenheimer, *The Criminal Responsibility of Lunatics: A Study in Comparative Law* (London: Sweet and Maxwell, 1909).

10. There are two important exceptions to this generalization; in both cases historians have focused in depth on a single dramatic criminal trial. See Michel Foucault, ed., *I, Pierre Rivière, Having Slaughtered My Mother, My Sister, and My Brother . . . A Case of Parricide in the Nineteenth Century,* trans. F. Jellinek (New York: Pantheon Books, Random House, 1975); Charles E. Rosenberg, *The Trial of the Assassin Guiteau: Psychiatry and Law in the Gilded Age* (Chicago: University

of Chicago Press, 1968). However, these studies are ignored in the medicolegal literature.

11. The importance of the M'Naghten Rules has led some medicolegal writers to look closely at the circumstances of M'Naghten's trial. See Jacques M. Quen, "An Historical View of the M'Naghten Trial," *Bulletin of the History of Medicine* 42 (1968): 43–51; West and Walk, *Daniel McNaughton*. But even here nonhistorical questions are paramount: Quen makes valuable suggestions about public perceptions of criminal violence at a time of Chartist agitation, but he does this to explain what he believes to be a reversal away from earlier liberal precedents (in Hadfield's trial in 1800, and in Oxford's trial in 1840) medicalizing the insanity defense. West and Walk's collection contains little which is not better covered in Walker, *Crime and Insanity,* and Nigel Walker and Sarah McCabe, *Crime and Insanity in England. Volume Two: New Solutions and New Problems* (Edinburgh: Edinburgh University Press, 1973). Whether any historical study can provide social prescriptions is, of course, a problem in itself.

12. Thus, to my mind, the most meticulous and persuasive argument for a legal clarification of the insanity defense is so indifferent to history as to have Prime Minister Pitt as M'Naghten's victim (in 1843!). See Herbert Fingarette, *The Meaning of Criminal Insanity* (Berkeley: University of California Press, 1972), p. 139. This is extreme; more typical is the attribution of intentions or actions to historical figures which conform to the point the writer wishes to make: e.g., Sir Roger Ormrod, in "The McNaughton Case and Its Predecessors," in West and Walk, *Daniel McNaughton*, p. 5, states that Erskine, Hadfield's defense counsel, "succeeded in demonstrating to the judges who tried that case the knowledge and understanding of the effects of such [paranoid] delusions which had been acquired quite recently by doctors studying mental disease." There is no evidence that Hadfield's verdict followed the demonstration of "medical" knowledge and, in 1800, it is very difficult to know what knowledge Ormrod has in mind. Hadfield had a distinct head wound and exhibited delusions which were easily perceived in a lay or commonsense way.

13. Fingarette, *Meaning of Criminal Insanity,* pp. 128–42, has argued, I think rightly, that something beyond the mens rea requirement is necessary to account for our intuitive willingness to accept the existence of a defense of insanity. But this issue was not thought out by earlier writers on jurisprudence. For nineteenth-century authority, see James Fitzjames Stephen, *A History of the Criminal Law of England,* 3 vols. (1883; reprint ed., New York: Burt Franklin, n.d.), 2:94–186. Cf. Walker, *Crime and Insanity,* pp. 15–73.

14. See [J. Blackwell], "[Report on the Treatment of Lunatics]," *Quarterly Review* 74 (1844): 416–47. For Oxford's and M'Naghten's trials, see William C. Townsend, *Modern State Trials,* 2 vols. (London: Longman, Brown, Green, and Longmans, 1850), 1:102–50, 314–402; Walker, *Crime and Insanity,* pp. 90–103, 186–87; West and Walk, *Daniel McNaughton,* pp. 12–81.

15. The question of the "growth" of crime has recently been tested in David Philips, *Crime and Authority in Victorian England: The Black Country 1835–1860* (London: Croom Helm, 1977).

16. E.g., Stephen, in evidence to the Select Committee on the Homicide Law

Amendment Bill, *Special Report*, 1874, British Sessional Papers, vol. ix, p. 7. Nevertheless, the defense was used for other offenses (especially arson), and it should be noted that among those formally designated "criminally insane" many had been arraigned for minor offenses, but were found insane on arraignment, while awaiting trial, or after conviction.

17. Their Lordships' questions, and the answers to them (the "Rules"), are discussed in Walker, *Crime and Insanity*, pp. 96–102. For contemporary authority, see William A. Guy and David Ferrier, *Principles of Forensic Medicine*, 4th ed. (London: Henry Renshaw, 1875), pp. 212–24; William Oldnall Russell, *A Treatise on Crimes and Misdemeanors*, 3 vols., 5th ed. rev. Samuel Prentice (London: Stevens, 1877), vol. 1; Alfred Swaine Taylor, *The Principles and Practice of Medical Jurisprudence* (London: John Churchill, 1865), pp. 1093–134.

18. The Criminal Lunatics Act (1800), Amended (1816); The Insane Prisoners Act (1840), Amended (1864); The Criminal Lunatics Asylum Act (1860); The Trial of Lunatics Act (1883); The Criminal Lunatics Act (1884). Cf. *Report of the Commission Appointed by the Secretary of State for the Home Department to Inquire into the Subject of Criminal Lunacy* (London: Her Majesty's Stationery Office, 1882).

19. *Report of the Commission*, pp. 4–6; Patricia H. Allderidge, "Criminal Insanity: From Bethlem to Broadmoor," *Proceedings of the Royal Society of Medicine* 67 (1974): 897–904; Walker and McCabe, *Crime and Insanity*, pp. 2–10. For the number and distribution of criminal lunatics, see *Report of the Metropolitan Commissioners in Lunacy, to the Lord Chancellor* (London: Bradbury and Evans, 1844), pp. 195–99, and Appendix G, p. 274; annual figures in the *Reports of the Commissioners in Lunacy;* Criminal Lunacy Commission 1882, *Report*.

20. Cf. Scull, *Museums of Madness*. The symbolic importance of the insanity defense for the professional aspirations of the alienists is not discussed by Scull.

21. Standard medical authorities for the view that insanity was brain disease included John Charles Bucknill and Daniel Hack Tuke, *A Manual of Psychological Medicine* (London: John Churchill, 1858); Wilhelm Griesinger, *Mental Pathology and Therapeutics*, trans. C. L. Robertson and J. Rutherford (1867; reprint ed., New York: Hafner, 1965); Henry Maudsley, *The Physiology and Pathology of the Mind* (London: Macmillan, 1867); Ray, *Medical Jurisprudence*.

22. E.g., Jacques M. Quen, "A History of the Anglo-American Legal Psychiatry of Violence and Responsibility," in *Violence and Responsibility: The Individual, the Family and Society*, ed. Robert L. Sadoff (New York and London: SP Medical and Scientific Books, 1975), pp. 17–32. The full text of Lord Denman's summing-up can be read in a number of ways, and his statement did not become an important precedent in liberalizing the insanity defense (even if alienists thought it *should* have done so). See n. 14 in this chapter.

23. The Insane Prisoners Amendment Act (1864) closed an administrative loophole which allowed doctors appointed by Townley's solicitor to certify his insanity, and thereby circumvent the capital sentence. Cf. [Henry Maudsley and C. L. Robertson], *Insanity and Crime: A Medico-legal Commentary on the Case of George Victor Townley* (London: John Churchill, 1864); Walker, *Crime and Insanity*, pp. 205, 207–9.

24. [Editorials], "[The case of Luigi Buranelli]," *Lancet,* pt. 1, 1855, pp. 441, 518–19, 540–41, 564–66, 589–91, 540.

25. Ibid., p. 540.

26. [J. C. Bucknill], "The Trial and Conviction of Luigi Buranelli for Murder. Plea of Insanity," *Asylum Journal* 1 (1855): 209–13.

27. *Lancet,* 1855, "Case of Buranelli," p. 566; cf. Forbes Winslow, *The Case of Luigi Buranelli Medico-legally Considered* (London: John Churchill, 1855; Supplement to vol. 8, *Journal of Psychological Medicine and Mental Pathology*).

28. Reported in Daniel Hack Tuke, "The Plea of Insanity in Relation to the Penalty of Death; Or, the Report of the Capital Punishment Commission Psychologically Considered," *Social Science Review, Sanitary Review, and Journal of the Sciences,* n.s. 5 (1866): 289–309, 301–2.

29. Quoted in Anon., "Criminal Jurisprudence of Insanity," *Asylum Journal of Mental Science* 2 (1856): 391–92 (p. 391).

30. Anon., "The Late Murder in Bedford-Row," *Medical Times and Gazette* 12 (1856): 166–68. This kind of case encouraged alienists to think that an intermediate verdict, between guilt and acquittal, would resolve controversy about the insanity defense: e.g., William Wood, "Lunatic Criminals—Their Responsibility," [Letter to the Editor] *Medical Times and Gazette* 12 (1856): 290. The judicial discretion to *"record"* the death sentence was abolished in 1861.

31. The Bethlem archives contain the Criminal Lunatic Books, 1810–1885. For Westron, see the Criminal Case Books, CBC/3, p. 176. I am grateful to the governors of the Royal Bethlem Hospital and to the archivist, Patricia Allderidge, for the facilities they have made available to me.

32. James Fitzjames Stephen, *A General View of the Criminal Law of England* (London: Macmillan, 1863), p. 394.

33. Printed in J. C. Bucknill, "Plea of Insanity—The Trial of William Dove," *Asylum Journal of Mental Science* 3 (1857): 125–34.

34. Caleb Williams, *Observations on the Criminal Responsibility of the Insane; Founded on the Trials of James Hill and of William Dove* (London: John Churchill, 1856), p. 13.

35. Bucknill, "Trial of Dove," p. 132.

36. Reported in Stephen, *View of the Criminal Law,* pp. 398–99.

37. The prosecution, quoted in Williams, *Criminal Responsibility of the Insane,* p. civ.

38. *Times* (London), 10 August 1854, p. 12, reporting the trial.

39. The postmortem reports for the criminally insane are preserved in the Bethlem archives. Cf. evidence of the medical superintendent at Bethlem, Dr. W. Charles Hood, in *Report of the Capital Punishment Commission* (London: For Her Majesty's Stationery Office, 1866), minutes 2777–84.

40. [Forbes Winslow], "Recent Trials in Lunacy," *Journal of Psychological Medicine and Mental Pathology* 7 (1854): 572–625. Dr. Winslow gave expert evidence in Mrs. Brough's defense; he is here responding bitterly to his critics.

41. Bucknill, *Unsoundness of Mind,* pp. 133–36.

42. This is not intended to be a philosophically satisfying account of legal decision-making, but to correspond to the relevant historical level of perception. For a legal view, see Anon., "Criminal Irresponsibility of the Insane," *Law*

Magazine 3rd ser. 1 (1872): 215–19. Cf. H. L. A. Hart, *Punishment and Responsibility: Essays in the Philosophy of Law* (Oxford: Clarendon Press, 1968), pp. 32–33.

43. See the alternative descriptions offered for the crimes of Dove and Brough cited above. See also the radically different descriptions of George Bryce (who killed a serving girl at Newcastle in 1864) that are given in Thomas Laycock, "On the Legal Doctrines of the Responsibility of the Insane and Its Consequences," *Journal of Mental Science* 10 (1864): 350–66, and in Anon., "[Legal Responsibility of the Insane]," *British Medical Journal*, pt. 2 (1864), pp. 227–28; cf. P. Riot, "The Parallel Lives of Pierre Rivière," in Foucault, *I, Pierre Rivière*, pp. 229–50.

44. It was not unusual for a jury to demonstrate sympathy by accepting an insanity defense in order to acquit a mother who had killed her young child: e.g., Anon., "Chelmsford—Friday, March 10. Charge of Murder.—Acquitted on the Ground of Puerperal Insanity," *Journal of Psychological Medicine and Mental Pathology* 1 (1848): 478–80. On the other hand, medical evidence could be ignored when judge and jury concurred in wanting retribution: e.g., case of Fooks (or Fowkes), who shot a neighbor, referred to in Anon., "Homicidal Mania and Moral Insanity," *Saturday Review* 15 (1863): 370–72, and Anon., "Regina v. Fooks. Dorset Spring Assizes, 1863," *Journal of Mental Science* 9 (1863): 125–37.

45. James Fitzjames Stephen, *A Digest of the Criminal Law* (London: Macmillan, 1877), pp. xxix–xxx, 15–16.

46. Taylor, *Medical Jurisprudence*, p. 1121.

47. Ibid., pp. xvii–lix.

48. Thomas Harrington Tuke, evidence to the Royal Commission on Capital Punishment 1866, *Report*, minutes 2455–56.

49. E.g., Phillips, *Law Concerning Lunatics*, p. 56, note.

50. See the different responses to the question of the integration of nervous levels in W. B. Carpenter, *Principles of Human Physiology*, 4th ed. rev. (London: John Churchill, 1853), pp. 763–861, and in Thomas Laycock, *Mind and Brain: Or the Correlations of Consciousness and Organisation*, 2 vols. (Edinburgh: Sutherland and Knox, 1860). For the neurophysiological context of these ideas, see Robert M. Young, *Mind, Brain, and Adaptation in the Nineteenth Century: Cerebral Localization and Its Biological Context from Gall to Ferrier* (Oxford: Clarendon Press, 1970).

51. For a systematic compendium of moralistic physiology, see W. B. Carpenter, *Principles of Mental Physiology*, 4th ed. (London: Henry S. King, 1876).

52. On criminal law and drink, see Russell, *Crimes and Misdemeanors*, pp. 114–16; Taylor, *Medical Jurisprudence*, pp. 1127–32; Walker, *Crime and Insanity*, pp. 177–82.

53. For a bibliography, see Arthur MacDonald, *Abnormal Man, Being Essays on Education and Crime and Related Subjects* ([Washington]: Bureau of Information, Circular of Information, no. 4, 1893); cf. R. A. Nye, "Heredity or Milieu: The Foundations of Modern European Criminological Theory," *Isis* 67 (1976): 335–55; Charles E. Rosenberg, "The Bitter Fruit: Heredity, Disease, and Social Thought in Nineteenth-Century America," *Perspectives in American History* 8 (1974): 189–235. The links between crime and insanity were developed in Britain particularly by Henry Maudsley and Charles Mercier. Arguments for a collective response to the biological determination of society have been examined

in recent work on the origins of the eugenics movement: e.g., Donald MacKenzie, "Eugenics in Britain," *Social Studies in Science* 6 (1976): 499–532; G. R. Searle, *Eugenics and Politics in Britain, 1900–1914* (Leiden: Nordhoff, 1976); R. Schwartz Cowan, "Nature and Nurture: The Interplay of Biology and Politics in the Work of Francis Galton," *Studies in the History of Biology* 1 (1977): 133–208.